Changing Practice in Health and Social Care

Edited by

Celia Davies, Linda Finlay and Anne Bullman

The Open
University

in association with
The Open University

SAGE Publications
London • Thousand Oaks • New Delhi

Compilation, original and editorial material
© The Open University 2000

First published 2000

SAGE Publications Ltd
6 Bonhill Street
London EC2A 4PU

SAGE Publications Inc
2455 Teller Road
Thousand Oaks, California 91320

SAGE Publications India Pvt Ltd
32, M-Block Market
Greater Kailash – I
New Delhi 110 048

British Library Cataloguing in Publication data

A catalogue record for this book is available
from the British Library

ISBN 0 7619 6496 7
ISBN 0 7619 6497 5 (pbk)

Library of Congress catalog record available

Typeset by Mayhew Typesetting, Rhayader, Powys
Printed in Great Britain by The Cromwell Press Ltd,
Trowbridge, Wiltshire

Changing Practice in
Health and Social Care

Changing Practice in Health and Social Care

This reader forms part of the Open University course Critical Practice in Health and Social Care and the selection of items is related to other materials available to students and to three further published texts:

- Evaluating Research in Health and Social Care
- Using Evidence in Health and Social Care
- Critical Practice in Health and Social Care

If you are interested in studying for this course, or related courses, please write to the Information Officer, School of Health and Social Welfare, The Open University, Walton Hall, Milton Keynes, MK7 6AA, UK. Details can also be reviewed on our web page http://www.open.ac.uk

Opinions expressed in the reader are not necessarily those of the Course Team or of The Open University.

Contents

Acknowledgements

The authors and publishers wish to thank the following for permission to use copyright material:

David Higham Associates for 'Entirely' by Louis MacNeice. The Open University Press for 'Introduction' and 'Conclusion' from Tony Butcher (1995) *Delivering Welfare*, for extracts from Jane Lewis and Howard Glennerster (1996) *Implementing the New Community Care*, for extracts from Neil Thompson (1995) *Theory and Practice in Health and Social Welfare*, for extracts from Tom Kitwood (1997) 'Requirements of a Caregiver' in *Dementia Reconsidered*, for extracts from Suzy Braye and Michael Preston-Shoot (1995) 'Understanding and Managing the Interprofessional System' in *Empowering Practice in Social Care* and for extracts from Ellie Scrivens (1995) 'Chapter 3 – The Accreditation Experience' in *Accreditation: Protecting the Professional or the Consumer*. Cambridge University Press for extracts from Julian Le Grand 'Knights, Knaves or Pawns?' in *Journal of Social Policy*, 26(2): 149–69. RCN Publishing Company for Christine Nash (1996) 'Applying Reflective Practice ' in *Emergency Nurse*, March 1999, 6(10): 14–18. Stanley Thornes Publishers Ltd for extracts from Francis M. Quinn 'Reflection and Reflective Practice' in *Continuing Professional Development*. Whurr Publishers Ltd for extracts from Rosemary Barnitt (1998) 'The Virtuous Therapist' in *Occupational Therapy: New Perspectives* edited by Jennifer Creek. Macmillan Press Ltd for extracts from Sarah Banks (1995) 'Social Work Values' in *Ethics and Values in Social Work*. Blackwell Publishers for extracts from Cheryl Cott (1998) 'Structure and Meaning in Multidisciplinary Teamwork' in *Sociology of Health and Illness*, 20 (1998) (pp. 848–73) © The Editors of *Sociology of Health and Illness*. Sage Publications for extracts from Mark Priestley (1995) 'Dropping 'E's: The Missing Link in Quality Assurance for Disabled People' in *Critical Social Policy*, 44/45, 15(2/3). Ashgate Publishing Ltd for extracts from 'Quality in Personal Social Services: The Developing Role of User Involvement' Peter Beresford, Suzy Croft, Clare Evans and Tessa Harding in *Developing Quality in Personal Social Services: Concepts, Cases and Comments* edited by Adalbert Ever, Rutta Haverinen, Kai Leichsenring and Gerard Wistow (1997) and for extracts from Luis Archer 'Looking for New Codes in the Field of Predictive Medicine' in *Ethics Codes in Medicine* edited by Ulriche Trohler and Stella Reiter-Theil

(1998). Taylor and Francis for extracts from David Thompson, Isabel Clare and Hilary Brown (1997) 'Not Such an "Ordinary" Relationship' in *Disability and Society*, 12(4): 573–92, and for extracts from Simon Biggs 'User voice, Interprofessionalism and Postmodernity' in *Journal of Interprofessional Care*, 11(2): 195–203. Web site: http://www.tandf. co.uk. Hodder Headline for extracts from Pam Smith and Ellen Agard 'Care Costs: Towards a Critical Understanding of Care' in *Caring: The Compassion and Wisdom of Nursing*, edited by G. Brykczynska. Routledge for extracts from Steven Shardlow 'Confidentiality, Accountability and the Boundaries of Client–Worker Relationships' (1995) in *Ethical Issues in Social Work (Professional Ethics)* edited by Richard Hugman and David Smith. Elsevier Science for extracts reprinted from *Social Science & Medicine*, 36(7): 849–56, article by Nick Black and Elizabeth Thompson 'Obstacles to Medical Audit: British Doctors Speak' (1993) and for extracts reprinted from *Social Science and Medicine*, 46(1): 23–8, Gray Southon and Jeffrey Braithwaite 'The End of Professionalism?' (1998). Arnold Publishers for extracts from Chris Corkish and Bob Heyman 'The Resettlement of People with Severe Learning Difficulties' (1998) in *Risk, Health and Health Care* edited by Bob Heyman. Blackwell Publishers Ltd for extracts from Diana Leat and Elizabeth Perkins 'Juggling and Dealing: The Creative Work of Care Package Purchasing' (1998) in *Social Policy and Administration*, 32(2): 166–81 and for extracts from Martin Barnes and David Prior 'From Private Choice to Public Trust' in *Public Money and Management*, 16(4): 51–7. The Policy Press at The University of Bristol for extracts from Margaret Harris 'Instruments of Government?: Voluntary Sector Boards in a Changing Public Policy Environment' in *Policy and Politics*, 26(2): 177–88. Butterworth Heinemann Publishers, a division of Reed Educational & Professional Publishing Ltd, for Della Fish and Colin Coles 'Seeing Anew: Understanding Professional Practice as Artistry' (1998) in *Developing Professional Judgement in Health Care*. Blackwell Science Ltd for extracts from Mike Saks 'Sociological Perspectives on Health, Illness and Health Care' in *Professionalism and Health Care* edited by S. Taylor and D Field. BMJ Publishing Group for extracts from Sue Dowling, Robyn Martin, Paul Skidmore, Lesley Doyal, Ailsa Cameron and Sharon Lloyd (1996) 'Nurses Taking on Doctors' Work: A Confusion of Accountability' in *BMJ*, 312, May 1996: 1211–14. Netherlands School of Social and Economic Research for Celia Davies 'Care and the Transformation of Professionalism' in *Care, Citizenship and Social Cohesion: Towards a Gender Perspective* (1998). School of Public Policy at the University of Birmingham for extracts from Michael Clarke and John Stewart *Handling the Wicked Issues – A Challenge for Government* (1997).

Entirely

If we could get the hang of it entirely
  It would take too long;
All we know is the splash of words in passing
  And falling twigs of song,
And when we try to eavesdrop on the great
  Presences it is rarely
That by a stroke of luck we can appropriate
  Even a phrase entirely.

If we could find our happiness entirely
  In somebody else's arms
We should not fear the spears of the spring nor the city's
  Yammering fire alarms
But, as it is, the spears each year go through
  Our flesh and almost hourly
   Bell or siren banishes the blue
    Eyes of Love entirely.

And if the world were black or white entirely
  And all the charts were plain
Instead of a mad weir of tigerish waters,
  A prism of delight and pain,
We might be surer where we wished to go
  Or again we might be merely
Bored but in brute reality there is no
  Road that is right entirely.

Louis MacNeice

Introduction

There is a deliberate ambiguity in the title of this collection of readings. Practice is changing but practice also can be changed. There is no doubt that things have changed for practitioners. Demands for recording, reflecting and researching have escalated. Those in the front line of services, in the public, private and voluntary sectors, are required to do more in the way of explaining and defending practice.

Is your planned intervention cost effective and can you demonstrate that this is the case? How exactly are you responding to user perspectives? What is your risk management strategy and what have you based it on? Can you devise better performance indicators for the new quality assurance system that we plan to put in place? Faced with such questions, it is not surprising if practitioners feel defensive, threatened and overloaded – in short, they feel under siege (Fish and Coles, 1998).

Service users have themselves contributed to this sense of siege. With access to more information than ever before, and sometimes supported by organized user movements, they too are challenging practitioners and demanding new kinds of response. Furthermore, where once it was social work that was under a media spotlight, run through the mill for abuse in residential care, challenged for its practices in child protection, now even doctors and other health professionals are under that media gaze, being challenged about their decisions and their competence.

But if practice is changing, practitioners are not passive puppets. They are often willing and eager initiators of change. This is 'changing practice' in the second of its two senses. There is more scope in today's services than there was in the past to respond to local need, experiment and foster good practice. Some have rejected familiar settings altogether; they are working on short-term contracts, offering specialist consultancy to the public, private and voluntary sectors, and creating portfolio careers. Others have found scope to redefine their jobs and create more team-based and user-centred practice. This in turn brings new challenges. How will you evaluate your new practice? How can you actively search out good practice elsewhere?

Changing practice, in both of the two senses above, means that those in the front line of services, and those in management posts supporting them to do so, need to find ways of putting new practice into words, and fostering its further growth. Professional bodies in nursing and social work, in the therapy professions and in complementary and alternative medicine have responded to this by encouraging and requiring continuing professional development. There is widespread recognition that no practitioner is a finished product at the end of initial education and training, that learning is lifelong and that the means need to be put in place to encourage and enable both personal and professional development to occur.

This collection of readings is designed to respond to and support these developments. It does not follow any particular set of professional requirements. These will quickly date. Instead it seeks to tease out some of the underlying ideas, knowledge, skills and attitudes which will help the continuing practitioner to respond to the myriad of changing demands. Today's practitioners can take very little for granted in what Donald Schön so famously called the 'swampy lowlands' of practice. (Schön, 1983: 42) They need to reflect and explore, to check out understandings and work with others to solve problems. These problems, furthermore, often cannot be resolved within the confines of a single occupational group. Nor, often, can they be resolved without listening to service users and carers and understanding how the actions of a range of service providers – in turn influenced by complex processes of policy change – are impacting on them. Underpinning this collection of readings, therefore, is what we would see as a newly emerging approach to professional development across the spectrum of health and social care that envisages a practitioner who is at once positive yet critical, analytical yet active.

The structure of the book

What kinds of readings would be helpful in this complex and demanding context? The book grew out of debates and discussions of an Open University course team preparing a wide-ranging third-level course in the field of health and social welfare, intending to provide some of the key foundations for interprofessional, continuing professional development. The principal selection criterion for this collection was that the chapters would support and enhance the concept of critical practice as developed in the course. However, the consultations we had in the process of developing the course with professional leaders and potential students, managers and service users showed that there was a wider need that this book could serve. Their comments centred around the demands of working with uncertainty and change, the sheer confusion of rapid policy change, the pitfalls as well as the potentials of developments such as team-working, quality assurance, performance review and a need to 'keep the faith' without cynicism or despair.

With all this in mind, we were convinced of the need to search out material that gave authentic voice to the complexity, uncertainty and dilemmas of day to day practice. We were committed to drawing examples from across the spectrum of health and social care. We could not hope to represent all occupational groups and all settings in this wide spectrum, but we did want to include items that would enlighten those from one particular area, about the different histories, traditions, values and practices of colleagues. We were also influenced by the words of Charles Handy – especially by his notion that learning and growth occur through actively analysing real situations, and of creating a 'cycle of discovery at work'.

> We need to be able to identify problems and opportunities. We need to be able to organise ourselves and other people to do something about them, and we need to be able to sit back and reflect on what has happened in order that we can do it all better the next time round. (Handy, 1995: 207)

Handy suggests that there are three skills involved in the kind of learning he had in mind – conceptualizing, co-ordinating and consolidating. We have built on this idea in ordering the material for this collection.

Six words beginning with the letter 'C' provide the overall organizing framework. Part I, *Contextualizing* brings together a number of articles to set the broad policy context in a way that has meaning and relevance for individual practitioners. *Connecting* takes the reader through questions of theory, values and practice, showing just how powerfully these can be connected in a world that still depressingly often divorces them from each other. Part III, *Collaborating*, has a particularly broad reach. It addresses collaborations across professions, as well as collaborations between practitioners and users. This section also explores different ways to foster collaboration; it takes into account both psychodynamics and organizational structures. Part IV on *Coping* relates closely to this. It deals with some of the most demanding challenges that practitioners face, from both difficult clients and demanding managers, and seeks to design ways to handle these without becoming defensive. The final two parts look forward. *Constructing* new professional identities is part and parcel of *Creating* new futures. Different visions of what each of these futures might entail are offered.

We have resisted the impulse to reproduce standard arguments, for instance about professionalism, care or barriers to teamworking. Instead, we have sought to take a fresh look at the subjects by integrating ideas from practice, education, management and social policy. We were helped here by the way that theorist-practitioners are now beginning to emerge and by the *rapprochement* that is occurring between the academic world and the world of practice.

Using the book

This book can be used in a number of ways. Some will want to adopt it alongside other Open University texts and pursue the concept of critical practice. Others will want to see it as a stand-alone collection, capable of being used by students in the further and higher education sectors, across a wide range of courses and at pre and post-registration levels. Here there are a number of possibilities. Each of the parts can be studied individually. Brief editorial introductions have been provided for each part, giving a rationale for the juxtaposition of chapters and guidance on how we see some of the key links between them. Alternatively, it is possible to use the book in support of more conventional themes treated in 'professional issues' courses for practitioners. The reader will find, for example, that reflective practice can be explored and examined, that there is material on user involvement and participation, and that teamworking and collaboration, quality issues, monitoring and inspection are all represented with classic thinking and up to date ideas. What a reader will not find here is the latest policy change or the details of service organization and management. We have deliberately looked for writers who are able to bring perspective by giving the longer view or teasing out underlying principles and issues. Threaded through all the parts – but most prominent perhaps in the last – are the questions: 'what kinds of services for health and welfare do we want to see in future?' and, 'how can we both prepare the people and create the structures to promote these?' Although the book is designed principally for health and social care practitioners, students of social policy, social welfare, the sociology of health and illness are likely to find much of value in the way that the analytical ideas combine with a vivid awareness of the realities of day to day practice.

It remains for us to acknowledge our debts. Firstly, if the book works in the many ways outlined, it will be due to the co-operation and help we have had as editors from colleagues. This collection would not have come about at all without the energies and commitment of the Open University K302 course team. Team members have particularly helped in the editing and preparation of the chapters. Those who made a direct input to this include: Ann Brechin, Maureen Eby, Roger Gomm, Jan Gibb and Gill Needham. We would like to acknowledge their contribution to finding the material for this reader and drawing attention to the importance of the themes that can be found in the various chapters and discussing with us, at innumerable team meetings, the way that students would be likely to respond. Secondly, we would like to acknowledge the contributions of three further team members: Hilary Brown, Linda Jones and Sheila Peace. Each contributed substantially to our thinking in the early stages. Circumstances, however, meant that they were unable to continue to remain involved. Thirdly, as the reader will see, the chapters included here are for the most part edited and shortened versions of previous work. We therefore wish to thank authors and publishers for permission to reprint material and we would like to think that readers will sometimes be stimulated by the material that is here to read the original writings in full and perhaps to follow up references that the authors suggest. Fourthly, a certain number of chapters have been specially commissioned for this volume. We are particularly indebted to the authors of these chapters. Often at short notice, they agreed to distil their thinking into the short compass of a reader article, or, in some cases, to take on something quite new, given the 'slot' that we were encouraging them to fill. They rose to our challenge with enthusiasm and often with rather more grace than we deserved as we tried to shape their thinking and speed up their timetables to fit the emerging ideas of the book. Last, but not least, we want to record our thanks to Kathy McPhee. As course team secretary, she added the demands of preparing this book to an already impossibly busy course production schedule and was always willing to do that bit more to ensure we met our targets.

References

Fish, D. and Coles, C. (eds) (1998) *Developing Professional Judgement in Health Care*, London: Butterworth Heinemann.

Handy, C. (1995) *The Empty Raincoat – Making Sense of the Future*, London: Arrow Books.

Schön, D. (1983) *The Reflective Practitioner: How Professionals Think and Act*, London: Temple Smith.

PART I

CONTEXTUALIZING: WORKING WITH CHANGING STRUCTURES

How can people who work in health and social care make sense of the policy changes that they have been living through? Those who started their careers in the 1960s and 1970s are acutely aware of the sea change they experienced with the creation of the mixed economy of social care and with managerialism and internal markets in health enshrined in the 1990 NHS and Community Care Act. As this book goes to press, legislation is once again working its way through parliament, an expression of the Labour government's search for a 'Third Way' – rejecting both the market principles and the principles that served the founders of the post-war welfare state in the 1940s.

The five chapters in this part, in their different ways, consider the changing context of service delivery. Linda Jones starts with a very necessary reminder that there are different voices in the debate about welfare and contrasting assumptions about what dependency is and when it is legitimate to be vulnerable and in need of help from welfare professionals. While these arguments cross party lines, patterns can still be discerned. Tony Butcher offers one vision of how such patterns might be seen. Looking from a mid-1990s vantage point, Butcher was able to sketch out what he calls the 'public administration model' and to suggest that each of its features has been transformed and has, in turn transformed the conditions under which welfare state professionals work. His old and new models neatly encapsulate some of the key changes in the way professionals work and draw particular attention to the withdrawal of trust which has been a feature of modern times.

Ideas do not always fit into neat boxes and change, as Jones has pointed out, is uneven and contested. The next two readings bring this message home. Jane Lewis and Howard Glennerster provide a lively account of some of the key circumstances that surrounded the community care changes expressed in the 1990 Act. Fiona Brooks takes the case of the myriad influences, including user influences, on maternity services. These chapters remind us that stakeholders are more or less powerful, depending on the issue and the time and that user movements have become a more common and more prominent feature of the policy landscape.

At first sight, the final chapter seems to cover the ground of the first two chapters again. Julian Le Grand's concern is a different one however, focusing as he does on the sometimes unconscious beliefs about human motivation that underpin welfare institutions. His trinity of 'knights, knaves and pawns' – especially his proposition that in recent years knights have been treated as knaves – will have an immediate resonance with many of those who have felt that their commitment to the public sector has been devalued, discounted and traded upon in recent years. His arguments for a 'robust strategy' deserve to be taken seriously by some of those policymakers who attended the inaugural lecture at the London School of Economics, where this theme was first unveiled.

How important is it to develop a sense of place in a policy history? Setting oneself in the wider scheme of things sometimes puts present-day frustrations in perspective. It also helps us see the cracks and the conjunctures – the opportunities there may be to move things on. If we are to make a reality of changing practice – in that second sense of actively making a difference – context counts.

1

L.J.C. Jones

Reshaping Welfare: Voices from the Debate

> There is no universal principle which defines for all time and for all
> nations the good society. . . . We have to fashion our own priorities in
> the light of our country's circumstances and our own hopes for the future.
> Our fellow citizens' aspirations are always important; but we can, collec-
> tively, change these values by making new aims and moralities possible.
> (Donnison, 1977: 58)

Welfare has always been a contested arena. Views about rights and
entitlements to welfare are strongly linked to wider political and
economic ideas about what makes for the 'good society' and these are
subject to change over time and between cultures. Even in the two
decades after 1950, when there was considerable agreement about
the legitimacy of state welfare planning, UK politics was marked by
'grumbling consensus', 'acrimonious debate' and frequent use of 'the
vocabulary of crisis' by both critics and defenders of the welfare state
(Deakin, 1987).

After the Second World War, Keynesian theories about state
management of the economy and related ideas about national efficiency and social cohesion, contained in the Beveridge Report of 1942,
became widely known and supported. Government, it was accepted,
had the duty and capacity not only to regulate the economy in order
to secure economic growth and maintain full employment but also to
provide a minimum 'safety net' for all citizens. Risks common to all –
sickness, unemployment, disability, growing old and frail – should be
met by collective provision of benefits, allowances and services,
funded through national insurance and taxation.

Not all contemporaries supported the establishment of this welfare
state. Winston Churchill warned his cabinet colleagues of the 'false
hopes and visions of Utopia and Eldorado' that would be created and
leading industrialists argued that production and prosperity should
be seen as higher priorities than party plans (George and Miller,
1994: 7–8). In contrast to this, some campaigners voiced concern
about whether the needs of women and children would be adequately
met by an insurance-based scheme that made them dependent on
men (Abbott and Bompas, 1943; Rhys-Williams, 1943), but these were

largely unacknowledged voices. State welfare and economic management carried the day, together with increasing faith in scientific
'experts' – economists, social scientists and state bureaucrats.

By the late 1970s 'this apparently solid edifice of common assumptions had been riddled through by a fusillade of criticisms from every
point of the political compass. In its place there was widespread
acceptance that the Welfare State was inefficient, unpopular and on
the verge of disintegration' (Deakin, 1987: 16). This chapter explores
these criticisms of state welfare and notes how they are embedded in
deeper (and still unresolved) conflicts about individual and collective
responsibility. It suggests that individualist ideology, despite being
only partially translated into policy, has resulted in significant shifts
in the social relations of care. In doing this, it highlights the views of
some of the politicians, journalists, academics and campaigners from
all parts of the political spectrum who attempted to shift public
perceptions and political priorities.

The 'road to serfdom': liberating the individual

One striking aspect of the welfare debate is that ideas and values
shifted within and across political parties. Conservative neo-liberal-
ism in the 1970s – the 'New Right' of Margaret Thatcher – had its
roots in nineteenth-century anti-state Liberalism, echoes of which
could be heard in post-1945 Liberal Party calls for a minimal state. In
the earlier twentieth century, however, 'New Liberalism' was largely
identified with the extension of collectivism. In contrast, before 1945
Conservatives were highly suspicious about state intervention but
they endorsed the post-war welfare settlement. Indeed, some leading
politicians, such as Sir Keith Joseph, were as enthusiastic for state
economic planning in the 1960s as were most of the Labour Party.

By the mid-1970s 'New Right' Conservatives had begun to attack
collectivism and claim that liberty, freedom of choice and individual
responsibility were paramount values. They drew on the ideas of
Friedrich von Hayek (1944) to argue that state planning could lead to
totalitarianism – the 'road to serfdom'. Powerful groups, in particular
trade unions, could pressure the state to spend and extend welfare,
favouring sectional interests at the expense of the general good. A
strong, but more restricted state was the answer, one that preserved
the freedom of individuals and recognized their importance in creating
economic growth. Prime Minister Margaret Thatcher commented, 'In
our party we do not ask for a feeble State. On the contrary, we need a
strong State to preserve both liberty and order' (quoted in Heald, 1983:
322).

The state's role in promoting equality, providing social welfare
and redistributing income and wealth, on the other hand, came under

question. The New Right formulated a new version of citizenship that challenged the collectivist assumptions of the post-war years, using the left critique of the failures of the welfare state and of the 'experts' who presided over it as ammunition. Central to this vision were individual responsibility, enterprise and choice, as against the debilitating and dangerous effects for the individual of 'nanny state' welfare provision. Above all, citizenship meant being self-reliant – in contrast to the benefits 'scrounger', the feckless welfare dependant and the 'underclass'.

> A state which does for its citizens what they can do for themselves is an evil state. In such an irresponsible society no one cares, no one saves, no one bothers – why should they when the state spends all its energies taking money from the energetic, successful and thrifty to give to the idle, failures and the feckless. (Rhodes Boyson, 1971: 63)

> [The] intellectual basis of [the collectivist trend] has been eroded as experience has repeatedly contradicted expectations. Its supporters are on the defensive. They have no solutions to offer present-day evils except more of the same. (Friedman and Friedman, 1980: 331)

The New Right also recast the social relations of care. Instead of relying on professionals, people were urged to stand on their own feet and re-make themselves as rugged individuals. As sovereign consumers they should make market choices, paying their way and looking after their own, with welfare professionals playing a subsidiary role.

> The sense of being self-reliant; of playing a role within the family, owning one's own property, of paying one's way, are all part of the spiritual ballast which maintains responsible citizenship, and provides a solid foundation from which people look around and see what more they might do for others and themselves. (Thatcher, 1977: 97)

> I believe that the volunteer movement is at the heart of all our social welfare provision. That the statutory services are the supportive ones, underpinning where necessary, filling the gaps and helping the helpers. (Thatcher, 1981 quoted in Ungerson, 1985: 214)

This emphasis on 'reforming the self' in Thatcherism has been described as a contest between a cast of characters – the 'enterprising self', 'sovereign consumer', 'active citizen' and 'conservative self' (Heelas, 1991: 73–5). All four were deployed, but it was wealth creation and the 'enterprising self' that triumphed.

From the 1980s, successive Conservative governments struggled to create the leaner but stronger state that would liberate enterprise and regulate but not provide every type of welfare service. Policy shifts included the selling of public sector housing to the private sector, allowing schools to opt out of local authority control, the competitive tendering of ancillary services in health and successive cutbacks and greater targeting of benefits. The 1990 NHS Health and

Community Care Act went one stage further, by creating competitive markets in health and social care that were designed to hold down costs and be more responsive to consumers. The outcome, however, was a complex and costly system that did little to extend freedom of choice to individuals and did not noticeably reduce government interference. Viewed retrospectively, the extent to which the New Right was able to undermine collectivism and de-commit from welfare provision was much less than its rhetoric claimed. But the ideology of consumer sovereignty and the enterprise society fundamentally influenced New Labour thinking in the late 1990s.

The crisis of costs

A key factor in the shift of political and public opinion about state welfare was the economic crisis of the early 1970s. In place of full employment and economic growth, the bedrock of the post-war settlement, the economy became characterized by economic stagnation and high inflation – 'stagflation' and even 'slumpflation' (Mishra, 1984). Unemployment rose and demand for welfare benefits grew. In these circumstances the tax base on which governments depended to finance welfare expenditure shrank, with little prospect of recovery other than through increased taxation or welfare retrenchment. The Keynesian approach, in which government management of the economy was able to ensure that demand was regulated and full employment was maintained, became increasingly discredited. At the same time, the weight of welfare expenditure and the general growth in state intervention began to be seen as partly responsible for this economic downturn. Doubts about the efficacy of state intervention grew as economic growth faltered. Rising living standards for people in work encouraged them to be more individualistic in their attitudes and less tolerant of further tax rises to support social welfare provision.

New Right thinking gained ground in this fertile soil as the political Left faltered in its belief that socialism could be achieved through welfare. Left-wing critics argued that the welfare state was faced with a crisis of legitimacy, in which not only the Keynes-Beveridge approach was questionable but also the possibility of further social change:

> The slumpflation of the 1970s has clearly underlined the unrealism of a socialist strategy based on manipulating distribution while leaving production in capitalist hands. Mass unemployment, cutbacks in social expenditure and tax concessions to the rich are a harsh reminder that 'welfare' is only tolerable so long as it does not interfere with the logic of capitalist production. The choice seems to be between capitalism and welfare capitalism. Pursuit of socialism through welfare has proved to be a myth. (Mishra, 1984: 24)

There was concern on all sides as the cost of benefits and services grew, far outstripping early expectations. While some UK welfare services, such as health, remained considerably cheaper than insurance-based schemes elsewhere, attempts to create earnings-related benefits or to extend universal benefits manifestly increased costs and were increasingly seen as impractical. The monetarist view adopted by Conservative governments after 1979 emphasized market deregulation, a stable money supply and the lowering of direct taxation. Welfare costs were a prime target for cuts and large sums were realized through efficiency savings, the selling of council housing and reductions in benefits. Although the main justifications given for cutting back the welfare state were ideological, the economic motive for the attack on welfare was always a central feature:

> There are powerful reasons why we must be ready to consider how far private provision and individual choice can supplement, or in some cases possibly replace, the role of Government in health, social security and education. Most of the reasons are economic. (Sir Geoffrey Howe, quoted in Riddell, 1983: 139)

The 'strategy for equality'

For many on the political Left the post-war settlement represented a first stage in the use of welfare to build a collective, socialist future: the so-called 'strategy for equality' (Tawney, 1966). These included Fabian Socialists in the Labour Party, who believed that change could be achieved gradually through insider pressure on government, and Marxists, who initially viewed welfare capitalism as a useful staging post on the way to revolution. Minimum entitlements to benefits were seen as merely a starting point in creating a society in which income and wealth were equalized and relative poverty eliminated. Campaigners for women's welfare, disappointed by the timidity and implicit sexism of the Beveridge Report, looked forward to a 'social contract' which would free women from unpaid drudgery and dependence on men (Rhys-Williams, 1943).

More than 20 years later there was little evidence of progress. A flourishing critique of the shortcomings of the Keynes–Beveridge welfare state developed, highlighting its failure to deliver greater equality and its marginalization of some social groups. For Black people, encouraged to settle in the UK but denied public sector housing and often benefits, the post-war welfare state offered little in the way of equal treatment (Williams, 1989). Feminist writers noted the continued stigmatization of women in welfare policy as dependants and 'natural' carers (Wilson, 1977; Land, 1978). They detailed how the assumption that women would provide unpaid care for children and for sick and aged relatives was written into the framework of the Beveridge welfare state.

A key issue for the political Left was poverty, the abolition of which had been a major objective in the original struggle to create the welfare state. The Child Poverty Action Group, an all-party pressure group, launched the first of a hard-hitting series of campaigns in the late 1960s on the theme 'Poor Get Poorer under Labour'. It questioned the 'central myth' that the Labour Party was dedicated to abolishing poverty and promoting equality and highlighted the 'Poverty Trap' created for low-paid workers as selective benefits were clawed back (Field, 1982: 30).

> Hundreds of thousands of trade unionists are not getting what they bargained for. It is now a fact that for millions of low-paid workers very substantial pay increases have the absurd effect of increasing only marginally their family's net income and in some cases actually make the family worse off. . . . The cause of the present state of affairs lies in the government's polarising pursuit of selectivity and a means-test society. The narrowness of its view of poverty has created a poverty trap. As a family's income increases not only does more tax have to be paid but entitlement to those benefits, available only to the poorest, is lost. (Field and Piachaud, 1971, in Field, 1982: 104)

In other words, benefits and services targeted at the poor reinforced their poverty. Studies of relative poverty in the UK concluded that redistribution towards the poor had been negligible (Townsend, 1979; Le Grand, 1982). Even free, universal health care had not appreciably narrowed the health gap between professional classes and unskilled workers since the 1940s (Townsend and Davidson, 1982). Nor was there evidence of greater equality: it was the middle classes, by and large, who had gained from state provision of education and health and the poor did not recoup these losses through selective benefits in social services and housing:

> Redistribution is not much of a reality and the social services can increas-ingly be seen to . . . reinforce rather than reduce poverty and inequality. (Townsend, 1979: 894)

> Public expenditure on the social services has not achieved equality in any of its interpretations. Public expenditure on health care, education, housing and transport systematically favours the better off, and thereby contributes to inequality in the final outcome. (Le Grand, 1982: 137)

Although Conservative politicians had shared some of the concerns about poverty and inequality in the post-war years, the debate about poverty and redistribution was sidelined after 1980. Instead, the critique by the Left provided useful ammunition for the New Right to justify its claim that state welfare had failed to deliver on its promises (Minford, 1984; Willetts, 1987).

An intellectual crisis

Alongside persistent criticisms of the limitations of the welfare state was a much more hesitant, and heavily contested, critique of its intellectual assumptions. The welfare state was rooted above all in the assumption that scientific knowledge could solve social problems, as demonstrated by the application of theories about economic development (Keynes) and social engineering (Beveridge). Within this framework 'experts' such as economists, social scientists and welfare bureaucrats were assumed to be acting in a disinterested way in the best interests of the public. This fitted in with a benign view of the state in which it was argued that 'sensible and decent men [*sic*] will use it for ends which are sensible and decent' (Tawney, 1966: 172). It explained the support for greater state intervention by many on the Left and Right in politics in the 1960s.

As we have seen, however, some social scientists suggested that piecemeal social engineering did not work and that the benefits system could create new problems (Field and Piachaud, 1971 in Field, 1982). A few critics also questioned the degree to which experts could identify with the poor or act in their interests. For example, Donnison (1971) noted the imperialism of welfare bureaucracies and their potentially self-serving agendas. This was the gentle beginning of left-wing and libertarian attacks on what were seen as the centralist and unresponsive bureaucracies which administered welfare and on the damaging impact of professional power (Illich, 1977). Service users were sometimes conscious of their exclusion and organized to combat it. Other critics included left-wing advocates of decentralization and community control of services (Hadley and Hatch, 1981), who also noted how services were producer driven, with professionals defining needs and services.

> The evidence from evaluations of professional interventions in education, health and social work hardly serves to explain and justify all the resources that have been devoted to them. A similar scepticism is merited by the great reorganisations of local government, health and the personal social services, in which much reforming zeal was invested. . . . Fresh assumptions and fresh guiding principles are required, and in particular a reappraisal of the role of the state in social welfare. . . . Our approach is a critical one. But what is being criticised is not the basic idea of making collective provision for social welfare: it is rather the forms by which this provision has come to be made. [The] possibility . . . sketched out here, is for a pluralist, decentralised and participative pattern of services. It would compensate for or correct the disbenefits of the economic system, but as much through promoting active involvement in those services as through passive consumption of them. (Hadley and Hatch, 1981: 2–3)

The New Right, however, pursued the attack on welfare professionals from the 1980s not through decentralization but by arguing that professionals would be more accountable to 'customers' through a market approach and through greater managerial control over services. While academics and reformers debated ideas about user participation, the Conservatives' 'sovereign consumer' model proved a powerful weapon in projecting its populist credentials. The use of devices such as customer charters, questionnaires and focus groups gave the public a limited but more active role in developing services. 'Care packages' created for clients by social services staff in the new social markets of the 1960s, for example, could take some account of individual preferences, although they were limited by financial constraints. The privatization of some services, such as transport and housing, was successfully marketed as widening choice.

Beyond the New Right: the 'third way'

The Labour government, elected in May 1997, signalled its adoption of a 'third way' in welfare, in which the cruder market model would be modified and public and independent sectors would work together to deliver a mixed economy of welfare. Co-operation and partnership – for example in primary care groups and in the 'duty of partnership' between local and health authorities – would replace market competition. Service users would have a greater voice in the development of welfare services and professional power would be controlled through clinical governance and 'best value' policies. After a decade of being marginalized, poverty and inequality began to move centre stage through the launch of New Deal anti-poverty programmes, where claims about redistribution were made.

In a political sense the New Right had collapsed in disarray even before its disastrous election defeat in 1997. However, several of its key assumptions survived and were integrated into Labour Party thinking. Foremost among these were cost containment, the assumption that welfare costs could not significantly grow and that direct taxation must be kept down. In addition, Keynesian approaches were abandoned and inflation was accepted as the major enemy. As the Labour Prime Minister, Tony Blair, commented in 1999, the 'wider vision for Britain' was 'an economy based on stable foundations, with low interest rates and sound public finances'. Behind this view lies more deep-rooted acceptance that welfare should demonstrate its efficiency and effectiveness, expressed in policies such as 'best value' in social services. While some of the cruder competition has been removed, New Right views about the value of markets in health and social care have been accepted, much to the anger of some of those on the Left.

Debates about welfare are still very much alive, therefore, highlighting the struggle to adapt the welfare state for a new generation. New challenges are apparent too, such as those presented by regionalization and by the creation of a separate assembly for Wales and a Scottish parliament. Following the 1999 elections, coalition government in the smaller nations of the UK is likely to result in significant restructuring and higher spending in the health and social care services. The Westminster government may come under considerable pressure from its counterparts in the rest of the UK to increase welfare expenditure and pay for it through higher taxation. And as the Labour government struggles to make its post-New Right welfare settlement stick beyond 2000, we can be sure that debates about individual and collective responsibility for welfare will continue.

References

Abbott, E. and Bompas, K. (1943) *The Woman Citizen & Social Security: a Criticism of the Proposals of the Beveridge Report as they Affect Women*, London: Women's Freedom League.

Blair, T. (1999) Speech, Health Conference, Birmingham, International Conference Centre, 13 April.

Boyson, R. (1971) *Down with the Poor*, London: Churchill Press.

Deakin, N. (1987) *The Politics of Welfare*, London: Methuen.

Donnison, D. (1991) *A Radical Agenda after the New Right and the Old Left*, London: Rivers Oram Press.

Donnison, D. (1997) *The Politics of Poverty*, Oxford: Martin Robertson.

Field, F. (ed.) (1982) *Poverty and Politics*, London: Heinemann.

Field, F. and Piachaud, D. (1971) 'The poverty trap', in Field, (1982) pp. 104–7.

Friedman, M. and Friedman, R. (1980) *Free to Choose*, Harmondsworth: Penguin.

George, V. and Miller, S. (1994) *Social Policy towards 2000: Squaring the Welfare Circle*, London: Routledge.

Hadley, R. and Hatch, S. (1981) *Social Welfare and the Failure of the State*, London: Allen and Unwin.

Hayek, F. von (1944) *The Road to Serfdom*, London: Routledge and Kegan Paul.

Heald, D. (1983) *Public Expenditure*, Oxford: Martin Robertson.

Heelas, P. (1991) 'Reforming the self: enterprise and the characters of Thacherism', in R. Keat and N. Abercrombie (eds), *Enterprise Culture*, London: Routledge.

Illich, I. (1977) *Disabling Professions*, London: Marion Boyars.

Land, H. (1978) 'Who cares for the family?', *Journal of Social Policy*, 7 (3): 257–84.

Le Grand, J. (1982) *The Strategy of Equality*, London: Allen and Unwin.

Minford, P. (1984) 'State expenditure: a study in waste', *Economic Affairs*, April–June.

Mishra, R. (1984) *The Crisis of the Welfare State*, Brighton: Wheatsheaf.

Rhys-Williams, J. (1943) *Something to Look Forward to: a Suggestion for a New Social Contract*, London: Macdonald.

Riddell, M. (1983) *The Thatcher Government*, Oxford: Martin Robertson.

Tawney, R.H. (1966) *The Radical Tradition*, Harmondsworth: Penguin.

Thatcher, M. (1977) *Let Our Children Grow Tall, Selected Speeches 1975–77*, London: Centre for Policy Studies.

Townsend, P. (1979) *Poverty in the UK*, Harmondsworth: Penguin.

Townsend, P. and Davidson, N. (1982) *Inequalities in Health: The Black Report*, Harmondsworth: Penguin.

Ungerson, C. (ed.) (1985) *Women and Social Policy: a Reader*, London: Macmillan.

Williams, F. (1989) *Social Policy: A Critical Introduction*, Oxford: Polity Press.

Willetts, D. (1987) 'The price of welfare', *New Society*, 14 August: 9–11.

Wilson, E. (1977) *Women and the Welfare State*, London: Macmillan.

2

T. Butcher

The Public Administration Model of Welfare Delivery

The welfare state that was created in the years immediately after the Second World War, and which was consolidated and expanded in the following three decades, was deliberately set up under a form of state organization which placed a great deal of emphasis on the bureaucratic ideal of efficient and impartial administration. It was what has been called an 'administrative model' of welfare delivery characterized by the familiar bureaucratic features of hierarchical structure, clearly defined duties, and rule-based procedures, in which tasks which could not easily be controlled by rules were carried out by professionally qualified staff who were given what has been referred to as 'bounded discretion' in the performance of their work (Hadley and Young, 1990: 12). Such an approach to the delivery of welfare was a deliberate move away from the provision by voluntary and charitable organizations that had been such an important feature of welfare provision for much of the nineteenth and early twentieth centuries. The Labour government which came into office in 1945 and established the apparatus of the welfare state as part of the post-war settlement, 'turned [their] backs on philanthropy and replaced the do-gooder by highly professional administrators and experts' (Crossman, 1976: 278). In the brave new world of post-war Britain, the public sector was entrusted with the primary responsibility for the delivery of social welfare. Faith was placed in the public sector as 'a way of guaranteeing provision that was comprehensive and universal, professional and impartial, and subject to democratic control' (Webb et al., 1976: 7).

The post-war Labour government regarded the state and its administrative apparatus as the main instruments of social change (Hadley and Hatch, 1981: 15). The institutions of public administration – central government departments, elected local authorities and the newly created National Health Service (NHS) – were seen as the

First published in *Delivering Welfare: The Governance of the Social Services in the 1990s*, T. Butcher (Open University Press, 1995), pp. 1–7, 156–61. Abridged.

most effective means of delivering the core social services of social
security, health care, education and housing, together with the
various local authority health, welfare and children's services which
were later to be consolidated as the personal social services in the
early 1970s.

What can be described as the public administration model, with its
emphasis on the efficient and impartial administration of services,
characterized the organization of the delivery of welfare in Britain for
most of the post-war period. Not only was the system created in the
years immediately following the Second World War based upon this
approach, but, as Hadley and Young (1990: 13) have shown, subsequent reorganizations of local government, local authority personal
social services and the NHS in the 1960s and early 1970s took many
of the principles of this model for granted. In recent years, however,
the public administration model, and the institutions associated with
it, have been the subject of critical debate, particularly since the
election of the Conservative Thatcher government in 1979. This
debate has been joined by critics on all sides of the political spectrum,
ranging from the group of thinkers described as the New Right,
through the welfare pluralists with their advocacy of the voluntary
sector, to the so-called New Urban Left. But it is the first group who
have been particularly influential: indeed one commentator has
argued that the general agreement that there is a case against large
state welfare bureaucracies is among the New Right's 'most striking
intellectual achievements' in the field of social policy (Deakin, 1987:
177). Since the election of the first Thatcher government, the welfare
state has been passing through an era in which traditional assumptions about the organizational arrangements for the delivery of
welfare have been fundamentally questioned and in which major
changes have been made in the organization and management of the
delivery agencies concerned. . . .

The public administration model of welfare delivery

The traditional public administration model which has underpinned
the delivery of welfare in Britain since 1945 has several distinctive
characteristics:

- a bureaucratic structure;
- professional domination;
- accountability to the public;
- equity of treatment;
- self-sufficiency.

These will be described in the following sections.

Bureaucratic structure

A major characteristic of the public administration model of welfare delivery is the emphasis on bureaucratic organization. Associated with the classic account outlined by the German sociologist Max Weber (1964) in the early years of the century, bureaucracy is a term used to describe a form of organization which in its 'ideal type' exhibits a number of characteristics, such as the hierarchical structure of offices, the clear specification of functions, rule-based procedures, and staff who act impartially without favouritism (see, for instance, Albrow, 1970).

Bureaucratic structure has been a major feature of the traditional pattern of organization in the delivery agencies of the welfare state. The traditional organization of the delivery of social services by both central government departments and local authorities has been characterized by the principle of hierarchy, the emphasis upon uniformity of treatment, and the division of responsibilities around particular tasks such as education and housing (see, for example, Stewart, 1986: 12–15). Thus the giant social security system operated by the Department of Social Security (DSS) has been described as 'the most bureaucratized, routinized and therefore "clericalized"' of the major social services (Pollitt and Harrison, 1992: 10). Writing in the mid-1980s about local authorities, the major delivery agencies of the welfare state, Stewart (1986: 15) argued that the principles of the bureaucratic mode had become 'written into the thought processes' of those who worked in local government. In his view, they had become not principles but assumptions that were rarely challenged. The form of bureaucratic structure traditionally found in the local authority departments concerned with the delivery of welfare has been what has been described as that of a 'professionalised bureaucracy', the professional staff of such organizations being allowed a certain amount of freedom in the way they deliver services (Taylor-Gooby and Dale, 1981: 206). As we shall see, this latter form of bureaucracy has also been a characteristic of the organization of the NHS.

The advantages of a bureaucratic system of organization are well documented: they are said to include such virtues as consistency, reliability and susceptibility to political control. A bureaucratic form of organization is also supportive of what we will later identify as two other key features of the public administration model, the values of accountability and equity (see Pitt and Smith, 1981: 139). By allowing for the detailed control of subordinate staff within a hierarchical structure, bureaucracy provides a means by which large organizations can carry out their functions in accordance with the requirements of public accountability (Greenwood and Wilson, 1989: 25). Bureaucracy's emphasis on the depersonalization of administration also means that the users of a bureaucratic organization's services are subject to 'formal equality of treatment' (Weber, 1964: 340).

Professional domination

Another major characteristic of the public administration model of welfare delivery has been the important role played by professionals in the delivery of social services. Although the biggest spending social service, social security, is a clear exception to this general rule, professionals have dominated the delivery agencies of the welfare state. Elected local authorities and the institutions of the NHS are dominated by professionals. It is doctors, teachers, social workers and other welfare professionals – described by one writer as the 'trusted instruments' of the welfare state (Donnison, 1982: 21) – who deliver welfare and, in many cases, make key decisions about resource allocation and other important issues. As Klein (1973: 4) has observed: 'The Welfare State is, in many respects, also the Professional State.'

The development of welfare professionalism was an inevitable concomitant of the expansion of state social services in the post-war period. As Wilding (1982: 14–15) puts it in his discussion of the nature of professional power in the field of social welfare:

> A commitment to welfare by government means a need for professionals – to advise on the organisation of services, to manage, man and mediate services, to decide questions of eligibility and need, to individualise justice, to raise standards of health and child care.

The three decades following the end of the Second World War represented what has been described as 'the high tide of professionalism' in the welfare state, with professionalism becoming 'the dominant occupational paradigm' (Laffin and Young, 1990: 17, 32). The two well-established welfare professions – medicine and education – consolidated their positions: indeed, the medical profession was given substantial representation in the administrative structure of the NHS established in 1948, as well as being allowed to continue to enjoy considerable professional autonomy in the way it delivered health care. Although not enjoying the same degree of influence and autonomy as the medical profession, the teaching profession was also given a substantial amount of freedom in the running of the post-war education system.

Other welfare professions developed within local government as local authorities were given responsibility for those services requiring what has been described as face-to-face 'professional style' involvement with the users of services (Cochrane, 1993: 14). Thus the new welfare responsibilities imposed on local authorities by the post-war legislation dealing with domiciliary and residential care, child care and community care 'pointed the way' for the growth of the social work profession in the 1950s and 1960s (Marwick, 1982: 62–3), culminating in the creation of a single professional social work organization, the British Association of Social Workers, in 1970. This particular process of professionalization was reinforced by the setting up of unified local authority social services departments a year or two later. . . .

Thus, in the words of one commentator: 'Professional power has marched hand in hand with public welfare' (Wilding, 1982: 70). Although it is difficult to generalize about the nature and extent of such power in the delivery of welfare, it is possible, using the typology constructed by Wilding (1982), to identify the different types of power exercised by welfare professionals. Firstly, welfare professionals exercise power in both the making of welfare policy and its administration. Secondly, the power of welfare professionals is underpinned by their generally accepted right to define the needs and problems of their clients. Thirdly, welfare professionals exercise power and influence in the allocation of resources, not only at the level of general planning decisions by central and local government, but also at the organizational level – hospitals, schools, etc. – and in routine decisions affecting the individual client. These last two forms of power both affect the way services are delivered and are examples of the way in which welfare professionals exert power over people – the fourth type of power. Finally, welfare professionals have power to control their area of work, through such devices as self-regulation of the profession.

These powers clearly derive in part from the expertise of welfare professionals and the important role that they play in both the making and implementation of social policy, but, as Wilding (1982: 67) observes, professional power is also buttressed by the bureaucratic nature of welfare delivery agencies. Being part of a bureaucratic organization releases welfare professionals from many of the constraints encountered if they work on their own in the private sector. Thus Wilding usefully quotes Klein (1973: 5): 'To the extent that the professional becomes part of an administrative machine . . . so his command over resources, and his ability to affect the consumer, is magnified.'

Accountability to the public

Another important characteristic of the public administration model of welfare delivery is accountability. The concept of accountability is an elusive one. One important aspect of what Day and Klein (1987: 1) describe as this 'chameleon word' is the existence of public accountability to elected representatives, at both the national and local level. As one textbook on public administration puts it: 'At its most elementary, public accountability simply requires that public bodies give an account of their activities to other people and provide a justification for what has been done' (Smith and Stanyer, 1976: 30–1). Thus the Secretary of State for Social Security is accountable to parliament for the operations of the DSS, whilst his cabinet colleague, the Secretary of State for Health, is accountable to parliament for everything that happens in the NHS. At the local government level, the directors of the local authority departments responsible for the delivery of education, housing and the personal social services report to committees of the elected local authority.

The accountability of the delivery agencies of central government, local government and the NHS is not confined to the political dimension. The armies of bureaucrats and professionals employed by the delivery agencies of the welfare state are also subject to what has been referred to as 'administrative accountability': the duty to account to non-political bodies which examine the fairness and reasonableness of administrative procedures – administrative tribunals and the various ombudsmen who operate at the level of central government, local government and the NHS (Oliver, 1991: 27). This particular form of accountability also includes the duty of local authorities and health authorities to account to the Audit Commission with regard to efficiency and value for money. Like other public bodies, the delivery agencies of the welfare state are also accountable to the courts, having to make sure that their activities conform to the requirements of legality. . . .

Equity of treatment

Another characteristic of the public administration model, with its emphasis on impartial administration, is that the personnel responsible for the delivery of social and other public services are, in the words of Greenwood and Wilson (1989: 9), 'expected to treat members of the public fairly without showing partiality to one at the expense of another'. Or as Glennerster (1992a: 32) has put it: 'Public organisations must be seen to be dealing fairly with all those who use the service. Like cases must be treated alike.'

Many of the services and benefits provided by the delivery agencies of the welfare state are specified in detail in legislation and there is a public expectation that delivery agencies and their staff will treat everybody equally and fairly. This value of equity 'puts a premium on stability, consistency and accuracy' in the operation of public bodies (Smith and Stanyer, 1976: 31). In parts of the social security system, this expectation is actually institutionalized in the form of the adjudicatory machinery provided by administrative tribunals. A range of ombudsmen also operate in an attempt to ensure that the users of social services are treated reasonably in their dealings with the various delivery agencies of the welfare state.

Self-sufficiency

Finally, another characteristic of the public administration model is what Stewart and Walsh (1992: 509), speaking of the public services in general, refer to as the assumption of self-sufficiency. Where a public organization is responsible for a function, it has normally carried out that function itself and employed those who deliver the service. As Pinker (1992: 273) has observed, it was 'taken for granted' in the years following the creation of the welfare state that the state had a dominant role to play as both the funder and provider of social services.

The two roles were not always combined. Before the emergence of a developed welfare state, government intervention in both education and housing had involved the separation of the funder and provider roles. Thus, in the nineteenth century, central government gave grants to voluntary societies to provide local education, whilst immediately after the First World War, government subsidies were given to private builders to provide working-class housing. But the need for closer quality control, together with demands for stronger financial and political accountability and equity in service provision, resulted in the fusion of the roles of funder and provider (Glennerster, 1992a: 32–3; 1992b: 15–16). The 'accepted way of thinking' about the delivery of welfare in the system that developed in the post-war period was that social services should be both financed and provided by an agency of the state (Glennerster, 1992a: 31). Thus welfare delivery agencies fulfilled the role of both funder and provider of most social services. The state provided and financed the core social services of education, housing, the personal social services, social security and health care. . . .

Reassessing the public administration model

We identified five key features of the traditional public administration model – its bureaucratic structure, the dominant role played by welfare professionals, the value of public accountability, the concern with equity and the notion of self-sufficiency – which characterized the organization of the delivery of welfare for most of the post-war period. The remaining sections of this chapter will briefly reflect on the status of these traditional characteristics in the light of the emergence of newer approaches to the delivery of welfare.

Bureaucracy

Welfare bureaucracies have been the subject of increasing attack from all sides of the political spectrum, ranging from complaints about inefficiency and waste in the use of precious resources to concerns about the failure of delivery agencies to be close enough to their customers in the delivery of those services.

A major consequence of such concerns has been the search for alternative forms of organizing the delivery of welfare. Thus, influenced by the proponents of the public choice school, with its preference for the dismantling of large centralized bureaucracies into smaller competing bodies, the 1980s and the 1990s have seen attempts to break up traditional public bureaucratic structures like local authority housing empires through such policy initiatives as the 'right to buy', the opting out of many local education authority schools to the newly created grant maintained sector, and the transformation of the majority of NHS hospitals and other health-care units into self-governing trusts.

What Hoggett (1991: 247) refers to as 'the demise of bureaucratic control' and its replacement by post-bureaucratic forms of welfare delivery has also included a movement away from the traditional 'top-down' hierarchies associated with bureaucratic arrangements for delivering welfare. One manifestation of this particular trend has been the devolution of managerial freedoms to smaller operational units within the organizations responsible for welfare delivery. There have been a number of developments in this area: local management has been introduced in schools; financial responsibility within the NHS has been devolved to hospital doctors through the Resource Management Initiative; fund-holding GPs have been established within the NHS; increased responsibility has been delegated to care managers in local authority social services departments; managerial and financial responsibilities have been devolved to chief executives in the newly created Benefits Agency and other executive agencies.

In some areas of the welfare state, notably community care and the NHS, we are seeing the abandonment of what has been referred to as 'control by hierarchy' and its replacement by 'control by contract' (Hoggett, 1991: 250). One advantage of the use of contract as a means of delivering welfare is that by separating the purchaser and provider roles, it moves away from the traditional organization in which those responsible for a service have tended to identify with those providing it, rather than with those using it (Stewart, 1993: 8). By setting out specific service targets, contracts are also a means of focusing attention on the quality of service delivery (see, for example, Longley, 1993: 43). However, the contract culture has limitations, notably the dilution of public accountability, as members of the public will not always be certain who is accountable for particular services. . . .

Professionals

The dominant role played by professionals in the delivery of welfare has also been challenged by the new paradigms of efficiency and consumerism. In this context, there have been a number of developments since the early 1980s. Perhaps the most significant of these has been the threat to the position of the medical profession, as manifested by the increased emphasis upon the role of managers in the NHS and by the replacement of consensus management with general management, what has been referred to as the 'shifting of the frontier' between doctors and NHS managers. The role of general management within the NHS has been reinforced by the internal market reforms, with general managers being given a major role in the new contracting process and hospital consultants being made directly accountable to managers, as well as being given responsibility for clinical budgeting. On the other hand, one must be careful not to exaggerate the implications of such changes for the medical profession: the contracting process is effectively dependent on medical advice (see Moon and Kendall, 1993: 186).

The position of welfare professionals has also been affected by the increasing concern with consumerism and customers. The introduction of the Citizen's Charter, together with the mini-charters published for the various social services, means that the environment in which welfare professionals, and other welfare delivery personnel, are working has changed. Detailed service standards and procedures whereby the consumers of social services can exert pressure on providers to improve the quality of services are now important features of the delivery of welfare. Performance indicators monitor the progress and compare the performance of different delivery agencies. League tables enable the users of services to compare the performance of competing delivery agencies.

The movement away from the professional mode of welfare delivery towards a more managerial mode has also involved what one commentator has referred to as 'creating managers out of professionals' (Hoggett, 1991: 254), requiring them to be more interested in the costs of services provided and the management of scarce resources. Thus the introduction of local management of schools, the devolution of financial control to hospital doctors and fund-holding GPs and the devolution of responsibilities to care managers in local authority social services departments have resulted in welfare professionals such as head teachers and their senior staff, doctors and social workers being required to manage the day-to-day operations of their particular operational units, including the handling of budgets and dealing with contractors. . . .

Accountability and the public

The notion of accountability has been a recurring theme in the debate about the delivery of welfare. The weaknesses in traditional approaches to accountability have been the subject of concern for

many years, with the accountability of elected representatives
(whether they be central government ministers or local government
councillors) having long been recognized as an inadequate mechanism for securing the public accountability of delivery agencies and
their personnel.

The 1960s and 1970s witnessed attempts to increase 'accountability
downwards' to the users of services through the introduction of new
complaints mechanisms such as the various ombudsmen institutions.
The same period saw moves towards the development of user participation in the social services. Such mechanisms have been seen as
ways of giving users 'voice' in the delivery of welfare (Bartlett and Le
Grand, 1993: 18). But it is the concern with the newer concept of
consumer accountability which has been such a significant feature
of changes in the arrangements for the delivery of welfare in the late
1980s and early 1990s. Recent initiatives have employed the concept
of 'exit' (Hirschman, 1970), whereby those consumers who are dissatisfied with the quality of public service provision can choose to
leave those services. Thus, in the field of social housing council
tenants have been given the opportunity to 'exit' from local housing
authorities through the 'right to buy' or by transferring to alternative
landlords. In the field of education, the Education Reform Act 1988
increases parental choice through open enrolment and allows parents
to ballot for state schools to opt out of local education authority
control.

Developments since the late 1980s have also seen the proliferation
of non-elected bodies with responsibility for the delivery of large parts
of the various social services formerly directly provided by elected
local authorities and by health authorities which, although not
elected, used to include local authority representation. What has been
described as the 'new magistracy' (Stewart, 1992: 7) can be found
on the governing bodies of grant-maintained schools, Community
Technical Colleges (CTCs) and further education corporations. The
boards of the new NHS trusts and the small number of housing
action trusts are also made up of appointed members. The creation of
such bodies has given rise to a debate about a so-called 'accountability crisis'. These new arrangements for welfare delivery have also
resulted in confusion about the location of responsibility. . . .

Equity and welfare delivery

A key theme in the restructuring of the delivery of welfare has been
the introduction of quasi-markets, a phenomenon which has major
implications, not least for the traditional imperative of equity, a key
component of the public administration model of welfare delivery.
Advocates of quasi-markets argue that the introduction of such
mechanisms enhances consumer choice, a claim which has been the

subject of much dispute. For example, under the new arrangements for community care and the NHS, choices about care are not made by the users of services, but by purchasers acting on their behalf – care managers, District Health Authorities (DHAs) and fund-holding GPs.

Furthermore, not all potential users of social services have the same capacity for making choices. People in lower socio-economic groups may have lower expectations about services and less information about alternatives than those in more affluent groups of society (Bailey, 1993: 21). The providers of particular services may also restrict the choices available to certain groups of potential users. It has been suggested that the new arrangements contained in the quasi-markets in health care and community care could tempt the providers of those services to engage in what has been described as 'adverse selection', with those people in most need of a service being excluded from its provision on the grounds of their costliness. Clearly these developments threaten the whole idea of social services under-pinned by the notion of equity, as does the emergence within the new NHS since 1991 of what some observers view as a two-tier system of health care, with fund-holding GPs being able to secure preferential treatment for their patients.

Self-sufficiency

The introduction of the purchaser–provider split in services such as the NHS and community care has also challenged the other major assumption which supported the organization of the welfare state for most of the post-war period: the concept of self-sufficiency. The idea that the delivery agencies responsible for the core services of the welfare state also normally provided those services has been under-mined by a number of developments. Local authority social services departments are increasingly engaged in relationships with private- and voluntary-sector organizations through contracts for the provision of community care. The notion of self-sufficiency is also challenged by the development of the enabling role in housing, education and the personal social services (Stewart and Walsh, 1992: 509), seen by some as presaging the end of local government. Yet, while some see these developments as a threat to the traditional self-sufficiency of local authorities as front-line delivery agents of the welfare state, others see them as a possible opportunity, opening up a broader enabling role than the one envisaged by the Conservative government and allowing local authorities to meet the needs of people in their areas (see, for example, Stewart, 1989: 177; Clarke and Stewart, 1988). Within the other major delivery agency of the welfare state, the NHS, the formerly self-sufficient DHAs now operate as purchasers of health care, buying services from a range of health-care providers, who include not only DHAs and NHS trusts, but also hospitals in the private sector.

Developments such as these are seen by some as empowering consumers. But unlike the private sector, where customers usually have
a choice of competing firms, most users of the social services are not
in a position where they can shop around and take their 'custom'
elsewhere. Also, although more responsive social services, more
sensitive staff and clearer standards are all essential components of
better-managed welfare delivery, consumerism and the customer
orientation by themselves are insufficient in the absence of adequate
resources.

Despite such reservations, the initiatives of recent years have
combined to create a system of welfare delivery in the 1990s which is
very different to the system which emerged in the late 1940s, was
consolidated in the 1950s and 1960s, and which still operated in the
1970s and early 1980s. A system dominated by central government
departments, local authorities and the NHS, and based upon the
practices and values of public administration – the public face of
welfare – is being replaced by a new set of practices and values,
based upon a new language of welfare delivery which emphasizes
efficiency and value for money, competition and markets, consumerism and customer care.

Such changes are the product of a deliberate attempt to restructure
the arrangements for the delivery of welfare. The issues that they
raise are part of a continuing debate about the governance of the
welfare state. It is a debate which will doubtless continue. . . .

References

Albrow, M. (1970) *Bureaucracy*, Pall Mall Press: London.

Bailey, S.J. (1993) 'Public choice theory and the reform of local government', *Public Policy and Administration*, 8: 7–24.

Bartlett, W. and Le Grand, J. (1993) 'The theory of quasi-markets', in J. Le Grand and W. Bartlett (eds) *Quasi-Markets and Social Policy*, Macmillan: London.

Clarke, M. and Stewart, J. (1988) *The Enabling Council: Developing and Managing a New Style of Local Government*, Local Government Training Board: Luton.

Cochrane, A. (1993) *Whatever Happened to Local Government?* Open University Press: Buckingham.

Crossman, R.H.S. (1976) 'The role of the volunteer in the modern social services', Sydney Ball Memorial Lecture 1973, in A.H. Halsey (ed.) *Traditions in Social Policy*, Blackwell: Oxford.

Day, P. and Klein, R. (1987) *Accountabilities: Five Public Services*, Routledge: London.

Deakin, N. (1987) *The Politics of Welfare*, Methuen: London.

Donnison, D. (1982) *The Politics of Poverty*, Martin Robertson: Oxford.

Glennerster, H. (1992a) *Paying for Welfare: The 1990's*, Harvester Wheatsheaf: Hemel Hempstead.

Glennerster, H. (1992b) *Paying for Welfare: Issues for the Nineties*, Welfare State Programme Paper No. 82, London School of Economics: London.

Greenwood, J. and Wilson, D. (1989) *Public Administration in Britain Today*, 2nd edn, Unwin Hyman: London.

Hadley, R. and Hatch, S. (1981) *Social Welfare and the Failure of the State*, Allen and Unwin: London.

Hadley, R. and Young, K. (1990) *Creating a Responsive Public Service*, Harvester Wheatsheaf: Brighton.

Hirschman, A. (1970) *Exit, Voice and Loyalty*, Harvard University Press: Cambridge, MA.

Hoggett, P. (1991) 'A new management for the public sector?', *Policy and Politics*, 19: 243–56.

Klein, R. (1973) *Complaints against Doctors: A Study in Professional Accountability*, Charles Knight: London.

Laffin, M. and Young R. (1990) *Professionalism in Local Government*, Longman: Harlow.

Longley, D. (1993) *Public Law and Health Service Accountability*, Open University Press: Buckingham.

Marwick, A. (1982) *British Society since 1945*, Allen Lane: London.

Moon, G. and Kendall, I. (1993) 'The National Health Service', in D. Farnham and S. Horton (eds) *Managing the New Public Services*, Macmillan: London.

Oliver, D. (1991) *Government in the United Kingdom The Search for Accountability, Effectiveness and Citizenship*, Open University Press: Buckingham.

Pinker, R.A. (1992) 'Making sense of the mixed economy of welfare', *Social Policy and Administration*, 26: 273–84.

Pitt, D. and Smith, B. (1981) *Government Departments: An Organizational Perspective*, Routledge and Kegan Paul: London.

Pollitt, C. and Harrison, S. (eds) (1992) *Handbook of Public Services Management*, Blackwell: Oxford.

Smith, B.C. and Stanyer, J. (1976) *Administering Britain*, Martin Robertson: Oxford.

Stewart, J. (1986) *The New Management of Local Government*, Allen and Unwin: London.

Stewart, J. (1989) 'The changing organization and management of local authorities', in J. Stewart and G. Stoker (eds) *The Future of Local Government*, Macmillan: London.

Stewart, J. (1992) 'The rebuilding of public accountability', in J. Stewart, N. Lewis and D. Longley (eds) *Accountability and the Public*, European Policy Forum: London.

Stewart, J. (1993) 'The limitations of management by contract', *Public Money and Management*, 13: 1–6.

Stewart, J. and Walsh, K. (1992) 'Change in the management of public services', *Public Administration*, 70: 449–518.

Taylor-Gooby, P. and Dale, J. (1981) *Social Theory and Social Welfare*, Edward Arnold: London.

Webb, A., Day, L. and Weller, D. (1976) *Voluntary Social Service Manpower Resources*, Personal Social Services Council: London.

Weber, M. (1964) *The Theory of Social and Economic Organization*, translated by A.M. Henderson and T. Parsons, Free Press: New York.

Wilding, P. (1982) *Professional Power and Social Welfare*, Routledge and Kegan Paul: London.

3

J. Lewis and H. Glennerster

Why Change Policy? Community Care in the 1990s

What was Mrs Thatcher's government trying to achieve when it introduced its community care reforms in the legislation it passed in 1990? Governments of all hues have been attempting to introduce something called 'community care' ever since at least 1948, and arguably earlier. So, what was the government up to? To understand the origins of the 1990 National Health Service and Community Care Act, or at least the community care part of it, it is important to try to review the rather confused tangle of events that preceded it. . . .

The immediate origins of the 1990 Act

Searching for the origins of the 1990 reforms takes us down an unlikely route. We have to go back to complaints made by the poverty lobby about the way supplementary benefits were being administered in the 1970s. Claimants' organizations argued that individual officers and local offices had too much discretion in interpreting claims. They called for more clearly defined legal entitlements. Paradoxically perhaps, government also saw a case for tighter legal controls, but from the opposite motive. Discretionary payments were rising fast and there was a view that by reducing the scope for discretion by individual officers this creeping growth could be checked. After an enquiry by the Supplementary Benefits Commission, it was concluded that the scheme should move to a more closely defined system of rules and entitlements.

What has all this to do with community care? One of the very small elements in the discretionary payments officers could make was to assist old people and others who were resident in a private residential or nursing home who found themselves in financial difficulties. This was a little-known and rarely used power. In 1979 the total sum

---

First published as 'The purpose of reforms', Chapter 1 of J. Lewis and H. Glennerster, *Implementing the New Community Care* (Open University Press, 1996), pp. 1–9. Abridged.

of money allocated in this way to individuals in distress was £10 million – out of a total supplementary benefit budget of about £2,000 million.

From November 1980 the rules under which people could claim board and lodging expenses were regulated by statute under parliamentary statutory instruments. These allowed someone who was a boarder to claim the full board and lodging charge plus an amount to cover personal expenses. A 'lodger' included not only those lodging with a landlady, say, in the normal sense of the word, but also those living in hostels and residential homes for the elderly and disabled and in nursing homes. A maximum sum for fee reimbursement was set, which had to be a reasonable charge for a facility 'of no more than a suitable standard' for the purpose in hand. It was fixed in relation to the normal levels of residential home fees in operation in a supplementary benefit office's area and became known as the 'local limit'.

There is still some dispute about how far politicians and officials were aware of what they were doing when they drew up these regulations, but their effects became all too clear before long. If you were a resident in such a home and you had no more savings or capacity to pay, the social security system would meet your fees. If you did have savings and hoped to hand them on to your children why not do so at once, become officially poor and let the social security system pay the fees? If this had not occurred to you, a thoughtful owner of the old people's home was likely to put you in the picture. One of the authors remembers just this happening to him when he finally arranged for his father to enter a home. Faced with advice that 'the social security can handle all this' he pointed out that his father had always had a dread of becoming dependent on the 'assistance' and would not wish to do so as long as his small pension and savings would suffice. The owner accepted the position with a rather quizzical look and a remark that few other people seemed to take that view.

Owners also soon caught on to the fact that the fees that were met were the average or normal local fee in the office's area. If all the fees in the area rose, so would the local limits and hence the sums payable to the owners by the local social security office.

Local authority treasurers and politicians began to ask why they should go on providing old people's homes if individuals could seek a home for themselves in the private sector and get the social security system to pay. Indeed, why not transfer the local authorities' homes into the private sector and get social security to pay the costs? Certainly there seemed no point in opening new local authority homes. Local authorities were, at this point, coming under great pressure to cut their spending, and central government grants were being reduced or stabilized while increasing numbers of people over 80 years old were needing care. Here was a way of getting another part of central government to pay, and serve them right.

The NHS was also under great budgetary pressure, trying to cope with the growing demands on its geriatric facilities. Geriatric medicine at its best in the UK has been very good. Hospitals sought to rehabilitate those old people who may have come in with a stroke or a cracked hip after a fall. Yet all their good work was useless if they could not discharge the elderly person because there was no domiciliary care or residential care to take them. If a hospital had an official arrangement with a nursing home or a hospice to take its patients, the patient could not claim any fees from the social security system. If, however, the patient went to a private home independently, the social security system would pay and resources would be freed for more NHS care in the hospital. It is not surprising that more and more patients began to be encouraged to make private arrangements funded by social security. As one geriatric consultant said to one of us, 'the social security route made an otherwise intolerable situation possible'. Many hospitals concerned with the mentally ill and the handicapped began to follow suit.

In short, the social security budget had inadvertently come to the rescue of families, local authorities and the NHS, all of them under tight budgetary limits and increasing demand. . . .

Rein in the runaway

At precisely this point the Treasury was undertaking a long-range review of public spending and the social security budget was its prime target. Here in the middle of this budget was the fastest-rising element in public spending and it seemed to have no ceiling. By the mid-1980s, the sum spent had risen from £10 million to £500 million.

The government began to try to recover from its mistake. In 1983 the amounts being paid for homes in some areas amounted to little over £50 but as much as £215 at the upper limit. New private homes were coming into being at a great rate and existing ones were expanding. It was not only officially registered homes that were covered. Homes with fewer than four residents also came within the scope of the regulations designed to cover board and lodgings. Social security officers were issued with simple instructions to decide whether such facilities were suitable for old people or not. They had no link with the local authority social workers who were doing the same with homes taking more than four people.

The government's first step was to introduce a freeze on the 'local limits' in December 1984. Then, in April 1985, the government introduced national limits on what could be paid for each resident, depending on the type of incapacity and type of facility. The regulations were generally tightened further in December 1985. None of this stemmed the rising tide of spending on the social security budget, which continued to accelerate.

External criticism

It was at this point that the recently created and independent agency responsible for overseeing local authority spending – the Audit Commission – stepped in. Its report was called *Making a Reality of Community Care* (Audit Commission, 1986). It was a cogent and highly critical document. It discussed the fragmented nature of the so-called spectrum of care that was supposed to be available, from hospital to domiciliary care. It pointed out that many agencies were involved and that many people were either getting the wrong kind of care or not getting care at all. It criticized funding arrangements that gave more central government support to hospital care than to local authorities, which were providing an alternative.

None of this was new. The same points had been made by the Guillebaud Committee nearly three decades earlier (Cmd. 9663, 1956). The Labour government had gone some way to tackle the issues in its joint planning and joint finance arrangements in the mid-1970s. Academics had certainly been critical in a similar vein (Wistow, 1983; Webb and Wistow, 1983, 1986; Glennerster, 1983). What was new was the exposure of what was happening to the social security funding of residential care. Under the heading 'Perverse effects of social security policies', the Audit Commission documented the rise in spending and argued that the government was being wholly inconsistent. It was telling local authorities that it wanted old people to stay at home for as long as possible because that was the most cost-effective and desirable thing to do but at the same time it was pushing large sums of public money into expensive residential and nursing home care. The government was going to elaborate trouble to set its local government grant levels, in line with demography, between one local authority and another, but it was happily handing out far more to some areas than others through its social security budget. As a result, the Commission claimed: 'there are now nearly ten times as many places per 1,000 people aged 75 or over in private or voluntary homes for elderly people in Devon and East Sussex than there are in Cleveland, for example' (Audit Commission, 1986: 3). These perverse incentives, the Commission concluded, must be removed. It reviewed a range of possible ways forward and recommended that a high-level review be undertaken: 'The one option that is not tenable is to do nothing' (p. 4).

Nothing

Yet, that is what the government did for the next four years. During that time social security expenditure rose from the original £10 million to over £2,000 million in 1991. There was one major stumbling block in the way of reform – and its name was Mrs Thatcher.

Simply to cut off the flow of social security money to new applicants would lead to the bankruptcy of many small private homes. Not only had they become an influential pressure group but they were exactly the kind of small family businesses of which Mrs Thatcher approved. It was also clear to nearly all of those involved in discussing the policy options that if government money was to be devoted to care in the community, however defined, there would have to be one budget holder, one gatekeeper, accountable for the decisions taken in respect of those old or disabled people who needed care. It was difficult to see any agency at that point that could perform the task except the local authority social services departments – and that was anathema to Mrs Thatcher. One of the authors remembers being drawn into discussions at this time with senior Conservative politicians to see if there was any other way out. At the end of a long discussion the conclusion was reached that there was no other way. Sighing, the chair looked up at a painting of the lady in question, who looked down on the assembled group, and said: 'But she will not have it.'

More advice

Sir Roy Griffiths, Mrs Thatcher's trusted adviser on the NHS, had already reported to her on the management of the NHS. He was called into service again. His terms of reference were: 'To review the way in which public funds are used to support community care policy and to advise me [the Secretary of State] on options which would improve the use of these funds' (Department of Health and Social Security, 1988). His essential job was to sort the money problem.

His eventual report, *Community Care: An Agenda for Action* (Department of Health and Social Security, 1988) was also clear:

> I recommend that public finance for people who require either residential home care or non-acute nursing home care, whether that is provided by the public sector or by private or voluntary organisations, should be provided in the same way. Public finance should only be provided following separate assessments of the financial means of the applicant and of the need for care. The assessments should be managed through social services authorities. (para. 6.39)

The social security payments to individuals for *care* should cease and the sums spent by transferred to local authorities to meet the needs of those who were in the vulnerable groups affected. It should be transferred as 'targeted specific grants', to ensure that the money was not spent on projects that had nothing to do with community care.

Then, in a section of the report on the duties of the state, Griffiths made it clear that the social services departments might be getting more funds under his scheme but that did not mean that their own budgets and facilities should expand. On the contrary, 'The primary function of the public services is to design and arrange the provision of care and support in line with people's needs', and such support could and should come from a variety of sources. A 'mixed economy' would encourage choice, flexibility and innovation in a climate of competition (para. 3.4). Two of the most influential advisers to Griffiths, Ken Judge, Director of the King's Fund Institute, and Herbert Laming, then Director of Social Services in Hertfordshire, had been advocating such an approach for several years. Moreover, there was nothing new about the idea as far as Conservative policy was concerned. Ever since 1980 local authorities had been statutorily obliged to contract out a growing proportion of their activities to private firms. Norman Fowler, Secretary of State for Social Services, had urged social service departments to follow suit and become 'enabling authorities' in his Buxton speech in 1984. (For an extended discussion of the antecedents see Wistow et al., 1994.)

Yet little had actually happened in the personal social services in most areas. Now the idea was being pushed to centre stage. Why? Certainly it reflected the temper of the times and the Conservative Party's third election victory in a row. The NHS, housing departments and indeed the rest of local government were being pushed in the same direction. The NHS was to become a 'quasi-market' too. But it is fairly clear that the main purpose was to get Mrs Thatcher to accept the Griffiths package. If the money being transferred to social services departments was *not* going to end up by further enlarging bloated local councils' social work staffs and *would* end up with private providers, her objections might be removed. So it proved. Griffiths's main proposals were accepted and a White Paper, *Caring for People* (Cm. 849 1989), embodied most of the ideas strengthening, if anything, the explicitness of the mixed-economy enabling model.

Lessons

This history is crucial to understanding the reforms and the way they were implemented. They were not primarily driven by a desire to improve the relations between the various statutory authorities, or to improve services for elderly people, or to help those emerging from mental hospital. They were driven by the need to stop the haemorrhage in the social security budget and to do so in a way that would minimize political outcry and not give additional resources to the local authorities themselves. Most of the rest of the policy was, as the Americans would say, for the birds. Like the Health Service reforms that were part of the same legislation, these were hurried ideas (Glennerster et al., 1994) pushed through to meet a crisis.

References

Audit Commission (1986) *Making a Reality of Community Care*, London: HMSO.

Cmd 9663 (1956) *Report of the Committee of Enquiry into the Cost of the NHS (Guillebaud Enquiry)*, London: HMSO.

Cmd 849 (1989) *Caring for People: Community Care in the Next Decade and Beyond*, London: HMSO.

Department of Health and Social Security (1988) *Community Care: An Agenda for Action*, London: HMSO.

Glennerster, H. (with Korman, N. and Marsden-Wilson, F.) (1983) *Planning for Priority Groups*, London: Martin Robertson.

Glennerster, H., Matsaganis, M. and Owens, P. (1994) *Implementing GP Fundholding*, Buckingham: Open University Press.

Webb, A. and Wistow, G. (1983) 'Public expenditure and policy implementation: the case of community care', *Public Administration*, 61 (Spring): 21–44.

Webb, A. and Wistow, G. (1986) *Planning, Need and Scarcity: Essays on the Personal Social Services*, London: Allen and Unwin.

Wistow, G. (1983) 'Joint finances and community care: have the incentives worked?', *Public Money*, 3 (2): 33–7.

Wistow, G., Knapp, M., Hardy, B. and Allen, C. (1994) *Social Care in a Mixed Economy*, Buckingham: Open University Press.

4

F. Brooks

Changes in Maternity Policy – Who, What and Why?

In the last three decades, the control of birth practices has become the site of an intensely polarized debate, one that has largely arisen from a vociferous critique of the medical model of childbirth, by women, feminists, academics, midwives and even the occasional obstetrician (Doyal, 1995; Annandale and Clark, 1996; Oakley, 1984; Savage, 1986). In terms of official policy, this debate was intended to be concluded by the Winterton Report (HOC, 1992) and the subsequent response for the Department of Health, *Changing Childbirth* (DOH, 1993). The latter document was received largely positively by the midwifery profession and consumer pressure groups as 'the most exciting and revolutionary report affecting the maternity services this century' (Walton and Hamilton, 1995). Maternity care, it was claimed, was about to become woman-centred, by placing the needs and wishes of women first (Summers et al., 1997). Baroness Cumberledge, launching the report for the government insisted that 'The report is not a charter for midwives. It is not a charter for obstetricians, pediatricians or GPs – rather, it is a charter for women' (Milhill, 1993: 2).

The representation of *Changing Childbirth* as constituting a revolution in user-centred health policy received further endorsement by the new Labour government. In a Department of Health (DOH) press release Baroness Jay, Minister of Health explained: 'The principles of accessible, responsive, user-focused services pioneered by *Changing Childbirth* are now mirrored by those of "The New NHS" White Paper' (4 February 1998).

This chapter sets out to explore the validity of the claim that there has been a radical shift in policy in this area. Current maternity policy, it will be claimed, has been shaped by the interdependencies and conflicts between a number of different stakeholder groups, among whom users are only one constituency. The chapter concludes that far from achieving women-centred care, maternity care remains a contested policy arena.

The *who* of maternity policy: participants and the process (1970–90)

The second half of the twentieth century has seen increased medical involvement in childbirth. Facilitated by technological change, obstetric surveillance and intervention has become possible for all births, with the result that the obstetric management of care has become an exercise in the management of risk. In the UK up to the 1980s, it was the obstetric discourse of childbirth as a pathological 'risky' event that was overtly endorsed by maternity policy. Both the Short Report (1980) and the earlier Peel Report (SMMAC, 1970) advocated enforced compliance with medicalized care and 100 per cent hospital delivery.

However, during the 1970s a 'groundswell of consumer complaints' had emerged criticizing maternity services (Munro, 1985). Dissatisfaction centred around unnecessarily high levels of medical intervention, poor communication, and the depersonalized and fragmented nature of care (Cartwright, 1979; Macintyre, 1982; Walker, 1985). Women's groups and feminists were especially critical of medicalized childbirth for having transformed women into passive bodies processed by a system over which they had little control and for constructing pregnancy as a process that can only be defined as normal in retrospect (Graham and Oakley, 1981; Rothman, 1987; Martin, 1987).

From the 1960s onwards user dissatisfaction fuelled both the emergence and the ranks of consumer-based maternity groups such as the National Childbirth Trust (NCT), and the Association for the Improvement in Maternity Services (AIMS), (Oakley, 1984). In presenting the case against medicalized maternity care, consumerist groups looked to the philosophy of the natural childbirth movement for support. Developed in 1930s as the brainchild of Grantly Dick Read (1933) the concept of natural childbirth is essentially concerned with the assertion of childbirth as a 'natural' rather than a pathological process, with an agenda to demedicalize, reduce intervention, and increase user control (Arney and Neill, 1982).

The discourse of the natural childbirth movement can be interpreted as problematic, in so far as it replaces the active management of labour with an essentialist discourse that renders pregnant women as instinctive beings who need to regress to their primitive state to achieve psychological control over labour (Brooks and Lomax, 1999). This prioritization of individual control over childbirth can leave those who do not achieve control feeling that they have failed to attain a proper standard of womanhood. Also, because it represents women as a largely undifferentiated group, it does little to acknowledge the broader social and economic context where many women are unable to exercise choice and control over their lives (Lupton, 1994).

Furthermore, evidence also suggests that black and ethnic minority women are particularly disadvantaged by the maternity services and are frequently subjected to negative cultural stereotyping, resulting in inappropriate care (Bowler, 1993; Bowes and Domokos, 1996). Their voices were not part of a consumerist movement discourse that reflected largely middle-class concerns of choice and control. It was the articulate middle-class voice of consumerist groups grounded in the natural childbirth discourse that constituted the impetus for a policy response. Consequently it is an individualized and personalized critique of medicalized maternity care that has been given prominence in the definition of woman-centred care within policy.

The Maternity Services Advisory Committee to the Secretaries of State for Social Services was set up in the 1980s in the wake of the Short Report (1980) and of continued and growing criticism. The Committee accepted from the outset that there was justification for user dissatisfaction. It made it clear that health workers could not make executive decisions on women's behalf. In essence, however, its message was of unwavering acceptance of the medical definition of every birth as only being normal in retrospect and it accepted that the hospital was the safest place for birth (Maternity Services Advisory Committee, 1984; part II: V). This commitment to the obstetric safety discourse was maintained, despite the fact that evidence was available at the time indicating the safety of home deliveries, and that the value of obstetrically managed childbirth derived from its selective rather than universal application (Tew, 1990; Pascall, 1997). The Committee, using the language of the natural childbirth movement, adopted informed choice as a means of repackaging the obstetric safety discourse, while at the same time retaining a distinction between acceptable professional expertise and unacceptable lay preference:

> Some mothers might prefer to have their babies at home despite the possible risks, feeling that these are outweighed by the benefits they perceive to themselves and their families. Doctors and midwives should discuss the reasons for each mother's preference, so that her final decision is an informed one. (Maternity Services Advisory Committee, 1984, part II: 23)

Women now needed only to be adequately educated, or informed, to appreciate the benefits of a hospital delivery and the value of technological intervention. The concept of 'informed choice' in effect extended medical surveillance beyond the pregnant body to women's sources of information and decision-making (Graham and Oakley, 1981; 70; Arney and Neill, 1982).

During the 1980s some concessions were made. Partners were 'allowed' to be present during childbirth; the organization of antenatal clinics was made more user-friendly; and efforts were made to change professional attitudes, such as encouraging doctors to be supportive and 'less dogmatic' about the care of maternity patients

(Graham and Oakley, 1981: 70). However, changes tended to be implemented piecemeal, and reforms were limited to humanizing the service rather than questioning it more fundamentally.

Midwives' changing places in the policy process

The 1980s also saw pressure for reform of the maternity services growing among the ranks of midwives. Official policy documents of the 1970s had presented midwifery as a key ally in the maintenance and reproduction of medicalized maternity care (SMMAC, 1970; Short Report, 1980). By the 1990s a very different construction has emerged: that of the midwife as the chief advocate for women and the provider of woman-centred care (DOH, 1993). To understand this dramatic transition, it is necessary to consider the way midwifery has been reconstructed during this period.

During the 1980s, the midwifery literature reflected an increasing concern that the medicalization of childbirth and in particular the move of the majority of maternity care provision into the hospitals had resulted in an erosion of the role of the midwife (Kitzinger, 1988). Although midwives delivered at least 85 per cent of all babies and an obstetrician was unlikely to be present at the birth, obstetrics controlled the formulation of care policy within the institutional setting of the hospital, thereby directing the nature of the work of other health workers (Arney, 1982; Kirkham, 1987). It appeared that within the hospital system midwives were becoming invisible and unable to provide continuity of care of choice for women (Brooks, 1990). If pregnant women were being processed as objects in a factory, midwives were the workers on the assembly line (Kitzinger, 1988).

A solution within the profession was framed as a reassertion of the traditional midwifery role, enabling midwives to be practitioners in their own right with separate skills but equal status to that of doctors. The growth of the Association of Radical Midwives (ARM), direct entry training and the move of some towards independent practice, were manifestations of this process. The justification lay in midwifery's traditional claim to be *with-women* (Campbell and Porter, 1997); that is the profession whose philosophy was most in line with women's needs and wishes. This model of midwifery is distinguished from the medical model by a focus on pregnancy as a normal event. Echoing the main themes of the natural childbirth movement, the midwife's role is to support women in exercising control over their care (Lewis, 1995). In 1986, the ARM published a *Vision* for maternity services: continuity of care, informed choice, community-based care and full utilization of the midwives' skills formed key elements of its proposals (ARM, 1986).

Undoubtedly, midwifery can represent a discourse that values women's subjective and situated knowledge and constructs pregnancy as a natural process (Brooks, 1990; Campbell and Porter, 1997). However, the notion that midwifery care represents an inevitable prioritization of women's needs requires scrutiny. In order to become a profession, midwifery must assert a unique body of knowledge and stake a claim to being the only provider that has access to that specific body of knowledge (Cartwright, 1979: 155). In striving for professional status in this way, midwifery is placed in a position of potential conflict with women. One illustration of this is the concern midwives have expressed about the threat of their own annihilation, in the face of members of the NCT teaching women and midwives about breastfeeding (Lewis, 1995: 638; Towler, 1982: 325). Consequently, the voicing of midwifery's concerns over medicalized care, and the emphasis on continuity of care as a solution to fragmented care needs to be interpreted not only as serving to form an alliance with women consumer groups, but also as operating to strengthen midwifery's claim to professional status within the context of obstetrically dominated maternity care.

It is in the light of this policy context – of professional groups operating with competing professionalizing strategies and a user voice that was largely defined by the articulate voice of consumerist groups grounded in the natural childbirth discourse – that I now consider the expression of maternity policy in *Changing Childbirth* (DOH, 1993).

Maternity policy in the 1990s: a radical departure?

The impetus to reconsider maternity policy occurred again in the early 1990s, when the continuing pressure from women, consumer groups and the midwifery profession for change in the maternity services combined with key elements of government philosophy. The Conservative government, keen to promote free market ideology in health care, sought to espouse individual consumer choice; challenge professional orthodoxy; and develop primary health care services while promoting cost efficiencies; all themes that are clearly apparent in the philosophy and objectives of *Changing Childbirth* (Sandall, 1995).

In March 1992 the House of Commons Select Committee produced the Winterton report (HOC, 1992) arguing that the medical model of care was not sufficient to drive the maternity service and that midwifery teams should be developed. The report was largely well received by the three Royal Colleges – of Obstetricians and Gynaecologists (RCOG), Midwives (RCM) and GPs (RCGP), whose joint statement was published in July (RCOG, 1992). Despite this, there is some evidence to suggest that Whitehall civil servants, believing that major change within the maternity services was not required, had advocated a negative response. They had attempted to load the later Expert Maternity Group with members of the RCOG, despite the Health Minister's desire for a high number of service users (Parliamentary Report, 1997). However, both the then Secretary of State for Health, Virginia Bottomley and Julia Cumberledge, Health Minister, appeared to be personally committed to achieving change within the maternity services, with Virginia Bottomley boasting that she was the first Secretary of State for Health who had experienced childbirth (Parliamentary Report, 1997). Consequently, despite opposition from within the Department of Health, the government set up the Expert Maternity Group, chaired by Julia Cumberledge, to inquire into the recommendations of the Winterton Report, the membership ultimately representing a compromise between Cumberledge and her departmental civil servants (DOH, 1993).

Changing Childbirth identifies four of the key principles of good maternity care:

- Women should be at the centre of decisions about their care.
- Services should be accessible to women.
- Services should be effective and efficient.
- Women should be involved in the planning and auditing of services.

In addition, there was to be a five-year target for providers to demonstrate 'a significant shift towards a community-oriented service', sensitive to local community needs. The role of the midwife, and continuity of care, were central themes of the report. Midwifery-led care was advocated, with obstetricians providing care in complicated pregnancies. These changes were to be supported by a five-year target, where 75 per cent of women were to be delivered by a midwife they knew during pregnancy, who could be the lead professional in normal pregnancies. *Changing Childbirth* in its promotion of midwifery and the normality of pregnancy does attempt to dismantle two of obstetrics's great bastions: the dominance of medical expertise and knowledge concerning pregnancy and the inherently pathological nature of pregnancy.

However, *Changing Childbirth* also offers considerable continuity with previous policy, and a version of woman-centred care that allows a prioritization of professional concerns and input. Support for this interpretation can be drawn from the status given to user views.

In the report, evidence derived from women service users' situated knowledge of childbirth is described as 'stories', whereas the accounts of professionals (or 'experts' according to the definition used in the report) represent 'testimony or evidence'. Moreover user 'stories' were frequently used to endorse the value of professional input, rather than as a means of identifying the direction of policy change:

> The experts heard many stories illustrating ways in which sensitive and flexible professional care can enhance the experience and safety of pregnancy and birth. (DOH, 1993: 11–12)

This suggests a prioritization of 'expert evidence' and a downgrading of consumer 'opinion' or 'stories'.

Two surveys were commissioned as a means of obtaining the views of women not linked to consumer organizations (MORI, 1993) and of Asian and Afro-Caribbean mothers (Rudat et al., 1993). These studies were given scant attention – a lack of weighting that raises questions over the basis for recommendations concerning the importance of achieving continuity of care, for example. Of the 1,005 women surveyed by MORI, 19 per cent indicated that continuity of care with a midwife or doctor was the most important issue to them, but not all mentioned that being cared for in labour by someone they knew was important. Although women's dissatisfaction with fragmented care has been highlighted in a number of studies (Oakley, 1984), does this alone sufficiently explain the weight and emphasis given to continuity of care by the expert group? Or is it that the preference by some women for continuity of care represents a fusion with the professionalizing strategy of midwifery?

The continued elevation of the medical discourse in *Changing Childbirth* can be illustrated by its treatment of the issue of safety (DOH, 1993: Part II). The document appears initially to problematize medicalized approaches to safety by pointing to empirical evidence identifying the safety of home deliveries (Tew, 1990; DOH, 1993: 9). Yet there remains a central emphasis in the report on medicalized definitions of safe maternity care:

> We believe, on the evidence that we have seen, that the service could be organised in a way which does not jeopardise safety, yet is kinder, more welcoming and more supportive to the women whose needs it is designed to meet. (DOH, 1993: Part II)

This continuing acceptance of the medical safety discourse was reported in the *British Journal of Obstetrics and Gynaecology* in reassuring tones. Obstetricians were urged to read the report carefully to dispel their doubts; home births were not *pushed* as an option, changes were to happen slowly and be subject to audit and finally, safety was to remain the 'foundation of maternity care' (Anderson, 1993: 1072).

In part because the definition of woman-centred care came from consumerist groups concerned with choice and control, far from proposing a radical reorganization of care, one of the primary concerns of the expert group appears to be to make the service 'kinder'. Yet the identification of safety as the foundation of maternity services suggests services are to be made user friendly rather than woman centred, with medicalized approaches to safety remaining unchallenged.

Implementation: policy marginalization

Virginia Bottomley announced the government's acceptance of the report in January 1994 and the intention to set up an advisory group to support the implementation. Circular EL(94) was issued to the NHS, setting out the action required to implement the report. This was followed in May 1994 by the provision of £349,000 in development funds to support pilot projects linked to *Changing Childbirth* and the establishment of a team of advisers for purchasers and providers.

Initially, the Royal College of Obstetricians and Gynaecologists perceived *Changing Childbirth* as heralding a revolution in which they were simply not prepared to participate. The objections of the College were largely focused on concerns that the obstetricians could face exclusion from 'normal deliveries' and that home births were presented as safe alternatives to hospital deliveries. The College was angered by its lack of influence over the proceedings of the expert group and after holding an extraordinary general meeting sought further discussion with the DOH (Dunlop, 1993). Perhaps in recognition of having lost part of the argument to midwifery, the College immediately sought to assert a role for medicine resulting from possession of a generic knowledge base. Doctors now needed to review every pregnancy not because pregnancy was inherently pathological but because they had skills in screening for other underlying conditions in women; conditions that midwives were not trained to screen for (Milhill, 1993). The College also sought to dilute the notion of lead professional by changing the terminology to *link* professional and by expressing concerns over the potential isolation of midwives (Dunlop, 1993).

However, in the main, the response to *Changing Childbirth* from the medical profession in the years since publication has been one of marginalization, with little debate being generated in the medical professional journals. The emphasis on informed choice and women's involvement in decision-making has more recently been employed to validate the promotion of increased medical intervention through elective Caesarean sections (Paterson-Brown, 1998). A further dilution of the agenda of *Changing Childbirth* has resulted from the report's ambiguous stance on many of its key terms including 'continuity of carer' and 'known midwife', thereby allowing for a multitude of interpretations (Sandall, 1995). Although care from a general practitioner is not required for a woman to gain a home delivery, in reality lack of support from GPs (concerns about potential litigation, lack of remuneration and time) remains a practical block to women choosing home delivery.

The marginalization of *Changing Childbirth* and its recommendations can also be seen to have occurred because the resources allocated for implementation have remained limited. Funds for *Changing Childbirth* were small and no additional moneys were allocated for 'rolling out' patterns of care demonstrated as successful by the pilot projects. Consequently, although the policy was intended to form part of a five-year development strategy (NHSME, 1994), in reality, change in the maternity service had to compete for resources alongside other strategic requirements. Time-limited pilot projects have also been demonstrated to be a problematic means of achieving mainstream change, at the very least because they require local funding and commitment to be continued (Rosser, 1997). The Department of Health made only a limited number of awards to midwifery pilot projects (Changing Childbirth Implementation Team, 1995). No pilot awards were made to team midwifery projects, the main means by which continuity of care was supposed to be developed.

Finally, midwifery has largely not achieved the position of lead profession in the delivery of maternity care; titles of articles in the midwifery journals illustrate the level of disillusionment among midwives; 'Changing childbirth: the best kept secret ever' (Troutt, 1996), 'Lies, damned lies and economics' (Rosser, 1997) and 'The death of *Changing Childbirth*' (Lewis, 1996). Midwives, it has been argued, face *burn-out* from increased case-loads and inadequate support to deliver team-based care (Sandall, 1995). The Royal College of Midwives had been accused by consumer groups of having 'fiddled while Rome has burned', too concerned with its own status to negotiate for women and midwives effectively (Beech, 1997). Institutional and medical opposition at a local level from GPs also appears to have been highly detrimental to the development of midwifery-led care.

Changing maternity policy – conclusions

Current maternity policy in the UK, including the most recent initiative *Changing Childbirth*, represents a humanizing of the medical model rather than a clearly identified alternative vision. In essence, the privileged position of obstetric discourses has been maintained and has provided a means of defusing more radical interpretations. This examination of *Changing Childbirth* exemplifies the continuing influence of professional power and of competing professional cultures on the provision of maternity care. The privileged position given to the medical perspective can be contrasted with the low level of user involvement in the construction and implementation of policy. Consequently it is an individualized and personalized critique of medicalized care that has been given prominence in the definition of woman-centred care within maternity policy from the 1980s onwards.

References

Anderson, M. (1993) '*Changing Childbirth*. Commentary I', *British Journal of Obstetrics and Gynaecology*, 100 (December): 1071–2.

Annandale, E. and Clarke, J. (1996) 'What is gender? Feminist theory and the sociology of human reproduction', *Sociology of Health and Illness*, 18 (1): 17–44.

ARM (Association of Racial Midwives) (1986) *The Vision: Proposal for the Future of the Maternity Services*, Ormskirk, Lancashire: Association of Radical Midwives.

Arney, W. (1982) *Power and the Profession of Obstetrics*, Chicago: University of Chicago Press.

Arney, W. and Neill, J. (1982) 'The location of pain in childbirth: natural childbirth and the transformation of obstetrics', *Sociology of Health and Illness*, 4 (1): 1–24.

Beech, B. (1997) 'Sounding off', *Modern Midwife*, 7(3).

Bowes, A.M. and Domokos, T.M. (1996) 'Pakistani women and maternity care: raising muted voices', *Sociology of Health and Illness*, 18 (1): 45–65.

Bowler, I. (1993) '"They're not the same as us": midwives' stereotypes of Asian women', *Sociology of Health and Illness*, 15: 157–78.

Brooks, F. (1990) 'Alternatives to the medical model of childbirth: a qualitative study of user centred maternity care', PhD thesis, University of Sheffield.

Brooks, F. and Lomax, H. (1999) 'Labouring bodies: mothers and maternity policy', in H. Dean and K. Ellis (eds) *Social Policy and the Body: Transitions in Corporeal Discourses*, London: Macmillan.

Campbell, R. and Porter, S. (1997) 'Feminist theory and the sociology of childbirth: a response to Ellen Annadale and Judith Clark', *Sociology of Health and Illness*, 19 (3): 348–58.

Cartwright, A. (1979) *The Dignity of Labour? A Study of Childbearing and Induction*, London: Tavistock.

Changing Childbirth Implementation Team (1995) 'New projects will develop: Changing Childbirth Initiative', *Changing Childbirth Update*, 3 (September): 2.

Dick Read, G. (1933) *Childbirth Without Fear*, London: Heinemann.

DOH (Department of Health (1993) *Changing Childbirth*, Report of the Expert Maternity Group, Part I, London: HMSO.

Doyal, L. (1995) *What Makes Women Sick: Gender and the Political Economy of Health*, Basingstoke: Macmillan Press.

Dunlop, W. (1993) '*Changing Childbirth*. Commentary II', *British Journal of Obstetrics and Gynaecology*, 100 (December): 1072–4.

Graham, H. and Oakley, A. (1981) 'Competing ideologies of reproduction: medical and maternal perspectives on pregnancy', in H. Roberts (ed.) *Women, Health and Reproduction*, London: Routledge and Kegan Paul.

HOC (House of Commons) (1992) *The Health Committee Second Report, Sessions 91–92, Maternity Services* (The Winterton Report). London: HMSO.

Kirkham, M. (1987) 'Care in labour', PhD thesis, Manchester University.

Kitzinger, S. (1988) (ed.) *The Midwife Challenge*. London: Pandora.

Lewis, J. (1995) 'Changing midwifery', *British Journal of Midwifery*, 3 (12): 636–40.

Lewis, P. (1996) 'The death of *Changing Childbirth*', *Modern Midwife*, 6 (6): 14.

Lupton, D. (1994) *Medicine as Culture: Illness, Disease and the Body in Western Societies*, London: Sage.

Macintyre, S. (1982) 'Communications between pregnant women and their medical and midwifery attendants. The 1981 Sir William Power memorial lecture', *Midwives' Chronicle and Nursing Notes*, November: 387–94.

Martin, E. (1987) *The Woman in the Body*, Milton Keynes: Open University Press.

Milhill, C. (1993) 'Danger seen in backing home births', *The Guardian*, 6 August. p. 2.

Maternity Services Advisory Committee (1984) *Care During Childbirth. Part II: V*, London: HMSO.

MORI (1993) *A Survey of Women's Views of the Maternity Services. Maternity Services research Study Conducted for the Department of Health*, London: MORI Health Research Unit.

Munro, A. (1985) 'Maternity care: a challenge to health authorities', *National Association of Health Authorities News*, 83 (May).

NHSME (National Health Service Management Executive) (1994) *Woman-centred Maternity Services*, (EL(94)9), Leeds: Department of Health.

Oakley, A. (1984) *The Captured Womb: A History of the Medical Care of Pregnant Women*, Oxford: Basil Blackwell.

Parliamentary Report (1997) *Midwives*. 110 (1319): 306.

Pascall, G. (1997) *Social Policy: A New Feminist Analysis*, London: Routledge.

Paterson-Brown, S. (1998) 'Should doctors perform and elective caesarean section on request? Yes, as long as the woman is fully informed', *British Medical Journal*, 31: 462–5 (15 August).

RCOG (Royal College of Obstetricians and Gynecologists) (1992) *Maternity Care in the New NHS: A Joint Approach*, London: RCOG.

Romalis, S. (1981) *Childbirth, Alternatives to Medical Control*, Austin: University of Texas Press.

Rosser, J. (1997) 'Lies, damned lies and economics: counting the cost of midwifery pilot schemes', *MIDIRS Midwifery Digest* 7 (2): 141–4.

Rothman, B. (1987) 'Reproduction', in M. Feree and B. Hess (eds) *Analysing Gender: A Handbook of Social Science Research*, London: Sage.

Rudat, K., Roberts, C. and Chowdhury, R. (1993) *Maternity Services: A Comparative Survey of Afro-Caribbean, Asian and White Women, Commissioned by the Expert Maternity Group*, MORI Health Research Unit, London.

Sandall, J. (1995) 'Choice, continuity and control: changing midwifery, towards a sociological perspective', *Midwifery*, 11: 201–9.

Savage, W. (1986) *A Savage Enquiry*. London: Virago.

Short Report (1980) *Second Report from the Social Services Maternity Committee: Perinatal and Neonatal Morality*, London: HMSO.

SMMAC (Standing Maternity and Midwifery Advisory Committee) (1970) *Domicilary Midwifery and Maternity Bed Needs: Report of the Sub-Committee*, London: HMSO.

Summers, A., McKeown, K. and Lord, J. (1997) 'Different women, different views', *British Journal of Midwifery*, 5 (1): 46–50.

Tew, M. (1990) *Safer Childbirth? A Critical History of Maternity Care*, London: Chapman and Hall.

Towler, J. (1982) 'A dying species? Survival and revival are up to us!', *Midwives' Chronicle and Nursing Notes*, September: 324–8.

Troutt, B. (1996) '*Changing Childbirth*: the best kept secret ever', *Midwives*, 1303 (109): 325.

Walker, J. (1985) 'Meeting midwives midway', *Nursing Times*, 23 October: 48–50.

Walton, I. and Hamilton, M. (1995) *Midwives and Changing Childbirth*, Hale, Cheshire: Books for Midwives Press.

5

J. Le Grand

Knights, Knaves or Pawns? Human Behaviour and Social Policy

In contriving any system of government, and fixing the several checks and controls of the constitution, every man ought to be supposed a knave and to have no other end, in all his actions, than private interest. By this interest, we must govern him and, by means of it, notwithstanding his insatiable avarice and ambition, co-operate to the public good. (David Hume, 1875: 117–18)

If it is accepted that man has a sociological and biological need to help, then to deny him opportunities to express this need is to deny him the freedom to enter into gift relationships. (Richard Titmuss, 1971: 243)

. . . Assumptions concerning human motivation and behaviour are the key to the design of social policy. Policy-makers fashion policies on the assumption that those affected by the policies will behave in certain ways and they will do so because they have certain motivations. Sometimes the assumptions concerning motivation and behaviour are explicit: more often they are implicit, reflecting the unconscious values or beliefs of the policy-makers concerned. Conscious or not, the assumptions will determine the way that welfare institutions are constructed. So, for instance, a welfare state constructed on the assumption that people are motivated primarily by their own self-interest – that they are, in the words of David Hume quoted above, *Knaves*[1] – would be quite different from one constructed on the assumption that people are predominantly public spirited or altruistic – that they are what we might term *knights* in contrast to knaves. Similarly, if policy-makers work on the assumption that people are essentially passive or unresponsive – neither knights nor knaves, but *pawns* – then again the policy concerned would be quite different from one designed on the assumption that human beings respond actively to the incentive structures with which they are faced.[2]

It might also be noted that these assumptions – or, more precisely, the relationships between the assumptions and the realities of

First published in the *Journal of Social Policy*, 26(2): 149–69 (Cambridge University Press, 1997). Abridged.

human motivation – are crucial to the success or otherwise of the policies concerned. Hume was keen to point out that policies designed on the assumption that people are knights are likely to have disastrous consequences if in fact they are predominantly knaves. But, as Richard Titmuss was anxious to emphasize in *The Gift Relationship* (whence came the second quotation at the beginning of the chapter), the same is true for policies fashioned on the basis of a belief that people are knaves if the consequence is to suppress their natural altruistic impulses.

We shall return to these points later. In the meantime, the importance of the beliefs about human behaviour involved in policy-making can be illustrated by comparing those implicit in the old-style welfare state and those implicit in the new, post-reform, welfare systems. Inevitably given their implicit nature, it is difficult fully to document any claims that one might wish to make about these beliefs by reference to explicit statements by policy-makers or others; hence such claims must at times remain more at the level of assertion than of scientifically established fact. However, it is hoped that the rather stylized set of pictures that are painted here have enough accuracy not seriously to distort the scenes that they are trying to represent.

Lowe (1993) has argued that there were two approaches to welfare that characterized the pre-reform British welfare state: the reluctant collectivists, pre-eminent among whom were Beveridge and Keynes, and the democratic socialists, who included Marshall, Titmuss and Crosland. Of these, he argued that:

> despite the predominant influence of Beveridge and Keynes in the early postwar years, it was the democratic socialists who gave the British welfare state its unique international reputation. At home these ideals also infused the welfare legislation of the 1954–61 Labour governments and provided the logic for further advances which the Conservative ministers struggled to refute. (Lowe, 1993: 18–20)

In Lowe's view, it was the social democratic approach, albeit tempered by that of the reluctant collectivists, which determined the evolution of the postwar welfare state: 'social democracy had history on its side' (ibid.).

What then were the assumptions concerning human behaviour implicit in the 'democratic socialist' welfare state? In trying to answer this question, it is useful to distinguish three sets of actors. First, there were those who operated the welfare state: the politicians and civil servants who devised its policies, the managers who administered it, and the professionals and others who delivered its services. Second, there were those who paid for welfare: taxpayers under the fiscal welfare system. Third, there were those who received the benefits of the welfare state: social security recipients, doctors' patients, school pupils and their parents, council house tenants and so on.

Democratic socialists assumed that the state and its agents were both competent and benevolent (Lowe, 1993: 23). Hence it followed that the first group – those who operated the welfare state – could be trusted to work primarily in the public interest (Donnison, 1982: 20–1). Professionals, such as doctors and teachers, were thought to be primarily motivated by their professional ethic and hence to be concerned only with the interests of the people they were serving. Similarly, politicians, civil servants, and bureaucrats and managers were supposed accurately to define social and individual needs in the areas concerned, and to operate services that did the best possible job of meeting those needs from available resources.

The second group – the taxpayers – were also assumed to be part of the collective view that 'social justice would be guaranteed by a predominant altruism' (Lowe, 1993: 19) and hence to accept a growing burden of progressive taxes (Donnison, 1982: 20–1). More specifically, it was assumed that the better-off would not only co-operate in collectivist enterprises such as national insurance and social services but also acquiesce in paying redistributive taxation that helped the disadvantaged, either because they empathized with the latter's plight or because they saw it as part of their civil responsibility to do so.

The democratic socialists did not assume that the third group – individuals in receipt of the benefits of the welfare state – were active altruists. Rather, the latter were considered to be essentially passive: pawns, not knights. Those who used social services were supposed to be content with a universal, often fairly basic, standard of service. So Titmuss, for instance, spoke of the desirability of 'one publicly approved standard of service' (1968: 195). In practice, with respect to the National Health Service, for instance, this meant that patients were supposed to live up to their appellation and be patient. They were to wait patiently in queues at GPs' surgeries or at outpatient clinics; if they needed further treatment, they had to wait for their turn on hospital waiting lists. When the time arrived for them actually to go to hospital, they were supposed cheerfully to accept being on a public ward, being served horrible food and, most significantly, being treated by doctors too busy, or too elevated, to have time to explain what was happening to them. As Klein has put it, in the early model of the NHS: 'it would be the doctor's judgement which would determine who should get what. . . . It was the experts who determined the need for health care, frame the appropriate priorities and implement their policies universalistically throughout the NHS' (Klein, 1995: 248).

Similarly, the parents of children in state schools were expected to trust the professionals, and to accept that teachers knew what was best for their children. The period between 1944 and 1975 was identified as the 'golden age of teacher control'. Moreover, as with the NHS, especially following the comprehensive reforms of the mid-1960s, parents were supposed to concur that 'the overriding objective in [education policy] was equality' (Lowe, 1993: 203) and hence to accept whatever degree of uniformity of educational provision attaining this objective required.

Council house tenants were expected to be grateful for the privilege they had been accorded in being granted a tenancy (Dunleavy, 1981: 28–33). Their accommodation was standardized, with heavy restrictions as to their freedom of action over what could be done with it. And again the experts were presumed to know best about the housing that people wanted. . . .

However, recent years have seen serious assaults on all of the assumptions that underlay the democratic socialist welfare state (Glennerster, 1995: 193–5; Lowe, 1993: 23–7; Timmins, 1995: Part V). The notion that, for the sake of the collectivity, everyone would passively accept standardized, relatively low levels of services was challenged by studies showing that in key areas of welfare the middle classes extracted at least as much if not more than the poor in terms of both the quantity and quality of service (Le Grand, 1982). More generally, it became increasingly apparent that many people – particularly, but not exclusively, the middle classes – wanted different kinds and different levels of service. Richard Titmuss himself may have enjoyed being in a public ward (Titmuss, 1974: 151) but many people did not. The length of waiting lists for medical treatment became a perennial political issue. Many of the better off put their children in private schools and took out private health insurance; many more subscribed to occupational pensions (although often this was a condition of service). The consensus supporting comprehensive education began to break down, with influential voices encouraging an end to teacher control over the curriculum, a return to selection, traditional teaching methods and a focus on excellence (Timmins, 1995: 318–29). As council estates declined and tenants felt increasingly powerless, owner-occupation became overwhelmingly the preferred form of housing tenure (Power, 1995: 212–14).

The assumption that knightly behaviour characterized those who worked within the institutions of the welfare state proved even more vulnerable. Fuelled in part by people's experience both of dealing with, and of working within, the welfare bureaucracies, scepticism grew concerning the belief that bureaucrats and civil servants necessarily operated in the public interest, and that professionals were only concerned with the welfare of their clients (Glennerster, 1995: 193). Instead, there was an increasing acceptance of the argument of the public choice school of economists and political scientists that the behaviour of public officials and professionals could be better understood if the assumption was made that they were largely self-interested (Lowe, 1993: 22–3).

The idea that knightly behaviour characterizes those who pay for welfare was also challenged. Goodin and Dryzek (1987), and, more comprehensively, Baldwin (1990), argued that the post-war growth of tax and social insurance funded welfare states in a wide variety of developed countries was not the outcome of altruistic gestures by the better off; rather it was directly related to the self-interest of the middle classes. Econometric studies by Peltzman (1980) and Pampel and Williamson (1989) came to similar conclusions. A more micro-level study undertaken by Winter and myself of changes in public expenditure and tax reliefs under the first Thatcher administration, based on the assumption that politicians were vote-maximizing, found a pattern of change that unequivocally favoured the better off (Le Grand and Winter, 1987).

Even more recently, taxpayer resistance to redistributive welfare has become an accepted political fact, on the left as well as the right. For instance, Piachaud argued in a recent Fabian pamphlet that 'there is now virtually no likelihood of further substantial redistribution of income through taxes and social security benefits' (1993: 3); a judgement he based not on technical impossibility of social undesirability, but simply on political feasibility. Field has gone further, claiming that politicians who argue that the middle class will support redistribution to the poor are a 'public menace, distracting from the real task' (1995: 1–2).

Finally, the idea that people in receipt of social benefits are pawns, and that they do not respond to any incentives or disincentives built into the system has also been vigorously assaulted. Again, although the assault began on the right, with Murray's book *Losing Ground* (1984) as a notable example, it has been taken up in other parts of the political spectrum; see, for instance, Etzioni's *The Spirit of Community* (1994) and the works of Deacon (1993) and Field (1995). . . .

Are people in fact knaves, knights or pawns – or some combination of all three? We have seen that there has been a shift in belief among many decision-makers and opinion-formers towards the view that, in most situations of relevance to welfare, the individuals concerned are more likely to be self-interested than public-spirited: but is this change in belief well founded?

Even to ask these questions is to invite the charge of over-simplification. Perhaps in consequence, few of the protagonists in the debate refer to psychological evidence concerning what does actually motivate people in different situations. It may be that such evidence does not exist; or, perhaps more likely, that such evidence that does exist is not amenable to simple interpretation. Nor, so far as I can ascertain, have there been many attempts to test the theories derived from the different assumptions by deriving predictions from the theories and testing them against the empirical record.

So for the moment I think we have to assume that we do not know whether, in welfare-relevant situations, people actually will behave as knights, knaves, pawns or indeed in some more complex fashion. What does that imply about the appropriate welfare strategy to adopt?

One possible implication is that, in a situation of ignorance concerning human motivation, it would be safest to adopt public policies based on the knaves strategy. For a knaves strategy will do little harm if people are actually knights; but a knights strategy could be disastrous if people are actually knaves.

That a knights strategy will fail if most people are in fact knaves is reasonably self-evident. That a knaves strategy could work even if most people are knights is perhaps less obvious, and is perhaps best illustrated by an example. Take a particular group of people involved in some welfare institution, say doctors in a hospital. Now suppose that most of these doctors are in fact knights, doing the best they can for their patients, often at considerable personal sacrifice. Moreover, the reward structure of the hospital is actually based on that assumption, with automatic payment of salaries and with no monitoring of doctor behaviour or performance review. But suppose, too, that there are a few consultants who are knaves, spending their time on the golf course or managing their investment portfolio, to the obvious detriment of their patients; behaviour that, despite the fact that it is only characteristic of a small number of doctors, is damaging the performance and reputation of the hospital as a whole, and thereby threatening its survival.

Now suppose in this situation that a system is introduced of performance-related pay. Since they are not motivated by economic self-interest, this will leave the knights' motivational structure untouched: they will still derive the same reward as before from doing good to patients. They will therefore carry on undertaking to the best of their ability all the activities that are part of what they perceive as their duty to patients. The knaves, on the other hand, will see that it is now in their self-interest to perform their duties properly and will react accordingly. What the new structure will have done, therefore, is bring the knaves into line, ensuring that they perform at least as well as the knights. Everybody, knights and knaves, are now performing to the best of their ability; and the hospital is saved.

However, in practice things may not always be that simple. The principal problem with the example is that it assumes there will be no impact of the introduction of the knave strategy on knightly behaviour. More specifically, the assumption is that, after the introduction of performance-related pay the knights will carry on as before; only knaves are affected. But this may not be the case: the intro-duction of a knave-directed strategy may make the knights behave more knavishly (Goodin, 1996: 41–2; Pettit, 1996: 72–5). A knightly doctor whose pay rises dramatically as a result of the introduction of performance-related pay might wonder whether she had not been selling herself short under the old regime or putting in an excessive effort. Further (again following Pettit, 1996), thinking about these questions may make her start paying attention to the promotion of her own self-advantage in the new situation. . . .

Now it could be argued that, in one sense, even if something like this does occur in these situations, it does not matter. Even if the introduction of a knaves strategy does have the consequence of turning knights into knaves, then, so long as the incentives for knaves are the right ones, performance will continue to improve. For the newly created knaves will respond to the self-interested incentive structure in the same way as the old established knaves; hence the outcome will be the same as if they had remained knights.

But there are two objections to this kind of argument. First, even if the eventual outcome is the same, there is something distasteful about setting up a system that turns knights into knaves. Our society regards altruistic or public-spirited behaviour as morally superior to self-interested behaviour and deliberately to encourage the latter at the expense of the former seems perverse. Second, the argument assumes that the knaves strategy is watertight; that there is no way of getting round the system in a way that furthers self-interest but on this occasion at the expense of the public good. So, for instance, a system of performance-related pay requires reli-able and accurate procedures for measuring and monitoring perform-ance; one that cannot be fiddled to indicate better performance than is actually happening. But – as is apparent from the example – watertight systems are not always easy to construct or maintain. So I am not convinced that the answer to the problem of our ignorance about human motivation lies in the wholesale adoption of knaves strategies.

A second possibility is to adopt or to continue with knights strategies, and to try by other means to ensure that people actually behave more like knights. . . . Through minimum wages and maxi-mum working weeks, legal welfare forces employers to pay decent wages and not to overwork their employees; the Child Support Agency compels errant fathers to meet their child maintenance responsibilities. . . . [This strategy] could also have a more positive role as an expression of social leadership. By indicating through the legal system social disapproval of the practices concerned, it could help internalize that disapproval within individuals, thus helping convert the knave into the knight.

Robust welfare policies

A third approach, and one that in some ways seems preferable to relying on strategies that appeal either only to knaves or only to knights, is to accept our ignorance about what actually motivates people and to try to design what might be termed *robust* strategies: strategies or institutions that are robust to whatever assumption is made about human motivation. Now this, of course, is far from easy. But, to show that it is not impossible, let me give illustrations, two of existing policies and two proposals for reform.

The first of the current policies concerns the schemes introduced in the NHS to improve the premises of general practitioners (GPs). There are two schemes: cost rents and improvement grants. The rules of the cost rent scheme are complex, but the effect of them is that a GP purchasing new premises receives an annual payment approximately equal to the interest that they would have paid if they had taken out a 100 per cent mortgage to finance their purchase. This is payable regardless of how the scheme is actually financed. Improvement grants are one-off cash payments to GPs to pay for up to two-thirds of the capital costs of improving surgery premises. They are available only to GPs who own their own premises.

Now these schemes appeal to both the knight and the knave in the GP. In each case, participating in the scheme results in an improvement in the premises concerned and thereby in services available to patients. Hence the knight is satisfied. However, in each case the GP owns the premises; hence the value of the property is enhanced and self-interest furthered. Both motivations work in the same direction.

It is no coincidence that these schemes have been very successful. For instance, a survey by Hambros (1992) found that £620 per annum per GP was being spent on the maintenance and refurbishment of GP suite in health centres. The comparable figure for spending through the cost rent and improvement grant schemes was £6,500.

The second example of an existing policy again concerns GPs, but this time in the role that some of them play as GP fund-holders. Under the scheme, GPs are allowed to keep any surplus on their funds, so long as they use it for any purpose that is beneficial to patients. Again this is a scheme that could appeal to the knight and the knave. The surplus could be invested in improving premises, thus benefiting both patients and GPs. Or it could be used to purchase new staff, thus easing the workload of GPs, and thereby both making them feel better off and enabling them to provide a better service, or perhaps a more relaxed one. Again both the knight and the knave are appeased.

A third illustration of a 'robust' policy concerns proposals for funding of long-term care. This I shall discuss in a little more detail. It is clear that, in order to provide an adequate level of finance for such care, it will have to rely in part on private resources, both in financial terms and in terms of time and effort provided by informal carers. The trick is in some way to mobilize those resources (or to continue to mobilize them) in a fashion that both generates enough combined resources (public and private) to provide an adequate level of care for those who need it, and does not seem punitive in implementation.

The problem with the current means-tested system in Britain is that it meets neither criterion. The level of provision of community care is universally regarded as inadequate. At the same time the means test, which requires the running down of assets until their value falls below a certain level, seems to penalize those who have had the foresight to save for their old age or for their children's inheritance, and is thus viewed as punitive and exploitative. Moreover, and of direct relevance to the theme of this chapter, it encourages people to behave knavishly: to engage in means-test avoidance, adjusting their means in such a way as to minimize the amount extracted by the state. What should be a noble act – the state helping those in need – becomes instead a sordid set of private activities of dubious morality and, often, even of doubtful legality.

One way of reforming the system is to introduce the version of legal welfare known as the *obligation alimentaire*, under which those who can afford it are legally obliged to provide financial support to their relatives in need of care. But this would involve extending the means test to relatives. Hence it would encourage people to behave knavishly, concealing their assets from 'the means-test man', as in the not dissimilar household means test that disfigured the British welfare state of the 1930s.

A more attractive alternative is the introduction of what might be termed a 'partnership' or 'matching' scheme. This would involve a minimum level of public funding coupled with a system of matching grants for expenditure over that minimum. Under this system each person assessed as being in need of care would be entitled to a minimum level of care met from public funds. This minimum, although adequate, would be basic. For the payment of care above the minimum, the government would undertake to match pound for pound the resources that individuals or their relatives can mobilize for their own care. To keep spending under control, there would be an overall limit on the total amount of grant that could be received by any individual.

There are unattractive features of such a scheme. In particular, it gives more to those who contribute more, and hence it is likely to be less progressive than any means-tested scheme it might replace. However, it does have the merit of avoiding any form of compulsory means tests, instead encouraging people voluntarily to contribute resources. More importantly from the point of view of this chapter, it could appeal to both the knight and the knave. It appeals to self-interest because it encourages people to provide for themselves. However, it also encourages relatives and friends to contribute resources to help people in need; and it appeals to a more collectivist spirit of altruism through the use of public money to provide the matching funds. . . .

Conclusion

The old welfare state was largely based on the assumptions that, in welfare-related situations, people would behave either like knights or like pawns. This chapter has discussed 'new' forms of welfare, some based on the assumption that people are knaves, some on the assumption that we can convert knaves into knights, and some on the assumption that we are ignorant about the mainsprings of human motivation. The last of these may not have the clarity, or even the moral appeal, of some of the others. But they are, I believe, more firmly grounded than the others and hence should offer a stronger foundation for a social and welfare policy aimed at what we all would like to achieve: the best possible health, education and welfare of all our citizens in the next century, be they knights, knaves or pawns.

Notes

This is a revised version of an Inaugural Lecture given at the London School of Economics on 12 July, 1995, under the title 'New Visions of Welfare'. I am grateful to Alan Deacon, Ken Judge, Rodney Lowe, Peter Taylor-Gooby, Nicholas Timmins, to an anonymous referee, and to many colleagues in the LSE Department of Social Policy and Administration and the Kings fund Policy Institute for helpful comments.

1 Hume was not the first to use the term in this way. That honour is probably due to Bernard Mandeville, who described an ideal constitution as one 'which remains unshaken though most men should prove knaves' (1731: 332, quoted in Pettit, 1996: 72).

2 Although I have generally tried to make my language gender neutral, it is possible that some of the terminology used in this chapter (especially that involving the terms knights and knaves) conjures up a world peopled entirely by men. This is unintended – and, if it distorts the argument, unfortunate. For it is not implausible that the balance of human motivation differs significantly between the genders. Hence it might be appropriate to design welfare policies quite differently depending on the gender balance of the groups involved. This is an issue that requires more exploration.

References

Baldwin, P. (1990) *The Politics of Social Solidarity: Class Bases of the European Welfare State 1875–1975*, Cambridge University Press: Cambridge.
Deacon, A. (1993) 'Richard Titmuss: 20 years on', *Journal of Social Policy*, 22: 235–42.
Donnison, D. (1982) *The Politics of Poverty*, Martin Robertson: Oxford.

Dunleavy, P. (1981) *The Politics of Mass Housing in Britain 1945–1975*, Clarendon Press: Oxford.

Etzioni, A. (1994) *The Spirit of Community: The Reinvention of American Society*, Simon and Schuster: New York.

Field, F. (1995) *Making Welfare Work: Reconstructing Welfare for the Millennium*, Institute of Community Studies: London.

Glennerster, H. (1995) *British Social Policy since 1945*, Blackwell: Oxford.

Goodin, R. (ed.) (1996) *The Theory of Institutional Design*, Cambridge University Press: Cambridge.

Goodin, R. and Dryzek, J. (1987) 'Risk sharing and social justice: the motivational foundations of the post-war welfare state', in R. Goodin and J. Le Grand *Not Only the Poor: The Middle Classes and the Welfare State*, Allen and Unwin: London.

Hambros (1992) *Report to the Department of Health: Review of Funding of Accommodation of General Practice in Health Care in England*, Hambros Bank Ltd for the Department of Health: London.

Hume, D. (1875) 'On the independency of parliament', in T.H. Green and T.H. Gross (eds), *Essays, Moral, Political and Literary*, vol. I, Longmans: London.

Klein, R. (1995) *The New Politics of the NHS*, 3rd edn, Longmans: London.

Le Grand, J. (1982) *The Strategy of Equality*, Allen and Unwin: London.

Le Grand, J. and Winter, D. (1987) 'The middle classes and the welfare state under Labour and Conservative governments', *Journal of Public Policy*, 6: 399–430.

Lowe, R. (1993) *The Welfare State in Britain since 1945*, Macmillan: Houndsmills.

Mandeville, B. (1731) *Free Thoughts on Religion, the Church and National Happiness*, 3rd edn, London.

Murray, C. (1984) *Losing Ground*, Basic Books: New York.

Pampel, F. and Williamson, J. (1989) *Age, Class, Politics and the Welfare State*, Cambridge University Press: Cambridge.

Peltzman, S. (1980) 'The growth of government', *Journal of Law and Economics*, 23: 209–87.

Pettit, P. (1996) 'Institutional design and rational choice', in Goodin (1996), ch. 2.

Piachaud, D. (1993) *What's Wrong with Fabianism?* Fabian Pamphlet 558, Fabian Society: London.

Power, A. (1995) *Hovels to High Rise: State Housing in Europe since 1850*, Routledge: London.

Timmins, N. (1995) *The Five Giants*, HarperCollins: London.

Titmuss, R. (1968) *Commitment to Welfare*, Allen and Unwin: London.

Titmuss, R. (1971) *The Gift Relationship*, Allen and Unwin: London.

Titmuss, R. (1974) *Social Policy*, Allen and Unwin: London.

PART II

CONNECTING: THEORY, VALUES AND PRACTICE

Under growing pressure to account for their judgements and actions, and to deliver more effective practice, professionals are being urged to deepen their understanding of what they do. They are being challenged to develop greater awareness and sensitivity to theory, to examine their own value systems and to reflect on practice. The eight chapters in this part explore different aspects of this challenge. Many of the contributors owe a strong debt to Schön's notion of the 'reflective practitioner' as one who engages creatively and thoughtfully with the realities of practice.

Part II opens with a strong affirmation of the indissoluble link between theory and practice. Rebutting the 'commonsense' view of theory as an armchair exercise of little relevance to the realities of day to day practice, Neil Thompson reminds us that theory and philosophy provide essential explanatory frameworks: without them, he argues, practitioners stand no chance of making sense of the complexities of practice. What he memorably calls the 'fallacy of theoryless practice' can place a real brake on change and improvement. He writes accessibly about the value, in areas like health and social care, of hermeneutics, critical theory and existentialism. Embracing uncertainty as a basic premise of human existence, he critiques technical rationality with its focus on problem solving to the neglect of problem setting.

The next two chapters examine the role of reflection in practice. Christine Nash offers a clear personal account of how she used both reflection and intuition in her approach to a new patient. She discusses how the use of reflective theory enabled her to question her practice and handle a difficult situation – in the process gaining valuable experience for the future. She urges practitioners to reflect on their practice regularly in order to make appropriate changes and to use reflection as a tool for developing others. A less sanguine note is struck by Francis Quinn. While valuing opportunities for reflection as part of a broader programme of experiential learning and professional development, he has reservations about the way in which reflection is being forced upon the nursing profession. After taking the reader through a number of models of reflection, he criticizes – on ethical, professional and pragmatic grounds – the way reflection has been operationalized. He concludes that reflection might better serve as a strategy for student learning rather than a system for use by qualified practitioners. It is enough that busy practitioners mentally reflect on their practice.

Adopting a psychodynamic approach to reflection, Tom Kitwood argues for the centrality of 'being' as opposed to 'doing' in care work. The capacity to be present is seen as a prerequisite for good, empathetic caring and the features of how such an approach is translated into interaction are explored in some detail. After examining some fundamental aspects of the psychology of caring, Kitwood suggests that when the hidden motives that draw people into care work can be owned, understood and integrated, these feelings can become a powerful resource along the difficult path of enabling therapeutic change.

Rosemary Barnitt, too, focuses on the personal side of professional development, reminding readers that the relationship between personal values and practice is not straightforward. In this provocative piece she asks whether therapists are altruists who sacrifice self-interest in the service of others, or whether they are self-centred, unprincipled and unfeeling. Reporting on her research into ethical dilemmas, she describes the tensions therapists experience about doing good to others versus doing good to themselves in a difficult practice context. Therapists, she suggests, are not free to make independent, personally virtuous decisions; instead they are forced into compromises as they take into account others' values and views.

The links between theory, values and practice, and between values, ideology and policy, are further developed in the final three chapters. Traditionally, Sarah Banks argues, the values of social work have emphasized the rights and interests of the individual user in line with the prevailing individualist ideology of Western capitalist society. Recent decades, however, have seen old assumptions under challenge from both the left and the right. Beginning in the 1960s, the radical social work movement, feminism and anti-racism have sharpened awareness of structural oppression, making social workers increasingly conscious of the context in which they practise. At the same time, the growth of the New Right introduced policies and ideologies contrary to traditional social work values. Social service users, argues Banks, should not be viewed as 'consumers' but as a totality. Towards this end, she concludes by setting out four basic principles for social work in the 1960s and beyond.

Concurring with this view that social workers operate at the sharp edge of discrimination, oppression and social exclusion, Sharon Pinkney contextualizes the growth of anti-oppressive theory in terms of social work practice. She shows how, in relation to race, an early emphasis on assimilation was replaced by multiculturalism, which in turn gave way to a more robust anti-racism in the 1980s. The chapter concludes with an exploration of how these shifts in thinking, theory and practice have been worked out through policy on the contentious arena of adoption placements.

Lorraine Culley focuses specifically on practitioners' theory, values and attitudes towards ethnicity and health in Britain. This persuasive piece argues for a more balanced and nuanced approach to a highly complex set of issues. At the level of theory, the author is critical of essentialist approaches that prioritize the role of culture in explaining health differences. Culture, she believes, should be seen as a complex and dynamic process rather than as a fixed set of attributes. Culley then pursues this line of thinking in terms of the interaction between health care practitioners and ethnic minority service users. Noting the many inadequacies in current practice, she urges practitioners to do more to embrace diversity and acknowledge the contingent and contextual nature of ethnicity.

All the contributors to this part agree that it is only through connecting with theory, values and practice that practitioners can truly become reflective. By critically reflecting on personal values and professional understandings, and then locating these within a broader ideological and policy context, practitioners will be better able to cope with complexity and challenge.

6

N. Thompson

Theory and Practice in Health and Social Care

A *theory* is a coherent group of general propositions or concepts used as principles of explanation for a class of phenomena – a more or less verified or established explanation accounting for known facts or phenomena and their interrelationship. If one thinks of knowledge as discrete bits of truth or discrete facts and observations like a pile of bricks, theory can be likened to a wall of bricks. In a theory the observations of the real world are ordered and put together in a certain way and held together by certain assumptions or hypotheses as bricks in a wall are held together by a material that cements them in place. Thus theory is a coherent group of general propositions, containing both confirmed and assumptive knowledge, held together by connective notions that seek to explain in a rational way the observed facts of phenomena and the relationship of these phenomena to each other.

Types of levels of theory

To develop a comprehensive typology of theories would be a major undertaking. However, we can usefully explore some of the major types and levels of theory in order to take our understanding of these issues forward.

A good way to begin this is to explain the distinction between grand theories and middle-range theories. A grand theory is one that attempts to explain more or less everything in society. That is, it goes beyond a simple level of explanation and becomes a philosophy of life, a particular view of the world, or to use the technical term, a *Weltanschauung*. Examples of grand theories would by psychodynamics, marxism and existentialism.

Middle-range theories are less ambitious in their claims and attempt to explain only a limited range of phenomena. That is, their

First published in *Theory and Practice in Health and Social Welfare* (Open University Press, 1995). Abridged.

focus is much narrower and their scope is not so all-embracing. Symbolic interactionism is a good example of a middle-range theory. It seeks to explain interpersonal interactions but remains silent on the questions of wider social issues. This raises two significant points:

- Middle-range theories are often unfairly criticized for being limited in the scope of their analysis. Such criticism is unfair in so far as it involves criticizing the theorists for not covering something they were not trying to cover!
- Middle-range theories are 'safer' than grand theories in two senses. First, they make fewer claims and are therefore less likely to be proven wrong. Second, by definition they have little or nothing to say about wider social factors such as power, inequality, oppression and disadvantage. They are therefore less likely to be seen as a threat to the powers that be and the status quo.

In addition to grand and middle-range theories, there are also micro-theories. These are on a very small scale and seek to explain only a very limited range of phenomena. Berger and Kellner (1981) are subtly critical of the tendency, in sociology at least, for such small-scale studies to proliferate at the expense of what they call the 'big questions':

> Good sociologists have always had an insatiable curiosity about even the trivialities of human behaviour, and if this curiosity leads a sociologist to devote many years to the painstaking exploration of some small corner of the social world that may appear quite trivial to others, so be it. Why do more teenagers pick their noses in rural Minnesota than in rural Iowa? . . . Far be it from us to denigrate such research interests! (Berger and Kellner, 1981: 15–16)

The distinction between formal and informal theory is also a helpful one, as it takes us another step forwards towards making sense of the complex world of theory. Curnock and Hardiker (1979) draw a distinction between formal 'theories of practice' and informal 'practice theories'. The former type of theory is 'official' theory in the sense that it is formally recorded in academic literature and forms the basis of much formal teaching. Informal 'practice theories', by contrast, are not officially recognized or formally codified. They constitute the 'practice wisdom' of a profession, the informal knowledge and assumptions which are 'built up through actual practice and "culturally transmitted" to new recruits to the profession' (Thompson, 1992: 12). This idea is captured, in a nursing context, by the notion of 'Sister says'. That is, much of this practice wisdom is learned by working alongside more experienced colleagues.

Both types of theory have advantages and disadvantages relative to each other. In terms of direct applicability to practice, informal theory scores more highly than formal theory in so far as it addresses more specifically and directly day-to-day practice issues. Such theory was born of practice and is therefore closely linked to the everyday concerns and realities of practitioners. Formal theory, by contrast, is at one remove from actual practice but scores highly in terms of being explicit and therefore open to question. It is possible to take issue with formal theory and challenge its basis; it can be adapted and extended by rational analysis, discussion and empirical investigation. However, informal theory, because of its status as received wisdom, is far less open to challenge:

> Whereas formal theory is open to debate, examination and counterargument, informal theory is relatively unassailable insofar as it is covert, implicit and taken for granted as 'obvious' or 'common sense'. In other words, informal theory has the status of dogma. Dogma is not based on evidence, coherent argument or experimental testing, nor is it open to critical analysis as it is taken for granted as 'obvious' or just 'common sense'. (Thompson, 1992: 18)

Both types of theory have a role to play but both also have limitations.

The fallacy of theoryless practice

Timms (1968: 23) makes the point that, 'We cannot conceive of practice without employing some kind of theory about what constitutes the practice, what indicates good or bad practice and so on'. The same point – that theory and practice are inextricably linked – is also made by Curnock and Hardiker (1979), Sibeon (1990) and a number of other writers.

When practitioners comment that they 'prefer to stick to practice', as if practice can be divorced from theory, they are reflecting the 'fallacy of theoryless practice' (Thompson, 1992). They are assuming, quite inappropriately, that complex actions can be divorced from thought. Underpinning their fallacy is the notion that theory refers only to formal 'book theory', that informal theory either does not exist or does not count. As we noted earlier, informal, 'uncodified' theory has an important part to play in guiding our actions and informing our practice.

If we do not recognize that frameworks of ideas and values are influencing how we act and interact, we are not in a position to question those ideas and ensure that they are appropriate and constructive. That is, we need to recognize the fallacy of theoryless practice so that we are not guilty of failing to review our ideas and lacking the flexibility to adapt or abandon them in the light of changing circumstances. In short, we need to be wary of the fallacy of theoryless practice, as it leads to dogmatism and stands in the way of the development of reflective practice. As Howe (1987: 9) comments:

> To travel at all is to hold ideas about the behavioural and social terrain over which we journey. To show no interest in . . . theory is simply to travel blind. This is bad for practice and unhelpful to clients.

The bias of theory

Theorizing is by no means a 'pure' activity, detached from the reality of the social and political world. That is, theory is inevitably embedded in the social context in which it arises and in which it should be used.

This is reflected in the biases apparent in traditional theory. For example, consider the feminist concept of '*her*story', the critique of the invisibility of women in (men's) accounts of history. . . . The relative absence of women in accounts of history reflects male dominance in society in terms of both the power struggles described in history texts and the authorship of those texts as primarily a male activity. History is therefore not neutral, but rather reflects the patriarchal structure of society.

Patriarchy is a very significant term in this context, as the 'law of the father' subordinates not only women but also children. Stainton Rogers and Stainton Rogers (1992) therefore argue that children, too, are largely 'invisible' in the accounts of history dominated by patriarchal ideology.

Pascall (1986) also challenges patriarchy when she applies a similar argument to social policy, indicating that women's voices are rarely heard, despite the fact that women make up the majority of welfare consumers and providers.

Williams (1989) echoes this view and reinforces the critique of traditional social policy as a male preserve. She also extends the argument to include a racial dimension by emphasizing the ethnocentric nature of dominant thinking in social policy.

What both Pascall and Williams are promoting is a critique of the biases inherent in traditional social policy analysis. This can also be extended to take account of issues of disability, age, sexual orientation and so on. The central point to be emphasized is that the theory base underpinning social policy reflects the biases and interests of dominant power groups and therefore indicates the operation of ideology.

What this tells us, then, in terms of our basic question of 'What is theory?', is that it is *not* an abstract academic exercise unconnected with the real world; it is, rather, a dynamic development of ideas linked to power structures in society and the interaction of dominant and countervailing ideological forces.

The distinctiveness of social science

Within social science, positivism manifests itself as a belief in the appropriateness of applying natural science methods and procedures to the study of society. What this fails to take into account is the fundamental differences between nature and society. As Giddens (1993a: 85–6) puts it:

> The difference between the social and natural world is that the latter does not constitute itself as 'meaningful': the meanings it has are produced by human beings in the course of their practical life, and as a consequence of their endeavours to understand or explain it for themselves. Social life – of which these endeavours are a part – on the other hand, is *produced* by its component actors precisely in terms of their active constitution and reconstitution of frames of meaning whereby they organize their experience.

To see social science simply as an extension of natural science is therefore a significant error, as it overlooks a central feature of social life: the fact that social processes and structures are produced or reproduced in and by human action.

A second significant difference is what Giddens (1993a) describes as a 'double hermeneutic'. By this he means a two-way interaction between the knowledge base generated by social science and society itself. . . .

A positivist approach to social science is inappropriate, as it ignores this active dimension of social science – the fact that social scientists and their work are part of the fabric of the society they study, part of the process of creating and recreating that society.

Alternatives to positivism

There are clearly many problems in adopting a positivist approach to health and social welfare. Perhaps the most significant of these is the tendency of the factors outlined above to result in *determinism*, a view of human action as being determined by factors beyond our control. . . .

We need to be careful, though, that we do not 'throw the baby out with the bathwater' by rejecting not only positivist science but science itself. The distorted version of science represented by positivism is referred to as 'scientism'. The question is, therefore, 'Can we reject scientism without also rejecting science?'. Giddens (1993b: 20) defines science as:

> the use of systematic methods of investigation, theoretical thinking, and the logical assessment of arguments, to develop a body of knowledge about a particular subject-matter. Scientific work depends on a mixture of boldly innovative thought and the marshalling of evidence to support or disconfirm hypotheses and theories. Information and insights accumulated

through scientific study and debate are always to some degree *tentative* – open to being revised, or even completely discarded, in the light of new evidence or arguments.

Clearly, research and theory development in health and social welfare can proceed on this basis without making any of the over-ambitious claims of scientism. There are, therefore, alternatives to positivism, in particular hermeneutical science and critical theory. I shall outline each of these in turn before focusing in particular on some key issues relating to the role of research.

Hermeneutical science

While positivism seeks to exclude the subjective dimension, hermen-eutics places subjectivity at centre stage. The objective, external world is meaningless without a subjectivity (a conscious human subject) to interpret it. Thus, for hermeneutical science, the object of study is not the objective world *per se*, but the interrelationship of the objective world with subjective actors who experience it. In fact, the term *experience* is a central one. . . . Behaviour is observed from the outside, while 'experience' refers to what happens within – and it is this internal, experiential dimension which has tended to be neglected in studies of health and social welfare. In short, hermeneutics is a science of the *person*, focusing on people as active subjects, rather than inert objects, puppets of external forces.

Hermeneutical science is a counterbalance to the positivist emphasis on objectivity and it achieves this by reintroducing the subjective or experiential dimension absent from scientism. This makes scientific investigation more difficult and more complex, and a different under-taking from traditional positivist studies. However this approach can be seen to be more in keeping with the demands of professional practice. As Schön (1992: 53) comments:

> Given the dominant view of professional rigor, the view which prevails in the intellectual climate of the universities and is embedded in the insti-tutional arrangements of professional education and research, rigorous practice depends on well-formed problems of instrumental choice to whose solution research-based theory and technique are applicable. But real-world problems do not come well-formed. They tend to present themselves, on the contrary, as messy, indeterminate, problematic situations.

That is, the reality of practice is far closer to the hermeneutical model of science than it is to the positivist.

Critical theory

The term 'critical theory' is used in two senses, narrow and broad. In its narrow sense, it refers to the work of theorists such as Horkheimer, Marcuse and Habermas (see Jay, 1973; Held, 1980), who sought to integrate elements of marxism (power, oppression, conflict, social structure) with elements of psychoanalysis (meaning, interpretation, desire). In its broader sense, critical theory refers to a range of theoretical analyses which seek to integrate hermeneutical (or 'phenomenological') issues with wider social or political factors. It is in this second sense that I shall be using it here.

It is also important to note that critical theory is currently a very active and rapidly developing theoretical perspective engaged with issues of 'postmodernism' and the critique of traditional forms of intellectual inquiry and theory building (Lash, 1990; Shotter, 1993). However, much of the work to date is of an exploratory or experimental nature and has yet to reach the stage at which the implications for practice are readily deduced.

Critical theory shares with hermeneutics a dissatisfaction with positivism's neglect of subjective factors. It accepts the basic tenets of hermeneutics but argues that the focus on subjectivity needs to be located in the broader context of society and politics. Although each of us is a unique individual, we also have to take account of the ways in which we are not unique, the commonalities we share with other groups in society and the differences between those groups. Critical theory recognizes the importance of subjectivity but also recognizes that each individual is 'socially located' in terms of class, race, gender and other social divisions.

Critical theory is often seen as a rebuttal of hermeneutics. However, it can also be seen as an *extension* of hermeneutical science, a development of this approach rather than a rejection of it. Critical theory continues the hermeneutical tradition of acknowledging the significance of experience. It sees subjectivity as a *necessary* condition for understanding human action, but it is not a *sufficient* condition.

Philosophy as a form of theory

Philosophy places great value on explanatory power and seeks validity not from empirical rigour, but from the strength of its arguments. This focus on explanatory power gives philosophy a higher degree of applicability to practice than a narrower, more technical theoretical approach. A greater willingness to tackle value issues makes philosophy of greater relevance, potentially at least, to the needs and concerns of practitioners.

This point relates closely to Schön's (1983) critique of 'technical rationality' as the basis of professional practice. He argues that the technical rationality of science is well suited to clearly defined, well-bounded problems but lacks the flexibility to deal with the indeterminacy and 'messiness' of the problems encountered in professional practice.

An important aspect of Schön's distinction between the high ground of science and the lowland of practice is the need to see problem-solving in the context of problem-setting. Professional practice is concerned with problem-solving. However, what is not so fully recognized is the process of problem-setting – the process by which a problem and its parameters are defined and interpreted. In general, there is relatively little attention paid to the 'swampy' process of problem-setting, while the 'technical rationality' of theory and research has tended to concentrate on finding solutions to the problems.

Existentialism

. . . Existentialism is one example of a holistic philosophy which has had some impact as counselling and psychotherapy, especially in the USA (May et al., 1958; Frankl, 1973), but a very limited impact on social work (although not quite so limited in the USA: see for example, Stretch, 1967; Krill, 1978).

Existentialism offers a 'philosophy of existence', a conceptual framework which aims to understand human existence in terms of freedom and responsibility, and the problems and complexities we encounter when we exercise such freedom (in the form of choices and decisions) and take responsibility for the consequences of our actions. It seeks to locate such freedom (the fundamental freedom of being responsible for ourselves) in the wider social context of the structure of society, in terms of social constraints and influences, for example class (Sartre, 1976), race/ethnicity (Sartre, 1948) or gender (de Beauvoir, 1972).

Existentialism emphasizes the dialectical interaction of individual factors (my choices, values, actions) and wider sociopolitical factors (the oppressions of sexism and racism). It is not a case of working out which dimension is more important, the personal or the social, but rather a matter of understanding existence as a constant interplay of the two, a dynamic process simultaneously personal and social.

Dialectical reason does not contradict or invalidate analytical reason, it goes beyond it. Analytical reason breaks things down into their component parts, and this is an essential first step in the process of understanding. It is, however, only a first step and needs to be followed by *synthesis* – the linking of those parts into a coherent whole. This process of synthesis, or as I shall call it 'totalization', is the hallmark of dialectical reason.

The basis of dialectical reason is conflict. The dialectic refers to the process by which conflicting forces come together and produce change. This process is perhaps best known in relation to marxism, as indicated by the term 'dialectical materialism'.

The process, in its simplest form, can be seen to work as follows: A particular force (the thesis) enters into conflict with another force (the antithesis) and, as a result of this interaction of conflicting forces, a new situation is produced (the synthesis). It is in this way that dialectical reason is cyclical – the synthesis, thus producing a new cycle of dialectical change. For marxism, the dialectic is the primary means by which we can understand history (although Marx himself did not express this directly in terms of thesis–antithesis–synthesis: McLellan, 1975).

This model can be seen to apply to interpersonal dynamics in which two or more people enter into conflict over a certain issue or set of issues, and from this a new position or understanding is achieved (a synthesis). However, this may then prove to be the basis of further conflicts of interest or perspective – and thus the basis of a new cycle of the dialectic.

Dialectical reason can therefore be seen to have two advantages over analytical reason:

1 *It can more easily account for conflict.* Indeed, it recognizes the central role of conflict of interests as a factor in social life.
2 *It can account for change.* That is, it is dynamic, rather than static. As such, it avoids the pitfall of presenting a 'snapshot' which can very quickly become out of date.

Like other philosophies, existentialism cannot offer simple, specific solutions. However, what it can offer is a valuable way of approaching practice. In particular, it provides a basis for responding to what Schön (1992: 51) refers to as 'the indeterminate zones of practice – the situations of complexity and uncertainty'. Existentialism provides a framework for accepting uncertainty as a basic premise of human existence. While positivism stresses the quest for certainty – and conveniently sidesteps issues of uncertainty – existentialism takes uncertainty as a central concept. As Laing (1967: 47) comments:

> We must continue to struggle through our confusion, to insist on being human.
> Existence is a flame which constantly melts and recasts our theories. *Existential thinking offers no security*, no home for the homeless. It addresses no-one except you and me. (Emphasis added)

This notion of uncertainty – of no security or guarantees – is an important one for understanding practice, particularly the 'swampy lowland where situations are confusing "messes" incapable of technical solution' (Schön, 1983: 42).

Conclusion

A major concern of this chapter has been the need to recognize the value of a philosophical approach. Some may see this as a contradiction, placing the 'scientific' activity of research alongside the decidedly unscientific enterprise of philosophy.

However, this does not present a problem when we conceive of the two as conflicting elements within a dialectical interaction. That is, we need to understand research-based investigation and philosophical investigation as forces which interact and produce a new synthesis. They are part of a dynamic process, rather than two static entities which do not sit comfortably together.

In some ways, theory and practice fit neatly together but, in other ways, there is a degree of tension and conflict between them – hence the need to see them in the context of the dialectic.

Dialectical reason is the basis of the particular philosophy presented here as an appropriate and helpful basis for guiding and informing health and social welfare practice, namely the philosophy of *existentialism*. Existentialism is particularly appropriate in so far as:

- its focus on uncertainty can help practitioners to deal with the 'swampy lowlands';
- the fundamental principle of freedom and responsibility discourages dependency;
- it incorporates both the personal/individual dimension *and* the social/collective dimension;
- it provides a basis for understanding and challenging oppression;
- an understanding of ontology helps us to deal with the issues of crises and loss which health and social welfare workers so frequently encounter;
- it is premised on dialectical reason and is therefore well equipped to deal with two of the major features of practice – change and conflict.

Of course, these benefits of an existentialist approach do not mean that existentialism should be seen as a panacea for practice. On the contrary, one of the implications of existentialism is that there can be no panacea, no easy answers, as human existence is characterized by struggle and challenge. However, what the philosophy does provide for us is an explanatory framework which helps to make sense of many of the complexities practitioners face. . . .

References

Curnock, K. and Hardiker, P. (1979) *Towards Practice Theory: Skills and Methods in Social Assessments*, London: Routledge and Kegan Paul.

De Beauvoir, S. (1972) *The Second Sex*, Harmondsworth: Penguin.

Frankl, V. (1973) *Psychotherapy and Existentialism*, Harmondsworth: Penguin.

Giddens, A. (1993a) *New Rules of Sociological Method*, 2nd edn, Cambridge: Polity.

Giddens, A. (1993b) *Sociology*, 2nd edn, Cambridge: Polity.

Held, D. (1980) *Introduction to Critical Theory, Horkheimer to Habermas*, London: Hutchinson.

Howe, D. (1987) *An Introduction to Social Work Theory*, Aldershot: Wildwood House.

Jay, M. (1973) *The Dialectical Imagination*, London: Heinemann.

Krill, D.F. (1978) *Existential Social Work*, London: Collier Macmillan.

Laing, R.D. (1967) *The Politics of Experience and the Bird of Paradise*, Harmondsworth: Penguin.

Lash, S. (1990) *Sociology of Postmodernism*, London: Routledge.

May, R., Angel, E. and Ellenberger, H.F. (eds) (1958) *Existence: A New Dimension in Psychiatry and Psychology*, New York: Basic Books.

McLellan, D. (1975) *Marx*, London: Fontana.

Pascall, G. (1986) *Social Policy: A Feminist Analysis*, London: Tavistock.

Sartre, J.-P. (1948) *Anti-Semite and Jew*, New York: Schocken.

Sartre, J.-P. (1976) *Critique of Dialectical Reason*, London: Verso.

Schön, D.A. (1983) *The Reflective Practitioner*, London: Temple Smith.

Schön, D.A. (1992) 'The crisis of professional knowledge and the pursuit of an epistemology of practice', *Journal of Interprofessional Care*, 6 (1).

Shotter, J. (1993) *Cultural Politics of Everyday Life*, Buckingham: Open University Press.

Sibeon, R. (1990) 'Comments on the structure and forms of social work knowledge', *Social Work and Social Sciences Review*, 1 (1).

Stainton Rogers, W. and Stainton Rogers, R. (1992) *Stories of Childhood*, Brighton: Harvester.

Stretch, J.J. (1967) 'Existentialism: a proposed philosophical orientation for social work', *Social Work*, 12 (4).

Thompson, N. (1992) *Existentialism and Social Work*, Aldershot: Avebury.

Timms, N. (1968) *The Language of Social Casework*, London: Routledge and Kegan Paul.

Williams, F. (1989) *Social Policy: A Critical Introduction*, Cambridge: Polity.

7

C. Nash

Applying Reflective Practice

One late shift, I came on duty and took over from a nurse from the previous shift who handed over to me a young woman whom I will call Ann. The patient had been seen and assessed by the A&E doctor and found to be having a threatened abortion. She was now awaiting transfer by ambulance to one of our neighbouring hospitals where she was to receive gynaecological care.

I introduced myself to Ann and asked if she had had everything explained to her and if she knew what she was waiting for. She replied that she knew she was having a miscarriage; she added that she had been trying a long while to conceive. To this response, I put my hand on her shoulder and empathized how sorry I was for her. She immediately embraced me and began to 'cry', saying that she wanted someone to give her a hug. When she let go of me I looked at her but could see no tears. She also said that she had some pain in her lower abdomen.

On the trolley with her was a small sports bag, which was closed, but seemed to be packed tight. The history from the ambulance crew was that she had collapsed while out shopping in the local town centre. I explained to her that I would find her notes and see what pain killers I could give her. I also said I would investigate how long the ambulance might be. For this she was grateful.

When I left the cubicle, I started to reflect on what had just happened. First, she was expressing great upset over the event, but she was relatively calm and showed no tears. This seemed very strange to me. Second, for someone who had collapsed while out shopping, she had a very near full sports bag. (I thought about how I shop, usually with lots of bags!) This bag reminded me of a bag carried by patients who know they are going to be admitted to hospital. Third, her pain did not seem genuine, even though Sofaer (1983) and McCaffery (1979) argue that pain is what the patient says it is.

On reading her notes, it seemed apparent that a pregnancy test had not been performed. She seemed to have been taken on her word

First published in *Emergency Nurse*, 6(2): 14–18 (RCN Publishing Company, March 1999). Abridged.

that she was pregnant. Also, she was a patient who lived outside our catchment area. I had a 'gut feeling' that her complaint was not genuine and decided to check her on our computer system. She had attended our hospital last month at exactly the same time of the month, with the same problem. On that occasion she had been admitted. So, could this bleeding be her period?

Further investigations led me to telephone her local A&E, where they confirmed that she was a regular attender. She suffered from Munchausen's syndrome and had been admitted – only two days previously – for exactly the same reason. She was fully investigated for the same problem and found not to be pregnant or having a miscarriage. Armed with this information, I went back to the doctor who saw Ann and presented my findings. He was impressed but also possibly embarrassed with what I had found. He in turn approached Ann and put it to her that there was no pregnancy and that she was not experiencing a miscarriage. He offered her counselling which she refused and left the department. Was it the use of reflection or intuition which led me to establish that Ann suffered from Munchausen's syndrome?

Reflection

Reflection is a process of deep thought; both a looking backwards to the situation being pondered upon and projecting forward to the future, being both recall and reasoning (Jarvis, 1987). Boud et al. (1987) defines reflection as the learner's response to the experience. After the experience, there occurs a processing phase: this is the area of reflection. Schön (1983), popularized the usage of reflection but he was by no means the first to introduce it into the field of nursing.

Schön (1987) describes two types of reflection, namely reflection-in-action and reflection-on-action. Reflection-in-action means to think what one is doing while one is doing it. It is usually stimulated by surprise which puzzles the practitioner concerned.

Reflection-on-action involves a cognitive post-mortem; the practitioner looks back on his or her experiences to explore again the understandings brought to the practitioner in the light of the outcomes. Cervero (1988), supports Schön's theory of reflection-in-action by defining it as the core of professional artistry. Professionals reflect in the midst of action without interruption; their thinking shapes what they are doing while they do it. However, Boud et al. (1985) argue that reflection is a subconscious activity and it is not until we formalize these thoughts at a conscious level that we can fully understand and learn from them.

Mezirow (1981), breaks reflectivity down into further categories:

- Affective reflectivity: Becoming aware of how we fell about ourselves and how we think and act.
- Dscriminate reflectivity: Assessing the effectiveness of our perceptions, being able to identify why we are reacting in this way and which relationships are affecting this action.
- Judgmental reflectivity: Realizing that we all make value judgements about perceptions.
- Conceptual reflectivity: Being able to critique our reactions to others.
- Psychic reflectivity: Acknowledging that we judge people based on limited information; recognizing the forces that influence the way we perceive, think or act.

As Boud et al. (1985) discussed, I was reflecting subconsciously and had used several stages of reflection (Mezirow, 1981). The use of discriminate reflectivity was apparent when I was assessing the effectiveness of my perceptions, which then influenced how I acted. Judgement reflectivity was present when I judged my perceptions and judged the woman's presentation. This judgement, and the fact that I felt her complaint was not genuine, made me investigate her attendance further. Psychic reflectivity also played a strong role. I made judgements about Ann using limited information. I had had only a short conversation with her, but felt uncomfortable about her. I recognized this perception and acted further. Only now, reflecting back on the scenario, am I able to formalize my thoughts and learn from them (Boud et al. 1985).

Reflection before action

Greenwood (1993) suggests that reflection before action is that of stopping and thinking before acting. This, he says, would help avoid errors. He feels people should plan what they intend to do, and how they intend to do it, before actually doing it. Van Manen (1990), agrees with Greenwood by saying that anticipatory reflection is consideration given to various approaches to patient care. But could this be classed as a form of reflection-on-action? Would the person be using past experience on which to plan what he or she is about to do?

Van Manen's (1990) description of reflection is a useful reflective tool to use in nursing practice. Not only does he describe anticipatory reflection, but also reflection-in-action, echoing the thoughts of Schön (1987). He describes reflection as thoughtfulness and mindfulness – ways of being involved in situations where we are actively engaged in a manner of consciousness that only later is open to true reflection. Lastly, he describes recollective reflection, which considers the success of practices and interventions.

It is important to reflect on positive and negative experiences. The experience described earlier in this chapter was a positive experience and incorporated several of the examples of reflective methods mentioned. In particular, those of reflection-in-action and on-action. The statement that reflection 'is usually stimulated by surprise which puzzles the practitioner' (Schön, 1987) was true in this scenario. The puzzle of the 'nicely packed bag', and the fact that 'no tears came when she cried', made me reflect on the situation further.

The use of Schön's reflection-on-action, combined with Van Manen's (1990) recollective reflective theory, enabled me to question my practice and how I handled the situation, and provided the opportunity to read up on Munchausen's syndrome. It has also helped me gain experience, so in the future I will be able to relate to it should I be faced with it again.

Intuition

It was not reflection alone which enabled me to suspect that Ann's miscarriage was not genuine; experience and intuition played important parts. Benner (1984) defines an expert as someone who has deep background understanding of clinical situations based upon past paradigm cases, and expertise as a hybrid of practical and theoretical knowledge. Whereas Jarvis (1992), defines experts as those who have acted frequently within a specified field of practice.

Boud et al. (1985) define experiences as an individual's total response to a situation or event: what he or she thinks, feels, does and concludes at that time and immediately thereafter. They also note that experience alone does not necessarily mean that learning has taken place.

To take this further, we can look again at the work of Benner. . . . Her model of skill acquisition (1982, 1987), based on ascending levels of proficiency, was originally developed by Dreyfus and Dreyfus (1980), and Benner (1982) and Dreyfus (1987) claim that this model can be generalized to nursing. According to the model, the nurse passes through five stages of career development: novice, advanced beginner, competent, proficient and expert.

English (1993) argues against Benner's theory that experience is gained through encounters with many situations, by saying that the incremental development is dependent on a combination of depth and range of clinical experience which is positively correlated with the length of time spent in nursing.

Cook (1996) argues there is a distinction between useful learning 'experience' and 'time in the job'. After five years in a post, one nurse may be a more experienced practitioner than one who has been in the post for ten, having better utilized the learning opportunities presented in every situation. Intuition is defined as understanding without rationale (Benner and Tanner 1987). They point out that intuitive judgement is what distinguishes experts' human judgement from the decisions or computations that might be made by a beginner or by a machine. Schön (1983) says that in daily practice practitioners make many judgements of a quality nature for which they cannot state adequate criteria, and display skills for which they cannot state the rule and procedures; this equates to intuition.

To relate back to the scenario, when Ann said she was upset and wanted a cuddle, I had a gut feeling about her presentation. The whole thing did not seem real to me. The fact that she had no tears and the 'nicely packed bag' heightened my suspicions and made me act further.

Easen and Wilcockson (1996), say that for a number of researchers, intuition has been postulated as a non-conscious reasoning process; with this I would agree. It was definitely a non-conscious act at the time, and it was not until the event was over that I could look back and review the intuitive process which had taken place. Again, Eraut (1996) argues that the speed of intuitive decision making is such that it can only be rationalized after the event. There is an apparent bypassing of the linear reasoning process.

Experience goes hand in hand with intuition. The expert nurse practitioner no longer relies on an analytical principle such as a rule or guidelines to connect their understanding of the situation to an appropriate action (Farrington, 1993).

Benner (1984) argues that the expert nurse with a wealth of experience has an intuitive grasp of each situation and zeros in on the problem without wasteful consideration of a large range of alternative diagnoses and solutions. Benner further states that intuitive grasp should not be confused with mysticism since it is available only in situations where a deep background understanding of the situation exists.

Intuition has been broken down into six key aspects by Dreyfus and Dreyfus (1986): pattern recognition, similarity recognition, common-sense understanding, skilled know-how, and deliberate rationality. These five aspects will be discussed further in relation to the scenario, but it has to be remembered that in real life these aspects cannot work separately, but must work altogether. A necessary combination of conditions for expert intuitive judgement (Benner and Tanner, 1987).

Pattern recognition is a perceptual ability to recognize relationships without pre-specifying the components of the situation. Easen and Wilcockson (1996) state that for pattern recognition to take place it is of primary importance to have a sound, relevant knowledge base. Such pattern recognition is rooted in past decision making and experience is essential for this linking of similar past events. This can be relevant to reflective practice too.

Patients with Munchausen's syndrome often attend hospitals out of the area where they live, and usually out of hours and/or when new doctors start. They also give false identification. In my scenario, Ann fitted some of the above.

Similarity recognition is an amazing human capacity to recognize 'fuzzy' resemblances despite marked differences in the objective features of past and current situations. An awareness that the patient reminds the nurse of similar or dissimilar patients or family raises new questions and possibilities. In Ann's scenario, she did not seem to respond in the same way that other women have when having a miscarriage. Unlike Ann, they are usually upset and in a great deal of pain.

Common sense understanding is a deep grasp of the culture and language, so that flexible understanding in diverse situations is possible. It is the basis for understanding the illness experience, in contrast to knowing the disease. Benner and Tanner (1987) explain that expert clinicians learn to use what one called 'stupid stuff – what (patients) look like, how they talk etc.' This was evident in the scenario with Ann: the packed bag, the way she presented, her response to her condition and the 'pain'.

English (1993) who critiqued Benner's (1982, 1984) work on the expert practitioner argues that fellow patients are often able to point out that there is 'something wrong' with another patient and he asks if they too are expert? Although he makes a valid point, it does seem a little sarcastic. If we all watch someone for long enough, we are able to detect change.

Skilled know-how is to live in a meaningful world where events stand out as more important or less important, complete with nuances.

Dreyfus (1979) states that the expert nurse will not consider all tasks as equally important nor will all observations be equally pertinent. When one can operate in a fully differentiated world, it becomes possible to respond effectively to a situation without resorting to rule-governed behaviours.

Deliberate rationality. Proficient and expert performers have a deep web of perspectives that causes them to view a situation in terms of past situations. Thus the expert has learned to expect to attend to certain aspects of the situation which once again, could relate to reflective practice. For example, in Ann's scenario, the nurse from the early shift homed in on the information given by the ambulance crew regarding the miscarriage. It was not until I came on duty and looked at the situation from a different angle that a different opinion was reached. Intuitive opinion is often devalued or disbelieved because of an apparent lack of concrete evidence.

Benner and Tanner (1987) and Easen and Wilcockson (1996) state that Western society values knowledge and understanding that is reached in a conscious, systematic and explicable way. In that sense intuition may be considered to be irrational.

In conclusion, when reflecting back on my experience with Ann, I feel I could not have changed any of my practice. The outcome of the scenario was positive in that Ann was not readmitted unnecessarily, but it was negative in that she refused any counselling or help. A letter was to be sent to her GP, but it was questionable as to whether the information she gave us was correct. There may be scope here to review practice in relation to follow-up for such patients.

It is difficult to pinpoint whether it was reflection or intuition which led me to suspect Ann's case was not genuine – or a combination of both. Cook (1996) states that A&E nurses have a 'sixth sense' which is made up of intuitive and reflective practice. I believe that intuition plays an important part in nurses' practice, but especially that of A&E nurses. It is a skill which is developed subconsciously over time in relation to experience gained, and not something that can be taught. Reflective practice on the other hand can be taught. It is a skill which is not always formally recognized at the time as we are using it. Unfortunately it tends to be used for negative experiences when one is asked to reflect and comment on a problematic work situation. We should all be encouraged to reflect on our practice regularly and make appropriate changes. We should reflect on positive and negative events and then use this as a tool, if appropriate, for helping to develop others.

References

Benner, P. (1984) *From Novice to Expert*. Menlo Park, CA: Addison Wesley.

Benner, P. and Tanner, C. (1987) 'How expert nurses use intuition', *American Journal of Nursing*, January: 23–31.

Boud, D et al. (1985) *Reflection: Turning Experience into Learning*. New York: Kogan Page.

Cervero, R. (1996) *Reflective Continuing Education for Professionals*, San Francisco: Jossey Bass.

Cook, A. (1996) 'Reflective intuition: defining A&E nursing', *Professional Nurse*, 11 (4): 238–9.

Dreyfus, H. (1979) *What Computers Can't Do: A Critique of Artificial Reason*, New York: Harper and Row.

Dreyfus, H. and Dreyfus, S. (1980) 'A five stage model of the mental activities involved in direct nurse education', *Nurse Education Today*, 12: 81–7.

Dreyfus, H. and Dreyfus, S. (1986) *Mind Over Machine: The Power of Human Intuitive Expertise in the Era of the Computer*, New York: Free Press.

Easen, P. and Wilcockson, J. (1996) 'Intuition and rational decision-making in professional thinking', *Journal of Advanced Nursing*, 24: 667–73.

English, I. (1993) 'Intuition as a function of the expert nurse', *Journal of Advanced Nursing*, 18: 387–93.

Eraut, M. (1994) *Developing Professional Knowledge and Competence*, London: The Falmer Press.

Farrington, A. (1993) 'Intuition and expert clinical practice in nursing', *British Journal of Nursing*, 2 (4): 228–33.

Greenwood, J. (1993) 'Reflective practice: a critique of the work of Argyris and Schön', *Journal of Advanced Nursing*, 18: 1183–7.

Jarvis, P. (1992) 'Reflective practice and nursing', *Nurse Education Today*, 12: 174–81.

McCaffery, M. (1979) *Nursing Management of the Patient with Pain*, New York: J.B. Lippincott and Co.

Mezirow, I. (1981) 'A critical theory of adult learning and education', *Adult Education*, 32 (1): 3–24.

Schön, D. (1983) *The Reflective Practitioner*, New York: Basic Books.

Schön, D. (1987) *Educating the Reflective Practitioner*, San Francisco: Jossey Bass.

Sofaer, B. (1983) 'Pain relief: the core of nursing practice', *Nursing Times*, 79: 38–42.

Van Manen, M. (1990) *Researching Lived Experience: Human Science for Action-Sensitive Pedagogy*, Toronto: Althouse Press.

8

F.M. Quinn

Reflection and Reflective Practice

Although reflection as a concept had been established in education since the turn of the century, it was the work of Donald Schön (1983, 1987) in the mid-1980s that put it well and truly on the agenda of professional practice in both the teaching and the nursing professions. The significance of reflection in nursing lies in its close relationship to learning in professional practice settings; experiential learning is learning that results from experience and is essentially learning by doing, rather than by listening to other people or reading about it. Reflection is seen as an important component of experiential learning because it constitutes a means of thinking about professional practice. . . .

Are models of reflection helpful for clarifying what reflection is?

Some models of reflection have established themselves as front-runners in nursing, particularly those of Kolb (1984), Schön (1983, 1987), Boud, Keogh and Walker (1985; Boud, Cohen and Walker, 1993) and Johns (1992). Models of reflection, while differing in their levels of explanation, envisage reflection as essentially a retrospective phenomenon consisting of three fundamental processes:

- **retrospection**: i.e. thinking back about a situation or experience;
- **self-evaluation**, i.e. critically analysing and evaluating the actions and feelings associated with the experience, using theoretical perspectives;
- **reorientation**, i.e. using the results of self-evaluation to influence future approaches to similar situations or experiences.

Kolb's experiential learning cycle

For David Kolb (1984) learning is a core process of human development that is clearly distinguishable from a simple readjustment to

---

First published in *Continuing Professional Development: a Guide for Practitioners and Educators* (Stanley Thornes, 1988), pp. 121–45. Abridged.

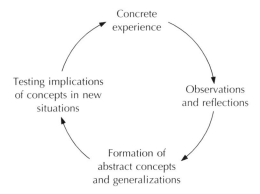

Figure 8.1 *Kolb's experiential learning model*

change. His experiential learning model (experiential learning cycle) is based upon the premise that development results from learning gained through experience. According to Kolb there are four generic adaptive abilities that are required for effective learning.

- **Concrete experience (CE)**: The learner must immerse him/herself fully and openly in new experiences.
- **Reflective observation (RO)**: The learner must observe and reflect on concrete experiences from a variety of perspectives.
- **Abstract conceptualization (AC)**: The learner must create concepts that integrate his/her observations into logical theories.
- **Active experimentation**: The learner must apply these theories in decision-making and problem-solving.

These four generic adaptive abilities consist of two pairs of opposites, which together form two primary dimensions of learning:

Concrete experience —— Abstract conceptualization
Active experimentation —— Reflective observation

Figure 8.1 shows the reflective cycle. The cycle commences with a concrete experience, either professional or personal, that is perceived by the individual as interesting or problematic. Firstly, observations and information are gathered about the experience, and then the individual reflects upon it over and over again. By analysing this reflection, insights begin to emerge as a kind of 'theory' about the experience. Implications can then be drawn from this conceptualization and used to modify existing practice or to generate new approaches to practice. . . .

Kolb's model does not have a great deal of empirical support, however, and it is unlikely that all learning situations will require an integrated approach using the four generic adaptive abilities.

Boud, Keogh and Walker's model of reflection

The Boud, Keogh and Walker (1985) model is a three-stage model to assist learners to reflect upon experiences.

- **Stage 1. Returning to the experience**: In this stage the learner mentally 'replays' the experience, describing what happened in a descriptive, non-judgemental way.
- **Stage 2. Attending to feeling**: This stage is about getting in touch with the learner's own feelings about the experience, utilizing any positive feelings about the experience and removing any feelings that may obstruct the reflection.
- **Stage 3. Re-evaluating the experience**: This stage is broken down into four substages, each of which is designed to enhance outcomes of reflection. In re-evaluating the experience, it is important that any new information arising from experience and reflection makes an **association** with the learner's existing knowledge and attitudes. These associations are then put together by **integration** into new ideas or attitudes, which are then tested by **validation** to determine whether there are any inconsistencies or contradictions. The fourth substage, **appropriation**, occurs when the new knowledge and attitudes become an intrinsic part of the learner's identity, and this will depend upon the significance placed upon any given experience and associated reflections. . . .

The Boud, Keogh and Walker model demonstrates a relatively rational approach to the process of reflecting upon experience, and as such as been adopted widely in nursing as a tool for teaching practitioners how to reflect. It is worth noting, however, that in a more recent paper (Boud, Cohen and Walker, 1993) the authors emphasize that systematic reflection is not the only way in which individuals learn from experiences:

> What we can say is that learning from experience is far more indirect than we often pretend it to be. It can be promoted by systematic reflection, but it can also be powerfully prompted by discrepancies or dilemmas which we are 'forced' to confront.

They go on to conclude:

> Much as we may enjoy the intellectual chase, we cannot neglect our full experience in the process. To do so is to fool ourselves into treating learning from experience as a simple, rational process.

The Gibbs reflective cycle

Figure 8.2 illustrates Gibb's (1988) reflective cycle. It is interesting to note that, although at first sight it looks similar to the Kolb cycle, it is

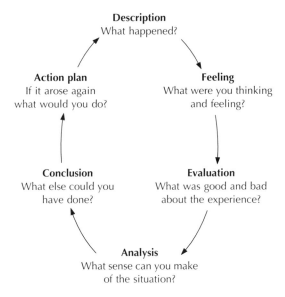

Figure 8.2   *The Gibbs reflective cycle*

actually much closer to the Boud, Keogh and Walker model. Gibbs uses the term 'description' rather than 'returning to the experience'; the emphasis on dealing with good and bad feelings is similar in both cycles; Gibbs's term 'analysis' is less specific than 're-evaluating the experience' in the Boud et al. model, but in his reflective cycle Gibbs makes more overt the action planning component of reflection. . . .

The Johns model of structured reflection

Johns (1992) uses the concept of guided reflection to describe a structured, supported approach that helps practitioners learn from their reflections upon experiences. The approach involves the use of the model of structured reflection, one-to-one or group supervision and the keeping of a structured reflective diary. The model of structured reflection involves a series of questions that help structure the practitioner's reflections. There is one core question and five cue questions, as shown in Figure 8.3.

Johns's model is more detailed than any of the models outlined above, and there are both advantages and disadvantages to this. The nursing literature indicates that nurses need to be taught how to reflect, and the detailed questions that practitioners are required to ask of themselves in the Johns model certainly provide a comprehensive checklist for reflection. The disadvantage of such a detailed structure is that it imposes a framework that is external to the practitioner, leaving little scope for inclusion of his/her own approach.

Core question: What information do I need access to in order to learn through this experience?

Cue questions

1.0 *Description of experience*
    1.1 *Phenomenon* – describe the 'here and now' experience
    1.2 *Causal* – What essential factors contributed to this experience?
    1.3 *Context* – What are the significant background factors to this experience?
    1.4 *Clarifying* – What are the key processes (for reflection) in this experience?

2.0 *Reflection*
    2.1 What was I trying to achieve?
    2.2 Why did I intervene as I did?
    2.3 What were the consequences of my actions for?
       – myself?
       – the patient/family?
       – the people I work with?
    2.4 How did I feel about this experience when it was happening?
    2.5 How did the patient feel about it?
    2.6 How do I know how the patient felt about it?

3.0 *Influencing factors*
    3.1 What internal factors influenced my decision-making?
    3.2 What external factors influenced my decision-making?
    3.3 What sources of knowledge did/should have influenced my decision-making?

4.0 *Could I have dealt better with the situation?*
    4.1 What other choices did I have?
    4.2 What would be the consequences of those choices?

5.0 *Learning*
    5.1 How do I **now** feel about this experience?
    5.2 How have I made sense of this experience in the light of past experiences and future practice?
    5.3 How has this experience changed my ways of knowing:
       – empirics?
       – aesthetics?
       – ethics?
       – personal?

Figure 8.3 *The Johns model of structured reflection*

It is also open to criticism on the grounds of complexity, although other models can be criticized on precisely the opposite grounds, i.e. they may appear simplistic and self-evident. . . .

Are there any reservations expressed about reflective practice?

It seems self-evident that, by reflecting upon practice, practitioners may gain insights into how their practice can be improved. Indeed, it is probably impossible to avoid reflecting on the past, particularly when the recollected situation or event has emotional overtones for the practitioner.

However, I would like to express some reservations I have about the way in which it is being promulgated in nursing. The impression gained from the literature is that the only effective nurses are those who actively and systematically reflect upon their practice, and that such reflection must be more than simply thinking about the situation or event. I have categorized my reservations under three headings: ethical, professional and pragmatic.

Ethical reservations

The theoretical basis for reflection, as interpreted by the nursing profession, is humanistic psychology as exemplified in the work of Carl Rogers (1951, 1969, 1983). It is therefore from the same stable as interpersonal skills training, encounter groups, and assertiveness training, all of which emphasize the paramouncy of the *self* and the importance of *feelings* over cognition, e.g. self-awareness, self-disclosure, self-actualization.

Criticism of this 1960s 'pop psychology' is beginning to emerge: Sigman (1995) suggests that during this period psychology diversified from the treating of problems to addressing issues of greater happiness. He argues that individuals' expectations turned away from contentment and self-acceptance towards personal growth and development. This constant striving for self-improvement may lead to feelings of self-disapproval and rejection of one's own personality, especially if the individual fails to achieve the self-improvement s/he is seeking.

The nursing literature suggests that reflection is more valuable if done in partnership with someone else, which leads me to believe that the approach is quasi-therapeutic: in other words, the principles have been transferred directly from client-centred psychotherapy and Rogersian counselling. The examples of reflective encounters given by Johns (1996) seem to me to be very much in this therapeutic mould.

The use of this approach may trigger powerful emotional responses such as guilt and anxiety, and as such we have to consider whether or not practitioners should be given a choice about participating in such activity.

Student nurses certainly appear to have no choice, as reflection is now a significant component of their pre-registration education. The following quotation from Fitzgerald (1994: 76) is illuminating in this respect: 'These are not particularly comfortable processes, which may lead students to personal distress and conflict.' Other writers, e.g. Rich and Parker (1995), identify the unease of some students with this approach.

Qualified practitioners too may have little choice, since reflection is seen as a crucial component of clinical supervision (Fisher, 1996) and of the Post-registration Education and Practice portfolio (UKCC, 1997). The question of choice is important also, given that there is currently little evidence for the effectiveness of reflective practice in nursing; indeed, the nature of reflective practice makes it almost impossible to evaluate with any accuracy. It is somewhat ironic, given the importance that nurses attach to informed consent in relation to patients and clients, that this aspect may have been entirely overlooked in the case of nursing staff and students.

It is interesting to note that the teaching profession, in its adoption of reflective practice, has placed much less emphasis on the emotional aspects of reflection, preferring instead to focus on the cognitive. This may well be because of the different goals and professional socialization of the two professions.

Professional reservations

The concept of victim-blaming is well established in the field of health promotion and refers to approaches that focus on the individual as the prime cause of his/her own ill-health, as opposed to the social, economic and political environment in which s/he lives. Similarly, reflective practice seems to put the onus on to the individual practitioner for the maintenance and improvement of standards of nursing care, which may divert attention from the responsibility of the organization to provide adequate staffing levels, effective staff development and adequate resources.

Another difficulty I find is that the literature of reflective practice seems to constantly devalue current nursing practice, thus undermining both the individual practitioner and the nurse manager. Most of the literature on clinical supervision suggests that the clinical supervisor should not be the individual practitioner's line manager, yet it is the latter who carries ultimate responsibility for the quality of care in a given practice context. This seems to imply that managers are not to be trusted, yet most nursing managers are themselves practitioners.

Relationships between nurse academics in colleges of nursing and practitioners in the field have been characterized by 'mutual distrust, little respect for each others' experience, even less empathy for each other, and often overt antagonism between the parties' (Quinn, 1994). The constant devaluing of current practice may undermine practitioners' confidence and lower their morale, resulting in a fall in standards of care, i.e. the exact opposite effect to what is intended by reflective practice.

Current models of reflective practice may also devalue physical care by overemphasizing psychological aspects. The devaluing of professional practice does not seem to occur to anything like the same extent in the literature of the teaching profession, which may lead one to conclude that the nursing profession may be going overboard in its critical approach to practice.

One could also advance the argument that reflection, particularly that done in partnership with a colleague or supervisor, could lead to the practitioner becoming dependent upon that individual, a well-documented phenomenon in the literature of counselling.

Pragmatic reservations

While reflection seems to be an important strategy for analysing individuals' practice, I have reservations about the practical implementation as proposed in the nursing literature. It is my belief that nurses already have too many professional development demands placed upon them, all of which are additional to their role in caring for patients. For example, nurses are required to engage in the following activities:

• Maintain a PREP portfolio as evidence for reregistration.
• Undergo clinical supervision.
• Undergo individual performance review (IPR) or appraisal.
• Undertake statutory training, e.g. moving and handling.
• Keep up to date by reading journals.

Given that current nursing practice is demanding, stressful and constantly changing, it may well be unfair and unrealistic to expect practitioners to reflect systematically on their practice unless they are given the time to do it during their working day. To quote one practitioner: 'After a hard day at work, the last thing I want to do when I get home is to start reflecting about it.' In the case of student nurses, there is also the potential for complicity, i.e. if written reflection is made a compulsory and assessed component of their education programme, students may invent reflections that meet the criteria laid down by their teachers.

The inference could be drawn that, if you are not a reflective practitioner in the way the term is interpreted in the nursing literature, you are not a good practitioner. Does this mean that practice was never any good before reflection was invented? It needs to be remembered that reflection, according to the nursing literature, is *ex post facto* and as such cannot affect the outcome of the situation being reflected upon. In effect, it can be seen as 'shutting the stable door after the horse has bolted'.

Of course, such reflection may influence the practitioner's approach to future situations, but this is a much less direct effect. What is needed, I suggest, is a shift of emphasis towards reflection-in-action and even reflection-before-action. Perhaps nurse education needs to emphasize much more the fact that nurses need not always respond to situations by 'thinking on their feet'. This can often lead to 'knee-jerk' reactions rather than carefully thought out responses. It is probably true to say that many situations in nursing do not require an instant response, and nurses might well benefit from the concept of 'taking time out' before making decisions in practice.

I am inclined to conclude that reflection as described in the literature should be seen as a strategy for student learning rather than a system for use by qualified practitioners in their everyday work. On the other hand, reflective cycles, e.g. Kolb (1984), Gibbs (1988), seem helpful, but can be done mentally without having to write everything down. However, to expect qualified, busy practitioners to be doing this on a regular basis is unwarranted given the present lack of evidence about its effectiveness. It is simply unacceptable for nurses to be branded as ineffective because they do not undertake the systematic process of reflection espoused by the proponents of reflective practice. Jarvis (1992) fired an early warning shot when he wrote: 'It might even be claimed that the idea of reflective practice is a bandwagon, upon which many professionals have jumped because it provides a rational for their practice.' Richardson (1990) also counsels against 'the danger of taking an abstract concept like reflection, and operationalizing it into behaviour that is generalizable, observable and teachable'. At the time of writing, another concept is beginning to dominate the world of health care – evidence-based practice. It remains to be seen what effect, if any, this will have on current notions of reflective practice.

References

Boud, D., Cohen, R. and Walker, D. (eds) (1993) *Using Experience for Learning*, Open University Press: Milton Keynes.

Boud, D., Keogh, R. and Walker, D. (1985) *Reflection: Turning Experience into Learning*, Kogan Page: London.

Fisher, M. (1996) 'Using reflective practice in clinical supervision', *Professional Nurse*, 11 (7): 443–4.

Fitzgerald, M. (1994) 'Theories of reflection for learning', in *Reflective Practice in Nursing*, ed. A. Palmer, S. Burns and C. Bulman, Blackwell: Oxford.

Gibbs, G. (1988) *Learning by Doing: A Guide to Teaching and Learning Methods*, Further Education Unit: Oxford Polytechnic, Oxford.

Jarvis, P. (1992) 'Reflective practice and nursing', *Nurse Education Today*, 12 (3): 174–81.

Johns, C. (1992) 'The Burford Nursing Development Unit holistic model of nursing practice', *Journal of Advanced Nursing*, 16: 1090–8.

Johns, C. (1996) 'The benefits of a reflective model of nursing', *Nursing Times*, 92: 27.

Kolb, D.A. (1984) *Experiential Learning*, Prentice-Hall: London.

Quinn, F.M. (1994) 'The demise of curriculum', in *Healthcare Education: The Challenge of the Market*, ed. J. Humphreys and F.M. Quinn, Chapman and Hall: London.

Rich, A. and Parker, D. (1995) 'Reflection and critical incident analysis: ethical and moral implications of their use within nursing and midwifery education', *Journal of Advanced Nursing*, 22: 1050–7.

Richardson, V. (1990) 'The evolution of reflective teaching and teacher education', in *Encouraging Reflective Practice in Education*, ed. T. Clift, W. Houston and M. Pugach, Teachers College Press: New York.

Rogers, C. (1951) *Client Centred Therapy*, Houghton Mifflin: Boston, MA.

Rogers, C. (1969) *Freedom to Learn*, Charles E. Merrill: Columbus, OH.

Rogers, C. (1983) *Freedom to Learn for the 80s*, Charles E. Merrill: Columbus, OH.

Schön, D. (1983) *The Reflective Practitioner: How Professionals Think in Action*, Basic Books: New York.

Schön, D. (1987) *Educating the Reflective Practitioner: Towards a New Design for Teaching and Learning in the Professions*, Jossey-Bass: San Francisco, CA.

Sigman, A. (1995) *New. Improved? Exposing the Misuse of Popular Psychology*, Simon and Schuster: London.

UKCC (1997) *PREP and You*, United Kingdom Central Council for Nursing, Midwifery and Health Visiting: London.

9

T. Kitwood

Requirements of a Caregiver

. . . In this chapter we will examine in some detail what dementia care requires on the part of a caregiver, and the kind of personal development that may be involved. First, we explore the caregiver's part in creating person-enhancing interaction. Then we will move on to a less obvious topic – that of hidden motives that often draw people into care work. I shall suggest that when these motives are 'owned', understood and integrated, they can become a powerful resource. This leads on to the topic of empathy, important in all interpersonal contexts, but doubly so in this field, where the recipients of care are so easily depersonalized. Finally, we will look briefly at the depth psychology of care work, and I shall make a contrast between the psychodynamic processes that impede, and those that facilitate, effective care.

The caregiver's part in interaction

The first requirement is deceptively simple, though profound in its implications. It is that the caregiver is actually present, in the sense of being psychologically available. In counselling and psychotherapy this is sometimes known as giving 'free attention'; being present with and for another person without distraction from outside or disturbance from within; perceiving the other with far less of the distortions, projections and judgemental reactions that so often get in the way of real meeting. Giving free attention is difficult enough in any context, yet it is widely agreed that this is essential for doing psychological work that really helps and heals. Some people fail to give free attention because they are caught up in the self-importance that is attached to their professional role. Those who have a lot of power, such as medical consultants or senior managers, are particularly liable to fall into this trap. Sometimes the problem centres on sheer overload; the immediate demands on the psyche are too great for it to

First published in *Dementia Reconsidered* (Open University Press, 1997), pp. 118–44. Abridged.

bear. More generally, however, people fail because they are strongly
driven by their vulnerability, anxiety or pain. If, as I have suggested,
dementia activates certain universal fears, there is a specially
important issue here. In colloquial terms people don't give free
attention because there is too much of their own emotional baggage
getting in the way. Being present cannot be learned as mere technique; the baggage must be faced and dealt with.

Having the ability to 'be present' is a gift to other people, and it is a
kind of liberation for oneself. It means being less troubled about the
past, less fearful about the future, and thus more centred on what is
immediately at hand. 'Being present' entails letting go of that
obsession with *doing* which often damages care work, and having a
greater capacity simply for *being*. It does not, of course, set a person
free from pain, either physical or mental, although it may lead
to better ways of dealing with pain. It is an absolute prerequisite of
good caring. For presentness is the quality that underlies all true
relationships. . . .

It has often been suggested that there are hidden (and generally
unacknowledged) motives that attract people to care work, and I
want to make some very positive suggestions on this topic. One of the
most illuminating ways of exploring the issues is through the idea of
a 'script', particularly as developed within transactional analysis. The
concept itself is a metaphor derived from the theatre. . . .

Scripts, when formed, are extremely resistant to change, because
they have been practised again and again. Presumably they are actually incorporated into nerve architecture. If a person were suddenly to
step out of the scripted way it would feel 'unnatural', and almost
certainly it would cause extreme anxiety. Also, of course, living outside the script is likely to cause upset to other people, because their
expectations would be violated.

> Alison, who is very committed to caring for others, is going through a
> period of feeling very insecure and troubled. Often she begins to cry for no
> apparent reason. One day she is visiting her 80-year-old mother, and she
> tries to speak about her distress.
>   'I'm so shaky and weepy, Mother. I don't know what's happening to me.
> Perhaps I'm suffering from depression.'
>   'Don't be so silly, You're not depressed. I can't be doing with you
> suffering from depression.'

Even in this tiny vignette we can catch a glimpse of Alison's script
and its origins – and possibly also of the underlying cause of her
current malaise. . . . Perhaps the commonest caring script is that of
the rescuer who tends to attract very dependent and needy people,
and who is drawn repeatedly into involvement with those who have
the corresponding script of victim. There is the guide, the kind of
person who has an almost uncanny ability to know what others are
thinking and feeling. There is the martyr, who is extraordinarily self-

sacrificing, whose normal way of life seems to involve an almost superhuman workload meeting the needs of others. And there is the hero, one who stands out strongly for a noble cause, esteemed from afar, but sometimes lonely and unsupported in personal life. . . .

Adults who have such scripts tend to have a chronically low level of self-esteem behind their everyday façade. They may have difficulty with psychological boundaries, tending to confuse their own desires and needs with those of others. Here, almost certainly, are the roots of co-dependency, where a person becomes compulsively involved with others who are very needy (Mellody, 1993). Some people with strong scripts of this sort, when they are in care work, have to endure a continual tension between their own privation and the needs of those who are in their care. If the underlying issues are not resolved there is serious danger of burn-out. A person may even turn, in deep resentment, against the very cause to which they had been so strongly committed, when at last the truth dawns that it will not meet their hidden need.

Scripts such as these do, however, have a very positive aspect. There is no place for a shallow cynicism, suggesting that all people who become caregivers are inadequate, or enter this kind of work for selfish motives. In each case the script meant developing resources of personality that are all too rare in a culture that is fixated on greed and egoism. Each script represents a creative choice, made in the face of difficulty. The child did not decide to become destructive, vindictive or utterly self-centred; the child did not decide to withdraw from social contact. Instead, the script entailed a resolve to help make the world a better place. It was a first step towards morality in the true sense; it was a vote for humanity, and for life itself. As Robin Skynner has pointed out, the inference is not that people with such scripts are unsuitable for care professions. It is, rather, that it is important to 'feed the goose that lays the golden eggs' (Schlapo-bersky, 1991: 155–69). . . .

Recovery from script

. . . Scripted behaviour tends to be blind, compulsive; in some deep sense it lacks direction, other than that it is patterned by anxiety and driven by unmet need. As recovery occurs a person comes to see more clearly what he or she is up to, and learns to interrupt familiar scripted scenes. Choices become more realistic and objective, taking a greater range of factors into account. If, in the light of new aware-ness, a person decides to continue in work as difficult and demanding as dementia care, it will be on the basis of clear and heartfelt choice, and not an unacknowledged compulsion. A script, thus transformed, can become a true vocation.

Anne is the manager of a day centre. She is highly committed to her job, and she is very good at it. She has a strong tendency to overwork, and twice she has had to take time off due to stress and depression. Through the help of a counsellor she came to recognize her script. She was the eldest daughter of eight children, five boys and three girls. In all her earliest recollections she was her mother's helper, and she had very few memories of play. Her father seemed to have featured scarcely at all in her childhood, except when he came home drunk. Gradually Anne came to realize that she may have received little real love as a child; but at the same time she felt great tenderness towards her mother, and valued the many caring and helping skills that she had learned. As her insight grew, she took steps to become more relaxed and playful. She began to learn pottery, and she joined a women's walking group. She negotiated a half day off per week, and stopped doing many hours of unpaid overtime. She began to feel much better about herself, and she believes that the quality of her work has greatly improved and deepened.

Points of pain and vulnerability

There is another kind of issue, also related to a person's past, but arising more directly from what happens in the care setting. It may be a matter of the way the organization itself functions. A manager, perhaps, is perceived in phantasy as if he or she were a powerful parent. Two or more members of staff might find themselves in competition for attention or reward – unconsciously recreating a situation of sibling rivalry. There may be problems over the actual roles: one careworker might be secretly resentful about being expected to do so much, or another might feel that he or she is not being given enough responsibility. Some members of staff might be very insecure in their role, and need a good deal of reassurance.

Morgan took a job as a care assistant at a time when he was unemployed; it was at least something to do. To his surprise, he enjoyed the work, and he began to feel committed to it. He even went, voluntarily, on two courses. However, he was never given feedback about his performance, and at times he felt that he was regarded as an intruder into a women's domain. As time went on he 'swindled and dwindled', until his confidence ebbed away completely. Eventually he left care work, but with great regret.

Prejudices of many kinds may get in the way of good care practice – ethnicity, age, social class or sexual orientation, or as in the example above, simply gender. When there are interpersonal difficulties in areas such as these, it is likely that jobs will be done less effectively. Situations will be perceived with less realism because they will be distorted by projections; truthful communication will be impaired. Far too much of the work of the organization will be given over to meeting the unacknowledged needs of members of staff. . . .

Whether or not there is a maladaptive script, everyone brings issues of a personal kind into their work; these are liable to be activated in an especially poignant way in a field such as dementia care.

The implication is that the most truly effective workers will be those who have a well-developed 'experiential self', who are familiar with the world of feelings, accepting of their own vulnerabilities, and able to live with a low level of psychological defence. . . .

To be blocked is to be out of vital contact with the psychological realities; to be overwhelmed is to be ineffective in any practical sense. Between the two extremes, but towards the low end, there is the range of greatest efficacy. Here a person is able to put his or her feelings and intuitions to good use.

The psychodynamics of dementia care

The central idea of all depth psychology is that we have motives, conflicts, imaginings, of which we are usually unaware. We can call these 'unconscious mental processes', although it would be more accurate to speak of neurological activity that is not being registered in consciousness and which, at that point of a person's development, cannot be; possibly the necessary brain 'circuits' are not available for use or haven't been fully formed as yet. Most of depth psychology has focused on what might be happening within the individual psyche, and rather less attention has been given to interpersonal processes. In this section I want to do both; first looking at the basis of empathy, and then at the nature of dementia care. Much of this is speculative. The most that can be said is that it is compatible with what can be observed, and that it seems to help some people have a better understanding of who they are and what they are doing. . . .

When we develop empathy with someone who has all their mental powers intact, we attend both to their words and to their non-verbal signals. Sometimes we notice discrepancies between the two kinds of message. A person might, for example, claim to be feeling 'perfectly OK', while showing clear signs of anxiety or inner turmoil. Gradually, keeping all the information in a kind of 'soft focus', we gain a sense of what they might be experiencing. A person who has highly developed empathic skill is able to retain his or her own feeling states, while also being aware of the feeling state of the other. In developing empathy with a person who has dementia the issues are similar, but not exactly the same. Words and sentences may not make ordinary sense, but yet have poetic meaning through metaphor and allusion. Non-verbal signals may be particularly clear. The full reconstruction of another's frame of reference, then, involves more than attempting to make sense piecemeal of the verbal and non-verbal signals that a person is conveying. It also involves drawing on feelings that are genuinely our own.

If this is the true foundation of empathy, it suggests that even the most difficult and painful memories can be turned to positive use.

Most people will find, if they dare to look, that they have had experiences that might resemble, to some small degree, what a person with dementia is going through: times of abandonment, of betrayal, of acute loneliness, of feeling powerless or terrifyingly incompetent, or being outpaced or outclassed. Everyone has had to endure a share of the malignant social psychology that is present in everyday life, and been made to feel more like an object than a person. As the 'experiential self' grows, these emotional memories become available. Even those privations, deprivations and injuries that underlie scripts such as those we have examined, can be transmuted into resources for care work.

Projective and empathic identification

Metaphorically we may say that every person, regardless of whether or not there is cognitive impairment, has a 'child' within; and at times this child can be needy, helpless or demanding. This is illustrated in Figure 9.1.

Suppose now that the caregiver remains in a state of denial and self-deception, unable or unwilling to recognize areas of damage and deficit, and steadfastly holding up a professional front. It is likely that such a person will be caught up in the defensive process of 'projective identification' first described by Melanie Klein (Segal, 1992): that is, the caregiver will 'see' aspects of his or her own self in the person who has dementia, and may even induce that person to act some of these aspects out; making them become more angry, more helpless, more confused, etc. as shown in Figure 9.2. . . .

The caregiver can maintain a state of self-deception, and at the same time misperceives the one who is being cared for. The needy child of the caregiver is looked after magically in the person who is cared for; the two are locked together in a way that hinders them both. This is illustrated in Figure 9.3. . . .

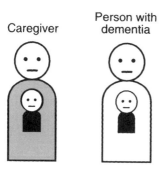

Figure 9.1

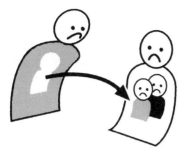

Figure 9.2

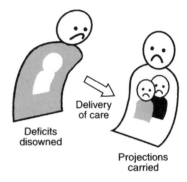

Figure 9.3

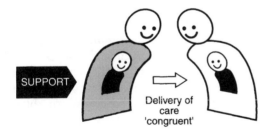

Figure 9.4

In contrast to this, let us imagine now that the caregiver has gone some way to developing his or her experiential resources; the script is being dealt with, and the child within is being recognized and cherished. The psychodynamics of this situation are shown in Figure 9.4. Now the caregiver and the one who is being cared for are both on the same human level, and far more able to appreciate what they have in common. Both carry a needy child within, and both are dependent on the support and comfort that is supplied by others. . . .

The child within the caregiver is being looked after in a more open and honest way, mostly outside the care setting. The process of caring is true, sincere, accurate, egalitarian, and the communication is congruent. The whole relationship might be described as one of empathic identification.

Two paths of personal development

When dementia care is seen in the kind of way that I have portrayed, it is indisputable that this work requires a very high level of personal and moral development on the part of those who undertake it. There can be no question of bolting on a body of knowledge, or of imparting a set of skills in a semi-automated fashion. We are looking for very intelligent and flexible action from a 'reflective practitioner'. The essence of what is required might be described as freedom from ego, so narrow, imperious, conformist, greedy, grasping and demanding. . . .

Two main paths of personal development are available to us at present. The first has been opened up by psychotherapy, and the second by meditation. They are not rivals, as several experts have shown (e.g. Watts, 1973; LeShan, 1983). An individual can be involved in both together, and it is also possible to combine them in some form of group process.

Psychotherapy attempts to deal with the issues that trouble a person, primarily by unravelling the content of those issues, and often by an exploration of their origins. If all goes well, and a relationship of trust develops, hidden feelings come out into the open, understanding increases, and there is a growth in self-esteem. . . .

In meditation, however, the approach is more indirect. A person undertakes exercises that are designed to strengthen the structure of the psyche, primarily through the cultivation of a still, serene centre that is not committed to inner talk. As this development occurs there is a gain in poise, awareness and flexibility. A person is more able to 'be present', and more able to act spontaneously and wholeheartedly. Wary and defensive postures that may formerly have served as a protection can gradually be laid aside. In meditation the aim, in a sense, is to learn how to 'not think'. . . .

Whatever route of personal growth is taken, the difficulty of the task should not be underestimated. We need to remember that, as with care work, the task is not 'purely psychological', but neurological too. To change long-standing habits and attitudes may actually involve the dismantling of existing nerve pathways, and the gradual formation of new ones. And these, we might reasonably hope, have more connections than the old, enabling a person to be more aware, more in touch with what he or she is undergoing, and with the processes of life.

I walk down the street
There is a deep hole in the sidewalk
I fall in
I am lost . . . I am hopeless
It isn't my fault
It takes forever to find a way out.

I walk down the same street
There is a deep hole in the sidewalk
I pretend I don't see it
I fall in again
I can't believe I'm in the same place
But it isn't my fault
It still takes a long time to get out.

I walk down the same street
There is a deep hole in the sidewalk
I see it is there
I still fall in – it is a habit
My eyes are open
I know where I am
It is my fault
I get out immediately.

I walk down the same street
There is a deep hole in the sidewalk
I walk around it.

I walk down another street. (Rinpoche, 1992: 31–2)

This passage was written by a Tibetan Buddhist, in the context of a discourse on meditation. It could equally well be an evocation of the difficult path of therapeutic change.

References

LeShan, L. (1983) *How to Mediate*, London: Aquarian Press.
Mellody, P. (1993) *Facing Codependency*, San Francisco: HarperCollins.
Rinpoche, S. (1976) *Keywords: A Vocabulary of Culture and Society*. London: Fontana.
Schlapobersky, J.R. (ed.) (1991) *Institutes and How to Survive Them: Selected Papers by Robin Skynner*, London: Routledge.
Segal, J. (1992) *Melanie Klein*, London: Sage.
Watts, A.W. (1973) *Psychotherapy East and West*, Harmondsworth: Penguin.

10

R. Barnitt

The Virtuous Therapist

. . . Statements about professional values and beliefs tend to extol emotional, attitudinal and behavioural perfection on the part of the therapist, rather than the messy realities of practice. For example, in 1992, Young and Quinn expressed their therapy values as follows: 'We value a therapeutic relationship of mutual co-operation with the patient' and 'We acknowledge the subjective perspective of the client' (1992: 62). These are carried over into the *Code of Ethics and Professional Conduct*, published by the College of Occupational Therapists in 1995, which states that occupational therapists are 'strongly committed to client-centred practice and the involvement of the client as an equal partner'. Whether these values are desirable is not open to question; however, it might be realistic to suggest that therapists who strive to perform at such levels are saints, martyrs or fools. In 1993, Joyce wrote, in an opinion article, that occupational therapists were a 'steady, compliant, professional group', when what was needed in today's climate was a 'radical occupational therapist operating anarchically' and not a therapist blessed with 'conservatism and moderation'. This caused outrage to some members of the profession and led to heated debate in the letters column of the professional journal.

Why is it that occupational therapists are so concerned with being seen to be virtuous? Can criticism such as Joyce's be put down to envy or defensiveness on the part of other professionals who cannot match occupational therapy standards? Recent research has suggested that, instead of criticizing therapists for 'being too nice', attention should be given to those therapists who struggle to live up to such ideals within 'rapid change in the health service' and 'autocratic management styles' that make working to high standards almost impossible, 'resulting in self-recrimination, frustration and disappointment' (Broom and Williams, 1996). Which is the real therapist: the moderate with conservative values, practising virtuously against the odds, or the passive reactionary who wants a quiet life?

First published in J. Creek (ed.) *Occupational Therapy: New Perspectives* (Whurr Publishers, 1998), pp. 77–98. Abridged.

During research into ethical dilemmas in therapy, a number of insights were gained into the thinking behind this issue of virtue. This chapter explores some of the issues related to altruism and virtue in occupational therapy.

What is virtue?

Lafollette (1997: 254) said that the notion of virtue had recently been 'reinjected into the public arena' but that for many people it remained a 'quaint' notion linked to chastity and humility: 'virtues possessed by the few – and usually the puritan'. Any understanding of virtue was linked to the social or political circumstances in which people lived. Related to these, Hill (1974) discussed the case of servility and whether this was a vice or a virtue. Hill argued that slaves were servile because this was a prudent way to behave to protect themselves and their families, whilst in less oppressive societies servility was seen as a vice. Hill also related virtue to the social or political influences on the role of women (which includes most therapists) in current society where, despite the rhetoric of equality, he suggested that women are still being taught to defer to men, as men's desires and interests are the more important. If this is still the case, it might help to explain the compliant relationship referred to by Joyce (1993), which is often between female therapists and male power figures in the health service.

A second aspect of virtue raised by Lafollette (1997) was that of the need for self-respect and of respect from others. Only if this condition was met could the individual, whether slave or woman, feel that he or she had rights and thus respect. However, attending to one's own needs and rights has also been viewed as synonymous with being an egoist, the person who is self-centred, unprincipled and unfeeling (Baier, 1993). Baier went on to explain that, in ethics, egoism has several versions: first 'the promotion of one's own good beyond the morally permissible'; second, that while people justify their behaviour as generally 'good', deep down it is still aimed at 'own' good, and, third, that a higher level of morality can be achieved where 'own' good 'and the common good are both addressed'. The final two versions of egoism given by Baier were ethical egoism and rational egoism. In the former, the greatest good is achieved by adopting moral standards (values and beliefs) and, in the latter, by being able to reason about and justify behaviour (reasoning and reflection). For therapists, the moral standards and behaviour required from the professional are laid down in codes of ethics whereas the capacity to reason and reflect is a primary objective of professional education.

A further debate about virtue is to what extent it lies within the individual, is internalized; and the extent to which it is subject to environmental factors and to social and political pressure. In the former case, the therapist could be held responsible for the personal morality of their actions, whereas in the latter case the therapist could claim social pressure to behave in certain ways not always consistent with their personal values. . . .

Virtue in occupational therapy

The claim might be made that the development of health professionals in the United Kingdom has partly been as a direct result of a lack of virtue in their predecessors. In nursing, this 'amoral' behaviour was epitomized in the description of Sairey Gamp, the nurse written about by Charles Dickens in *Martin Chuzzlewit* as a venal drunken woman. Descriptions of such 'camp followers', women who served as prostitutes while tending the sick and wounded, are found in accounts from the Napoleonic wars. The crusade that corrected these vices started when Florence Nightingale selected women with intelligence, education and strength of character to accompany her to nurse wounded soldiers in the Crimean War (Showalter, 1987). Similarly, in physiotherapy, which emerged as a profession approximately 70 years after nursing, the techniques of massage were developed to counteract the 'sinful massage provided by the oldest profession'. The 'new' masseuses were committed to demonstrating their 'skill and propriety'. This was as a result of newspaper exposures in the 1890s of 'immoral massage establishments' (Robinson, 1994). The point is seldom made that prostitutes and 'sinful masseuses' possibly provided a much-needed service before ladies of good works decided to clean them up. In occupational therapy, the link between questionable practices and the start of the profession is not as direct as for nursing and physiotherapy; however, its roots are clearly linked into the development of 'lay therapists' who provided domestic activities in the asylums of the late nineteenth century. Prior to this, in the majority of institutions, lunatics were considered as 'unfeeling brutes, ferocious animals that needed to be kept in check with chains, whips, straight waistcoats, barred windows and locked cells'. This image was later modified to become 'objects of pity whose sanity might be restored by kindly care' (Showalter, 1987: 8). This 'kindly care' was seen to be the imposition, or reinstatement, of domestic routines and moral habit training. In the 1990s, over a hundred years later, occupational therapists still have a major belief that domestic routines are an important part of therapy and refer to the imposition of routines previously lacking as 'habilitation' and reinstatement as 'rehabilitation'.

With the development of the professions of nursing, physiotherapy and occupational therapy, the original individual goodwill or virtue that energized practice has slowly become institutionalized. This is seen through the introduction of registration schemes, criteria for professional suitability, control over education and the introduction of standards for behaviour and codes of ethics. While all of these systems can be seen to ensure safe practice and control over the selection, education and employment of therapists, this does not necessarily mean that therapists are virtuous, morally excellent people who use their powers to do good. In 1993, Joyce wrote that occupational therapists were 'sensible, thoughtful and caring people who put the patient first'. However, Joyce then went on to criticize therapists for being unimaginative and safe in their practices, and suggested that what was needed by patients was 'preparing people for the jobs market . . . and filling the vast vacuum of leisure time', which Joyce said was beyond the grasp and competence of an occupational therapist. This opinion caused consternation in the profession, with a principal concern being that 'they' did not understand the role of the occupational therapist. Overall, little mention was made of the fact that some therapists also have difficulty with this. It may not be sufficient for a therapist to behave impeccably and have high standards that demand recognition by others, at the same time as being unable to explain their role. A curious contradiction is evident here. On the one hand, therapists receive a full professional education and find it easy to obtain employment (apparently with a job description), and managers bewail the fact that staff are difficult to recruit, whilst, on the other hand, therapists complain that no one has defined the unique skills of occupational therapy and that colleagues do not understand the therapist's role.

Some of these issues currently facing occupational therapy are due to the relatively early stage of development of the profession. It could be argued that occupational therapists in the profession are currently at an adolescent stage where the search for meaning, and need for an internalized self-image and self-esteem, is pre-eminent and absorbs professional energy. This links to theories of moral development where a stage is reached at which people are concerned with whether they exist, and are dependent on the views of others to validate themselves and their practice (Rest and Narváez, 1994). This also links with the third stage of moral development described by Kohlberg (1984) in which an individual is concerned with the morality of interpersonal concordance: be considerate, nice and kind and you will make friends. In other words, 'be virtuous; your behaviour will be beyond reproach, and you will gain respect'.

In a hard-driving and unpredictable world, it is perhaps not surprising that therapists' vulnerability is starting to show. The changing ethos of the health and social services has run counter to some therapists' beliefs. Virtue has been out of fashion (Lafollette, 1997) and skills that are currently valued include the operation of power, manipulation, confrontation and aiming for personal rather than social benefit. These values are viewed by some therapists as neither particularly desirable nor respectable. However, there is some indication that social values are changing again (Heater, 1990).

Therapists have to some extent been hampered in their professional growth and influence on health and social policies by the hierarchical patient referral arrangements that have existed for four decades between doctors and therapists. In the 1940s and 1950s, therapists worked on the basis of referrals from doctors. Some dissatisfaction with this was noted in the letters pages of the professional journal in the 1960s and 1970s, with complaints about inappropriate referrals, lack of respect for the therapist's opinion and lack of understanding of what the therapist could offer. However, this was muted compared to physiotherapists who made formal complaints to the government of the day when, in 1962, a White Paper was published (Robinson, 1994) which stated that 'Doctors should prescribe physiotherapy with the same precise therapeutic indications . . . as they have been prescribing drugs'. In 1995, similar differences in political strength have appeared between the two professions, with the College of Occupational Therapists accepting that supervising students should be done with goodwill as part of professional responsibility, while the Chartered Society of Physiotherapy has stated that without financial recognition students will not be supervised.

In view of these differences, occupational therapists could be seen as either very wonderful people who happen to be around at a difficult political time or not very wonderful people who cling to outdated values and have not yet developed the skills of radical politics. Some of these issues came up during data collection for a series of studies being carried out into ethical dilemmas in therapy. The following section deals with the values and beliefs of qualified therapists that were identified during a study of ethical reasoning. . . .

Ethical reasoning in therapy

. . . Sixteen therapists, eight occupational therapists and eight physiotherapists, were asked to tell the story of an ethical dilemma which they had experienced at work. The resulting transcripts were subjected to a number of readings to analyse different features of ethical reasoning (Barnitt, 1996). This led to a set of themes which fitted Lafollette's (1997) definition of virtue as self-respect and respect for others, and included altruism, social desirability, and social influence. It could be assumed that as a therapist the individual operated from the notion of altruism, from 'selfless disinterest', however, as a 'normal' human the individual might also hold selfish motives and have a need to be accepted by fellow professionals as well as clients, relatives or carers.

Young, in 1996, wrote a somewhat cynical but possibly realistic statement about the current state of morality in Western parliamentary life: 'It is not exactly an amoral world. It merely gives dissembling a higher priority than other worlds.' In the present research, a tension was identified in the research stories between describing events that implied ownership of professional integrity, the selfless disinterest referred to above, events which indicated fallibility and 'loss of face' and normal human failings.

The following sections give examples of areas of practice in therapy where the tension between behaving ethically and compromise were most evident.

Being seen to behave well

Baron (1988) described behaviour when dealing with difficult decisions as sometimes leading to a 'neglect of consequences of a choice for the feelings of others', and 'failure to recognise the conflict between self-interest and the interests of others'. Contrary to this, therapists in the research described situations where they indeed recognized these conflicts but, despite this, the need to retain a sense of worth and positive self-esteem proved too powerful. For example, narrators tended to allocate blame for 'wrong' actions to other participants, particularly other professionals, whilst allocating praise for 'right' actions to themselves. On occasion, this self-justification was quickly followed by insight into the device, for example with regard to a potentially risky discharge from hospital: 'It's easier to say that the doctor should make the decision than accept that responsibility myself' and 'I am aware that I keep saying "I was unable to do" . . . while underneath I know that I'm relieved that I don't have to make that decision and I can put the responsibility and blame on someone else.'

Being responsible for morally right but unpopular actions

In a perfect world, a therapist would decide which decision or course of action was best, or most moral, and then implement it. In practice, therapists are confronted with many situations where this is not possible, for example providing mobility or independence aids when there are resource shortages. Hard decisions have to be made about who is most deserving, and the therapist has to cope with criticism or formal complaints from those who have gone without. During the interviews, the therapists were concerned to establish early on that, given the opportunity, they operated from 'right thoughts' and 'right actions'. However, all had found themselves in circumstances where they had had to either compromise these 'right actions' or become subject to unpopularity with the peer group or managers. An example of the former was where a therapist was asked to be signatory for treatment, usually electroconvulsive therapy (ECT) for a patient admitted compulsorily to hospital. If the therapist refused, usually because the patient's rejection of this treatment was known from previous admissions, the therapist could be subject to hostility from other staff who had to cope with the patient's difficult behaviour. There was also anxiety that refusing to agree to the treatment might have been the wrong decision and the patient would have recovered with it. However, there was then the anxiety that, if the therapist did agree, a patient once recovered might feel that their trust had been betrayed, and this lack of trust could negatively influence all other aspects of therapy.

Overall it appeared that, where the therapist respected the patients' wishes and believed the resulting actions were right, self-esteem was retained, but this could be at the cost of anxiety over the risks involved and loss of social support. An example of this was where elderly people, living in their own homes, were deteriorating physically or mentally and becoming a risk to themselves or others, but insisted on staying where they were. The therapist might come under pressure from neighbours, and staff in other services, to coerce or recommend that the elderly person be removed to residential care. If the therapist honoured the elderly person's wishes there was a risk that a major disaster might occur, whereas if the therapist honoured the neighbours' and colleagues' wishes, this could affect the sense of worth of both the client and the therapist.

In these difficult circumstances, therapists argued responsibility in two opposing directions. The first was doing what was right even if it led to unpopularity: 'my colleagues don't know how to size me up. They say that they can't work out how I make decisions because I don't describe it in the way they understand. It doesn't make me popular but I have learnt to live with that.' Second was compromising what was right, justified as 'if I make too many enemies amongst my colleagues they can influence what I will be able to do with other patients. I would gain the moral high ground on this occasion but the consequence could be long term.'

Inconsistency in applying professional values

A number of subjects extolled the virtue of one ethical principle at one point in the story and then justified the opposite argument later in the story. A classic example was the strongly argued case for patient/client autonomy as a general ethical principle that should be adopted when working with a patient, followed by an equally strong case for professional judgement overruling the patient's autonomy in the particular case being described. Justification for this could be that the patient was judged as 'incompetent', that the patient was not capable of giving 'informed consent' because the issues were complex and could not be fully understood, or that the patient or relatives would make requests which could not be met.

An example from occupational therapy concerned the therapist's sense of responsibility for influencing a patient's decision to 'keep her from harm' and 'I've had a lot of experience of this and have a pretty good idea of what she needs'. This particular patient had a mental health problem and wished to come off medication to see if she could manage without. Later in the interview the therapist said 'You should never say you have seen it all before as this is too risky; you should say to yourself "this is the one who may be different". Anyway you must respect this patient's wishes even if they conflict with yours.'

An example from physiotherapy concerned a patient who had a neurological condition and the therapist made a decision to override the patient's refusal of treatment on the grounds that the patient was not competent to refuse. Later in the interview she said, 'You should always respect the patient's wishes in these circumstances. He's probably had physiotherapy before and knows what he is refusing. Our professional code states clearly that the patient is entitled to refuse.'

Consideration of choices

The therapists were asked in the interview if there was any other way of thinking about the ethical dilemma they had described. From the transcripts it was apparent that participants gave little consideration to alternative approaches. This could be for a number of reasons: that therapists did not consider choices much anyway, that choices had been considered initially but by the time the story was told to the researcher the therapist was happy to support the choice selected, or that the nature of the ethical dilemma was so stressful that the therapist had 'shut down' on their usual range of problem-solving skills. There is some evidence that the level of emotion generated by an ethical dilemma reduces reflective decision making and leads to a limited range of solutions (Eraut, 1985).

Helplessness

Concerns over the wish to behave well and yet not be in conflict with others, when added to uncertainty over which actions would lead to the best outcome, led the therapists to describe a sense of help-lessness. This was raised in particular with regard to the high level of uncertainty confronting the therapist when deciding how to act to resolve an ethical dilemma. Feelings of anomie were present in a number of stories: 'I felt trapped in the events and there was nothing I could do to alter them. I'm normally quite positive and try to make the best of things but this time I felt useless.' 'You felt that the whole situation had spiralled out of control, there were so many people and levels involved. All you could do was stand on the sidelines feeling helpless.'

Other respondents expressed their anxiety through anger. This was particularly true when the events had not been resolved and dissonance was still present when the story was retold for this research. Statements about the need to find a solution and end the tension were present in most narratives. As some of the events spanned several months, these periods were remembered vividly as 'living through hell', 'didn't sleep for several nights' and 'I thought of nothing else morning, noon and night'.

In the face of the overwhelming demands therapists face when dealing with ethical dilemmas, is it reasonable to expect them to be 'virtuous'?

Discussion

A major theme emerging from the research was the expressed wish of participants to be, and to be seen to be, virtuous. This was explained in a number of ways: the need to retain personal integrity; to conform to the wishes of the professional group and wider social, legal and political groupings, and to avoid the pain of exposure for absent or wrong actions and resultant punishment, guilt and shame. Each of these reasons could be positive or negative, behaving well for the right reasons – selflessness – or for the wrong reasons – selfishness.

Gilbert (1989) described a pattern of beliefs held by people who want to be therapists. He saw them as basically desiring to co-operate with others because of the need for relationships that are central to personal meaning. This can be seen as positive where co-operation is possible but it also brings the risk of rejection and abandonment when conflict arises. Some of these fears emerged in the research described, with therapists, when faced with unresolvable dilemmas, becoming anxious about their competency or loss of respect and good relationships with colleagues. Gilbert also said that therapists were more likely to come from, or gravitate towards, moralistic religions, and that by choosing a co-operative profession they were likely to find themselves in conflict-ridden or moral-dilemma-prone settings. He went on to say that co-operative therapists might come from families that placed a high value on duty but low value on affection. This would lead them to seek work that gave opportunity for esteem and recognition and would be highly achievement oriented. These therapists would be looking for appreciation rather than dominance. This theme of the desire for recognition and appreciation of effort was found in the present research.

Kagan, in 1984, questioned the notion of virtue and said that altruism and virtue were human inventions: 'they are prepared to invent and believe in some ethical mission . . . humans want to believe there is a more or less virtuous outcome'. However, as humans do believe in virtue it cannot be ignored, and the therapists in this research had no difficulty in describing good behaviour and good outcomes. They also described a number of altruistic beliefs, such as the belief that therapists were there to help patients, that at times the patient's needs were superordinate to the therapist's and that, by behaving well, the therapist might have to accept blame for an unwelcome outcome. Gilbert (1989) wrote that therapists had a right to make provision for their own good, at the same time as doing good to, or avoiding harm to, others. Where both were possible, happiness ensued and the event was unlikely to be described as a moral dilemma. Where only one party had good done to them guilt might ensue if the therapist was the party who had benefited most; and anger and frustration would be encountered where neither party benefited, or both suffered. These latter cases were likely to be described as moral dilemmas. . . .

A number of subjects in the research referred negatively to their professional skills and personal competency when these were under threat during a dilemma. Beck (1967) referred to the 'deception of competency' where people deny their competency – 'am I good enough for this?' – or say they are no good because of a fear of being discovered as inadequate. Therapists described feelings of doubt about their professional skills when these did not lead to a 'successful' outcome: 'did I do the right thing?' 'could I have done more?' A number of the dilemmas made the participating therapists feel helpless and damaged their confidence. Tillich (1977) described this existential guilt as 'negative self-evaluation to live up to one's own potential, it is a kind of self-condemnation for lack of courage in life'. The therapists who made unpopular decisions and who carried out unpopular acts were more likely to describe anger and frustration rather than helplessness when telling the dilemma story, whereas those who went along with social pressure, the popular act, were more likely to describe feelings of helplessness when the decision ran counter to their values.

Are therapists aiming for virtue, to act honourably to the highest ethical standard for their patients in all situations, or are they aiming to attend to their own needs in the hope that both interests will be served? Ellard (1993) said that there is always a tension between the two and that health professionals have to learn to live with paradox. He quoted from Galen's *De Placitas* (quoted in Burns, 1977), in which a distinction is made between medicine and one's motives for practising it. The only obligation on the physician was to be competent, whereas motives such as glory, money or philanthropy were all acceptable. Perhaps therapists have been excessively influenced by Christianity, particularly Calvinistic ideas of moral behaviour with the threat of punishment for poor attitudes and behaviour. Such standards require constant renegotiation in the light of cultural, especially political, change in healthcare contexts. The notion that therapists wish to be virtuous and act to the highest moral good may just be a myth, widely promulgated in codes of practice because this is the 'flavour of the age'. It may be no accident that there is an increased interest in professional misconduct procedures, and standards and codes of practice, at a time when it is increasingly difficult to 'behave well' because of rapid change in technology and resources. Certainly, the therapists in this research appear to have been healthily selfish in wanting to do good, if this were possible, but also wanting to retain face and self-esteem, keep out of trouble (on the whole) and not carry guilt or shame after the event. As one participant said, 'Ten years ago I was supposed to care for my patient, now I'm supposed to be efficient and work within resource restrictions. Does this mean that I should get a new set of morals, or are the old ones still supposed to work?' . . .

Whether therapists are altruists and 'sacrifice self-interest in the services of others' (Thompson et al., 1994: 46–7), or whether therapists are 'self-centred, unprincipled and unfeeling' (Baier, 1993) has been the subject of this chapter. From the research reported, it can be seen that therapists struggle with the tension between doing good to others and doing good to themselves, and are not all the well-behaved, conformist individuals described by Joyce. A further struggle was found between the therapist and the context of the dilemmas that they faced. Therapists were not free to make independent, personally virtuous decisions, as on many occasions they had to take into account other participants' wishes, in particular those of people who were more senior in the health hierarchy and patients, relatives and carers who claim increasing rights over services. . . . The capacity to develop ethical reasoning further, in conjunction with experience, should be built on during professional development. The influence of explicit statements about values and beliefs of the profession leading to virtuous behaviour and laid down in professional codes of ethics did not appear to have much influence, as few of the therapists had read or used them.

The conclusion is drawn that therapists make claims to be virtuous, but in practice describe the same healthy selfishness of any group or individual who wants to survive in health care. Becoming the radical anarchists suggested by Joyce (1993) will have to wait until the profession has matured further.

References

Baier, K. (1993) 'Egoism', in P. Singer (ed.) *A Companion to Ethics*, Oxford: Blackwell, pp. 197–204.

Barnitt, R.E. (1996) 'An investigation of ethical dilemmas in occupational therapy and physiotherapy', unpublished PhD thesis, University of London.

Baron, J. (1988) *Thinking and Deciding*, Cambridge: Cambridge University Press.

Beck, A.T. (1967) *Depression: Clinical, Experimental and Theoretical Aspects*, New York: Harper and Row.

Broom, J.P. and Williams, J. (1996) 'Occupational stress and neurological rehabilitation', *Physiotherapy*, 82 (11): 606–14.

Burns, C.R. (ed.) (1977) *Legacies in Law and Medicine*, New York: Science History Publications.

College of Occupational Therapists (1995) *Code of Ethics and Professional Conduct for Occupational Therapists*. London: Ethics Committee, College of Occupational Therapists.

Ellard, J. (1993) 'Medical ethics – fact or fiction?' *The Medical Journal of Australia*, 158: 460–4.

Eraut, M. (1985) 'Knowledge creation and knowledge use in professional context', *Studies in Higher Education*, 10 (2): 117–33.

Gilbert, P. (1989) *Human Nature and Suffering*, Hove and London: Lawrence Erlbaum Associates.

Heater, D. (1990) *Citizenship: The Civic Ideal in World History, Politics and Education*, London: Longman.

Hill, T.E. (1974) 'Servility and self-respect', *The Monist*, 57: 1.

Joyce, I. (1993) 'Occupational therapy: a cause without a rebel', *British Journal of Occupational Therapy*, 56 (12): 447.

Kagan, J. (1984) *The Nature of the Child*, New York: Basic Books.

Kohlberg, L. (1984) *The Psychology of Moral Development*, vol. 2. San Francisco: Harper and Row.

Lafollette, H. (ed.) (1997) *Ethics in Practice: An Anthology*, Cambridge, MA: Blackwell Philosophy Anthologies.

Rest, J.R. and Narváez, D. (eds) (1994) *Moral Development in the Professions: Psychology and Applied Ethics*, Hillsdale NJ: Lawrence Erlbaum Associates.

Robinson, P. (1994) 'Objectives, ethics and etiquette', *Physiotherapy*, 80 (January): 8A–10A.

Showalter, E. (1987) *The Female Malady: Women, Madness and English Culture 1830–80*, London: Virago Press.

Thompson, J.E., Melia, K.M. and Boyd, K.M. (1994) *Nursing Ethics*, Edinburgh: Churchill Livingstone.

Tillich, P. (1977) *The Courage To Be*, London: Fountain Paperbacks.

Young, H. (1996) 'Parliamentary morality', *Guardian*, 17 February: 21.

Young, M.E. and Quinn, E. (1992) *Theories and Principles of Occupational Therapy*, Edinburgh: Churchill Livingstone.

11

S. Banks

Social Work Values

This chapter will explore the philosophical foundations of the key values that have been traditionally stated as underpinning social work, and look at the extent to which recent developments in the policy and practice of social work are influencing the values of the profession. . . .

Focus on the individual user as a person: 1960s and 1970s

In the 1960s and 1970s the literature on social work values tended to focus on issues related to the rights and interests of the individual user. The emphasis was very much on the *nature of the relationship* between the social worker and user, and in particular on how the social worker should treat the user. The kinds of principles articulated were about respecting the user as a person who had a right to make her/his own choices; not judging the user; accepting the user for what she/he is; and respecting confidentiality of information given to the social worker by the user (Biestek, 1961; CCETSW, 1976; Butrym, 1976). These kinds of principles have often been termed 'Kantian' after the eighteenth-century German philosopher, Immanuel Kant, who developed an ethical theory 'based' on the principle of 'respect for persons' (Banks, 1990). At the heart of this set of values were the notions of *individualism* and *freedom*. Both these notions are, of course, at the core of prevailing ideology of Western capitalist societies, and hence it is not surprising to find them predominant in the social work literature. What is surprising is the fact that so much of the literature on values in social work gave so much emphasis to the one-to-one social worker–user relationship, in abstraction from the agency and societal context in which it took place. Agency and societal considerations (for example, agency demands for confidential information, societal requirements for the control of 'deviants') were

First published in *Ethics and Values in Social Work* (Macmillan 1995), pp. 25–46. Abridged.

seen as constraints or limitations on the key principles of respecting the individual user's rights to choice and privacy.

Growing awareness of structural oppression: 1970s and 1980s

During the 1970s there was a growing awareness amongst social workers that treating each user as an individual, and seeing the problem faced by that user (such as poverty, homelessness, mental illness) as personal problems was, in effect, 'blaming the victims' for the structural inequalities in society. A range of literature was published advocating 'radical social work', which acknowledged social workers' role as agents of social control on behalf of an oppressive state, and called on them to raise the consciousness of the people they worked with, to encourage collective action for social change and build alliances with working class and trade union organizations (Bailey and Brake, 1975; Brake and Bailey, 1980; Corrigan and Leonard, 1978). This literature of the 1970s did not discuss issues of ethics and values *per se*. This was probably partly because a lot of this thinking was based on Marxist perspectives. Marx himself discussed morality as a 'bourgeois illusion' – part of the prevailing ideology promoted by the ruling classes to control and dominate (Marx and Engels, 1969; Lukes, 1987). Secondly, a key theme of radical social work (although not always expressed very clearly) is 'praxis' – the notion of 'committed action'. On this view it makes no sense to regard values, theory and practice as separate.

Although the radical social work literature of the 1970s and early 1980s did not itself seem to influence the literature on social work values and ethics of the same period, the broadening of the understanding of oppression created by the feminist and anti-racist movements of the 1980s has now found its way into the lists of social work values. While the contributions from feminist and anti-racist theorists are often highly critical of the Marxist-inspired radical social work (Dominelli and McLeod, 1989; Day, 1992; Ahmad, 1990; Shah, 1989; Dominelli, 1988), they can nevertheless be seen to have grown out of, and alongside, the radical social work movement of the 1970s, and the collections of articles on radical work in the 1980s have included substantial contributions from feminist and Black perspectives (Brake and Bailey, 1980; Langan and Lee, 1989). A concern for anti-oppressive practice is reflected in the list of values produced by the Council for Education and Training in Social Work (CCETSW, 1989), an extract of which is shown in Table 11.1.

Jordan (1991) points out the contradictions between the traditional or Kantian values contained in the first part of the list (which includes variations on respect for persons, user self-determination and

Table 11.1   *The values of social work*

---

1   Qualifying social workers should have a commitment to:
  - the value and dignity of individuals;
  - the right to respect, privacy and confidentiality;
  - the right of individuals and families to choose;
  - the strengths and skills embodied in local communities;
  - the right to protection of those at risk of abuse and exploitation and violence to themselves and others.
2   Qualifying social workers must be able to:
  - develop an awareness of the inter-relationship of the processes of structural oppression, race, class and gender;
  - understand and counteract the impact of stigma and discrimination on grounds of poverty, age, disability and sectarianism;
  - demonstrate an awareness of both individual and institutional racism and ways to combat both through anti-racist practice;
  - develop an understanding of gender issues and demonstrate anti-sexism in social work practice;
  - recognize the need for and seek to promote policies and practices which are non-discriminatory and anti-oppressive.

Source: CCETSW (1989)

confidentiality) and the statements about structural oppression in the second part of the list. The individual freedom which social workers have a commitment to promote is, he claims, dependent on the structural inequalities in society which they also have a duty to challenge. He argues that the liberal values on which the first set of principles is based (including property rights and traditional personal morality based on notions of freedom of choice) are amongst the strongest intellectual defences of the privileges of wealth, whiteness, and maleness upon which structural oppression is based (Jordan 1991: 8). This reasserts the point that social workers in the radical tradition had been making earlier: that the agenda of structural change conflicts with the individualist premises upon which social work is based.

While the respect-for-persons doctrine would entail that a user who was Black, for example, should be treated as an individual with rights, choices and desires, with no pre-judgements or prejudice based on irrelevant factors like skin colour, it would, in effect, be a 'colour-blind' approach. For being Black would be regarded as irrelevant, whereas the position adopted by anti-racist social workers would be to regard being Black as relevant, to see the user as a member of an oppressed group and to take this into account in the social work relationship. It is in the former colour-blind sense that many institutions, agencies and individuals may adopt and implement equal opportunities policies and claim to be 'non-racist'. the brief statements saying everyone will be treated equally 'irrespective of race, gender, religion, etc.' are good examples of this in that they do not recognize institutional or structural discrimination and therefore do not recognize the need for positive action to promote change.

The profession of social work in Britain, on paper at least, has moved beyond the colour-blind approach, and most literature and policy statements recognize institutional discrimination and express a commitment to change it. They recognize, for example, that Black people are under-represented in senior and professional posts, that social services departments are not meeting many of the needs of Black users, and that action needs to be taken to redress this imbalance. An essentially reformist position can be adopted which seeks to make changes to the law, to policies and their implementation to improve the situation. This would entail focusing not just on the individual, but on the individual's position in society and working towards greater fairness and procedural justice in the distribution of rewards and punishments – basically a utilitarian outlook. However, the recognition and challenging of structural oppression – the recognition that the very rules and structures within which society operates reflect basic inequalities in power and that therefore fundamental and revolutionary change is required – is at odds with the emphasis on individual freedom of both Kantianism and utilitarianism; it calls for a more radical analysis and approach. . . .

The influence of the ideologies of the New Right: 1980s and 1990s

Simultaneously with the growing concern with structural oppression in the 1980s, has been the growing influence of the ideologies of the New Right in legislation and policies relating to the public sector. This has been reflected in the growth in contracting out of services to the private sector; reduction in the power of professional groups and of the role of the welfare state; an emphasis on individuals' right to choose as the consumers of services; and a focus on individuals' rights and responsibilities as citizens to complain, or to care for their children or relatives. This does not seem to have changed the value statements of the profession. Perhaps this is not surprising since we have already noted that the value statements have tended to be somewhat divorced from the reality of social work practice. A more important reason is that aspects of the New Right ideology appear superficially congruent with the key principles of the profession. Individuals' rights to choose and to complain could be seen to be part of the notion of respect for persons. The rights of users to information about their case, to be able to see their social work files, to know their rights to services and how to complain if they are not satisfied all fit in with the principle of treating users as rational, self-determining agents and can serve to protect them against the exercise of excessive parentalism or illegitimate power by social workers or social work agencies.

However, the focus of the New Right ideology is not on the user as a whole person, but just one narrow part of being a person: namely in the role of 'consumer'. 'Consumer rights' are not the same as 'users' rights to self-determination', for the former are limited to the person in the role of a consumer of services, a certain type of treatment, and a certain standard of goods. What is meant, in theory at least, by users' rights to self-determination relates to users as whole people – their rights to make choices, take decisions, to develop potential in a much broader sense than that of consumer.

Calling the user a consumer also serves to hide the fact of social worker as controller. It implies an active role and the possibility to exercise choice. It covers up the role of welfare as control – what some have called the 'new authoritarianism' which is based on the notion of the user as dangerous, as a risk to be assessed, as deviant and an outsider. This is another aspect of the policies and ideologies of the new right which is obviously contrary to the traditional social work values of respect for persons – the re-emergence of the Victorian distinction between the deserving and undeserving poor; the determination to punish and control those on the margins of society, the 'outcasts' or the 'underclass'. Some of these trends are reflected in the implementation of recent legislation relating to child protection and community care. While aspects of this legislation could be regarded as progressive in the promotion of children's rights and user participation in service delivery, other aspects are about treatment and control – the user as a problem to be technically assessed, clinically managed and processed through a proceduralized system. These policies and procedures are now based much more explicitly than in the past on the utilitarian values of procedural justice and the promotion of public welfare. They have generated not only procedures for assessment of risk and need, but also a host of codes of practice laying down users' rights, agency responsibilities and procedures for making complaints or for access to records, for example. . . .

Ethical principles for social work in the 1990s

Our discussion of the social work literature on ethical principles suggests that there is not one commonly agreed and coherent set of principles for social work. However, by looking at the literature and at the actual practice of social work, I think it is possible to determine four basic or first order principles which are relevant to social work:

1 respect for and promotion of individuals' rights to self-determination;
2 promotion of welfare or well-being;

3   equality;
4   distributive justice.

None of these principles is straightforward in meaning or implications for practice.

Self-determination

This could be categorised as being:

- *negative* – allowing someone to do as he or she chooses;

or

- *positive* – creating the conditions which enable someone to become more self-determining.

Recent emphasis on user participation (allowing users to have a say) and empowerment (developing users' skills and self-confidence so they can participate more) are manifestations of negative and positive self-determination. Self-determination in both senses has been for a long time one of the fundamental principles stated for social work practice, often phrased as 'client self-determination'. Yet while the social worker may sometimes be able to focus largely on one individual user and take on the role of advocate for the user's rights, often the social worker has to take into account the rights of significant others in a situation. In the interests of justice, it may not always be morally right to promote the user's rights at the expense of those of others.

Welfare

Promoting someone's 'good' or welfare is also open to interpretation depending upon what our view is of what counts as human welfare, and whether we adopt our own view of what a person's welfare is, or the person's own conception of their welfare. It is dependent on cultural views about what are the basic human needs and what is a good quality of life. Much of modern social work is explicitly about ensuring that the best interests of particular user groups are served (for example, children in child protection work). Codes of ethics generally stress the social worker's duty to work in the user's interests. Often it is the social worker's view of what the user's interests are that is regarded as important. However, as with self-determination, whilst in some cases it may be clear-cut that it is the user's interests the social worker should be protecting, in other cases the social worker has to consider the interests of significant others and the 'public interest' (for example through preventing re-offending in work with young offenders). These various interests may conflict.

Equality

According to Spicker (1988: 125), equality means 'the removal of disadvantage'. This can be interpreted in many ways including:

equal treatment – preventing disadvantage in access to services, including treatment without prejudice or favour. For example, it should not be the case that a middle-class white man seeking resources for his elderly mother is dealt with more quickly than a Black woman seeking similar support.

equal opportunity – the removal of disadvantage in competition with others, giving people the means to achieve socially desired ends. For example, a social worker may arrange for an interpreter for a Bengali-speaking woman so that she can express her needs in detail and have the same opportunity as an English-speaking user to receive the services she requires.

equality of result – in which disadvantages are removed altogether. For example, the residential home that would provide the best quality care for two older users with similar needs is very expensive. The user with a rich son who is prepared to pay is able to go to this home; the user who is poor is not. To achieve equality of result might entail the social services department paying the full fee for the poorer user, or, to avoid stigmatization, the state providing free high-quality care for all people with similar needs.

Social workers are concerned to promote all three forms of equality, although equality of treatment is much easier to achieve than equality of opportunity or result. Equality of treatment would follow logically from the principle of respect for persons. Equality of opportunity and of result require some more positive action to redress existing disadvantages, and may require additional resources or changes in government policy. To aim for equality of result may require structural changes in society – challenging certain people's existing rights to wealth, property and power. It is this type of principle that underpins some of the more radical and anti-oppressive approaches to social work.

Distributive justice

This is about distributing goods according to certain rules and criteria. The criteria for distribution may vary, and include the following:

- according to people's already existing rights (e.g. property rights);
- according to desert;
- according to need.

Although justice and equality are linked, a concept of justice based on property rights or desert may result in inequality. Rawls's (1972) concept of justice, for example, is based on two principles: equality in the assignment of basic needs and resources; and social and economic inequalities only to the extent that there are compensating benefits for everyone, especially the least advantaged. Although distributive justice *per se* is generally not listed amongst the social work principles, it is perhaps one of the most fundamental principles in the work (insofar as it is in the public sector) in that social workers are responsible for distributing public resources (whether counselling, care or money) according to certain criteria based variously on rights, desert and need. I would argue that this principle is in operation in much social work decision-making and is becoming more central in the present climate as resource allocation becomes a more common role for social workers.

Conclusions

In this chapter we have . . . suggested that the traditional social work values tend to focus on the *content* of the social worker – user relationship. Whereas, for social work, the *context* in which it is practised, as part of a welfare bureaucracy with a social control and resource-rationing function, also places ethical duties upon the social worker which may conflict with her duties to the user as an individual. These conflicts can be seen to reflect the tensions and contradictions of the welfare state. . . .

References

Ahmad, B. (1990) *Black Perspectives in Social Work*, Birmingham: Venture Press.

Bailey, R. and Brake, M. (eds) (1975) *Radical Social Work*, London: Edward Arnold.

Banks, S. (1990) 'Doubts, dilemmas and duties: ethics and the social worker', in P. Carter et al. (eds) *Social Work and Social Welfare Yearbook, 2*, Buckingham: Open University Press.

Biestek, F. (1961) *The Casework Relationship*, London: Allen and Unwin.

Brake, M. and Bailey, R. (eds) (1980) *Radical Social Work and Practice*, London: Edward Arnold.

Butrym, Z. (1976) *The Nature of Social Work*, London: Macmillan.

CCETSW (Central Council for Education and Training in Social Work) (1976) *Values in Social Work*, London: CCETSW.

CCETSW (1989) *Requirements and Regulations for the Diploma in Social Work*, London: CCETSW, (Paper 30).

Corrigan, P. and Leonard, P. (1978) *Social Work Practice under Capitalism: A Marxist Approach*, London: Macmillan.

Day, L. (1992) 'Women and oppression: race, class and gender', in M. Langan and L. Day (eds) *Women, Oppression and Social Work*, London: Routledge. pp. 12–31.

Dominelli, L. (1988) *Anti-Racist Social Work*, Basingstoke: Macmillan.

Dominelli, L. and McLeod, E. (1989) *Feminist Social Work*, Basingstoke: Macmillan.

Jordan, B. (1991) 'Competencies and values', *Social Work Education*, 10 (1): 5–11.

Langan, M. and Lee, P. (eds) (1989) *Radical Social Work Today*, London: Unwin Hyman.

Lukes, S. (1987) *Marxism and Morality*, Oxford: Oxford University Press.

Marx, K. and Engels, F. (1969) 'Manifesto of the Community Party', in L. Feuer (ed.) *Marx and Engels: Basic Writings on Politics and Philosophy*, Glasgow: Collins/Fontana. pp. 43–82.

Rawls, J. (1972) *A Theory of Justice*, Oxford: Clarendon Press.

Shah, N. (1989) 'It's up to you sisters: black women and radical social work', in M. Langan and P. Lee (eds) *Radical Social Work Today*, London: Unwin Hyman. pp. 178–91.

Spicker, P. (1988) *Principles of Social Welfare*, London: Routledge.

12

S. Pinkney

Anti-Oppressive Theory and Practice in Social Work

Before examining the background to anti-oppressive theory and practice in social work, we need to make an early attempt to define the terms. The argument here will emphasize the way language and discourse has become central in shaping our understanding of difference. Contestation has been a central part of the construction of the terms of these debates and at times distinct and often contradictory theories of difference have emerged. It is important to capture this within this account and also acknowledge that the project remains unfinished in the late 1990s.

As a starting point we can establish that the attempt to construct anti-oppressive theory and practice in social work emerged as part of the recognition of the specificities of oppression in relation to gender, 'race', class, age, sexual orientation and disability. The focus has been on the development of an understanding of oppression itself as well as an examination of its specific manifestations and consequences in relation to the policies, procedures, legislation and practice of welfare.

I will examine where anti-oppressive practice emerged from and then consider it in a specific area of practice. Lastly I will discuss future possibilities for a renewed agenda of critical practice in social work.

Where did anti-oppressive practice emerge from?

This account mainly concerns itself with challenges which came from those groups of people who had been marginalized within the conception, planning and delivery of social services (Lewis, 1998b). They emerged from various directions, including service user groups, such as the disability movement and HIV-positive groups, the social work profession itself and from academics. Together these challenges have been described as part of the 'new social movements' which taken together constitute the social basis for new forms of trans-formative and emancipatory political and social change (Oliver, 1990; Williams, 1992). They contrasted with 'challenges from the centre' which included child abuse inquiry reports, legislation, policy and procedures. These challenges differed in that they were largely shaped by the New Right critique of social work during the 1980s and 1990s (Clarke, 1993).

It would, however, be too simplistic to see these changes as arising only from that direction, since previous Labour governments had made it clear that reform was necessary as welfare spending was too high. The shifts which took place therefore had a wider resonance across various political parties and policy-making bodies (Pinkney, 1998). It is a story about the way discourses are multi-layered, involve contestation and are dynamic rather than static. This approach makes it possible to trace the threads of the emergence of anti-oppressive practice throughout the policies, practices and theory of social work.

The challenge of social class

During the 1960s and 1970s community social work methods had been favoured. There was an emerging critique of the individualistic casework method of social work, which was viewed as flawed in its assumption that it was the individual who needed to change, rather than locating problems at the structural or societal level. 'Patch' based social work, where social workers worked from and often lived within the communities where they worked, gained popularity over this period; the idea being that social workers would develop local expertise, become involved in a range of local community organizations and work towards structural change. This body of theory and practice became known as 'radical social work'. Most of these critiques were based upon a Marxist economic and materialist analysis which viewed social class as the main vehicle for oppression (Corrigan and Leonard, 1978; Brake and Bailey, 1980) and saw the social work role as seeking to combat that oppression.

Gender and social work

Parallel to these developments, the women's movement was gathering strength and feminist perspectives exerted a powerful challenge to the oppressive organization, theories and practices of social work. Here feminist social workers drew attention to the role of patriarchal power relations within the organization of social work as well as in work with service users and drew attention to the cultural domination of 'mother blaming' within social work theory and practices. The 'dysfunctional family' and family therapy perspectives which had been the dominant discourse in social work education, training and practice, came in for specific criticism (MacLeod and Saraga, 1988).

As a result many social services departments (SSDs) incorporated feminist perspectives into their child abuse policies. The London Borough of Islington was one of a number of authorities who led the field in acknowledging feminist critiques in their practices and policy regarding sexual abuse (Boushel and Noakes, 1988), following the Cleveland inquiry (Secretary of State, 1988; Campbell, 1988). Despite subsequent criticisms and a partial retreat, it was clear that feminism had posed a considerable challenge to the way social services were conceptualized and delivered (Langan and Day, 1992; Dominelli and McLeod, 1989; Hanmer and Statham, 1988).

'Race' and social work

The development of a critique of 'race' and social work can be seen to have three distinct though often overlapping phases.

One of the most dominant racialized discourses which informed social work theory as well as practice, and which reflected views held in wider society was that of assimilation. Within this perspective the responsibility was placed upon 'black and minority ethnic people' to integrate with the majority and accept its cultural norms and values as if they were their own.

During the 1970s and 1980s 'black' perspectives and voices began to demand to be heard (Cheetham et al., 1981; Ahmed et al., 1986; Coombe and Little, 1986). The shift which took place as a result was towards multiculturalism as a perspective. This approach differed from assimilation because it accepted there would be a diversity of identities and that these should be recognized as valid and celebrated. Multiculturalism has been seen as an uneasy accommodation of competing conceptions of the relationship between 'race' and 'nation'. It was, in part, a result of the struggles to articulate a position for minority ethnic groups that was not reducible to that of 'immigrant' (Lewis, 1998a).

Multiculturalism gave way to anti-racism during the 1980s. Here the nature of power and the way racism was pervasive and served to structure discrimination against 'black' people were to the fore. Anti-racism drew attention to both individual and institutional racism. Racism awareness training was one of the more controversial ways white practitioners examined their attitudes towards racial difference (Katz, 1978). Racism was also seen to be embedded within institutions such as social services, education and the police. The approach of anti-racism was therefore two-pronged in that it sought to increase awareness of and challenge individual racism, but also to challenge racism within institutions.

Before we trace these challenges into anti-oppressive social work legislation and practice, it is important to add another more recent perspective, which presents a further challenge to the way social work is conceptualized, organized and delivered.

Essentialism and social work

Stuart Hall has consistently argued for a mode of analysis of class, 'race', ethnicity, gender and sexuality which is non-essentialist (Hall, 1988 in Morley and Chen, 1996). The arguments against essentialism are important and need to be carefully considered in relation to their usefulness to social work theory and practice. Essentialism is 'the belief that social behaviour is determined by some underlying process or "essence" which works itself out in social contexts' (Clarke and Cochrane, 1998: 28). Essentialism implies a permanency of condition or identity, which will determine people's behaviour, attitudes and thinking. Examples would include categorizing people according to 'race', disability, or sexuality. Linked with essentialism is the homogenization of groups of people, which results in a denial of diversity and difference, assuming instead that all people who are socially constructed as 'black', 'disabled' or 'homosexual', for example, share similar experiences and aspirations. The result is that a series of exclusions is established which then closes down the possibilities for representations of difference within those groups (Lewis, 1998a).

If we consider these ideas alongside the new social movements discussed above, we can see that they shed important light on the issues raised there. The 'radical social work' movement was criticized for being largely male dominated and ignoring the gender dimensions in social relations. Similarly, the feminist movement was criticized for representing a white and invariably middle-class group of women, making the experiences of 'black' and working-class women invisible. The disability movement exerted considerable pressure on the accepted and dominant orthodoxy of the medical model of disability but is itself being challenged for representing the voices of only a small, articulate minority who are constructed as 'disabled'. Older people, who make up the largest proportion of people with disabilities, are seldom represented (Hughes, 1998). From these examples it is possible to see how essentialism carries within it a series of exclusions.

Adoption placements

One clear example of how these shifts in thinking had a direct impact on social work practice and the lives, opportunities and identities of service users is the case of adoption placements, which has produced heated, polarized and at times hostile debate, expressed within the media as well as within social work and allied professions.

During the 1960s and 1970s assimilationist policies within most SSDs led to the routine adoption and fostering of black children with white families. This became known as trans-racial adoption. Small argued that the other factor which led to this policy was that the numbers of white babies placed for adoption had fallen and so black children became the 'donor' group for white childless couples (Small, in Ahmed et al., 1986). One of the arguments put forward very powerfully from anti-racist and 'black' perspectives was that this 'colour-blind' approach ignored the fact that 'black' children within the care system might have any specific needs, such as developing strategies for dealing with racism. One consequence of the shift in approach from assimilation towards multiculturalism was that social work gradually move away from trans-racial adoption and towards 'same race' placements.

Research on identity and psychological self-construct had argued that 'black' children had been damaged and confused by their placements within white families and communities. Maxime, a clinical psychologist, wrote accounts of black children who experienced difficulties in accepting themselves as black (Maxime, in Ahmed et al., 1986). Earlier arguments that there weren't enough black families coming forward to foster or adopt were countered by evidence from the first black adoption agency, New Black Families Unit, which started to tackle the issue of recruitment of black families in 1980. They demonstrated that once communities were approached and given information about the gaps in adoption and fostering the numbers of applications increased dramatically (Small et al., in Ahmed (1986).

As a result of increasing pressure from the anti-racist movement the Central Council for Education and Training in Social Work (CCETSW) carried out a formal survey of teaching on 'race', child care, child abuse and the law. As a result of the survey and its findings in particular on 'race' CCETSW published its second edition of Paper 30, *Rules and Requirements for the Diploma in Social Work* (1991). The paper contained a number of anti-racist requirements. In addition, Paper 30 obliged social work students to make links between 'race' and other forms of oppression, based on gender, disability, age, class or sexual orientation (CCETSW, 1991b). By this time some were beginning to see that anti-racism was problematic because of its limited capacity to link 'race' with other forms of oppression such as gender (Ahmed, 1991 and Mullard, 1991 in CCETSW, 1991b). These emerging critiques can be seen as an important development within anti-racism to a position which resists racism, refuses essentialism and seeks to make links between oppressed groups.

The legislative framework also changed dramatically at this time. The Children Act 1989 was introduced after two decades of fierce criticism and hostility levelled against social work in general and feminist and anti-racist perspectives in particular. Most relevant here was that the Act required that the child's 'race', religion, language and culture should be taken into account when assessing or making a placement for a child. In relation to anti-racist social work practice, Ahmad (in Macdonald, 1992) argued that this provided an important opportunity for enhancing anti-racist social work. This was interpreted widely as support for the same race placement policy, which by then was firmly established in social work theory and practice.

In the late 1980s and 1990s anti-racism came in for severe criticism from a different direction. The Conservative government and the media launched a severe attack which was to have lasting consequences for the theory and practice of social work. The potential for resistance to anti-racist perspectives in social work had been anticipated, although the extent and nature of the attack was greater than expected. Melanie Phillips, writing in the *Observer*, led a particularly strong attack on anti-racism and on CCETSW's Paper 30, claiming that '. . . the urge to stop oppression has itself become oppressive. Indeed it would hardly be an exaggeration to describe what is going on as totalitarianism' (Phillips, 1993). Within the general assault upon anti-oppressive social work, Phillips and others were critical of the 'same race' placements policy. The argument put forward was that a fixation on racial matching meant that black children waited longer to be placed when there were available white families. Part of the attack was an appeal to 'commonsense' reasoning, with those opposed to same race placements constructed as having it, whereas those in favour were viewed as dogmatic and misguided. The debates became strongly linked to those around 'political correctness'.

The immediate result of this hostility varied. CCETSW's response was to backtrack on Paper 30 and disband its Black Perspectives Committee (Dominelli, 1997). The authorities which had employed anti-racism as a strategy during the 1980s came under increasing pressure and many abandoned or retreated from their policies during the late 1980s and early 1990s. The backlash against so-called 'loony left' London boroughs and councils was evident in the media as well as from central government. Most councils maintained equal opportunities policies but abandoned other initiatives which came from the anti-racist and feminist social work movements. At best, SSDs became silent on these issues – the picture which emerged from this period was one of confusion and acrimony, with debates becoming increasingly polarized.

The 'unsettling' of the same race placement policy therefore came about as a result of pressure from several directions. As outlined above, the New Right and the media played a significant role in undermining the policy. Alongside these perspectives, however, critiques of a different kind were emerging. These 'insider' critiques questioned the essentialism implicit within the same race placement policy. These arguments need to be clearly distinguished from those arising from the New Right.

Gilroy argued that 'Anti racist orthodoxy now sees [black families] as the only effective repositories of authentic black culture . . . "same race" adoption and fostering for "minority ethnics" is presented as an unchallenged and seemingly unchallengeable benefit for all concerned' (Gilroy, quoted in Macey, 1995: 133). Macey recognized that anti-racism as a form of separatism was undoubtedly a response to racism within society, but that the result was a form of 'intellectual paralysis' which worked against critical and analytical debate (Macey, 1995). The earlier work on 'identity confusion' was also challenged on the basis that it relied on largely outdated theories of identity. Phoenix and Owen argued that:

> There is no evidence, for example, that 'race' is privileged over gender or social class as social identities and it is now common for psychological approaches to view identities as plural rather than unitary and as dynamic rather than determined by particular characteristics. The challenge posed by new theories of identities is to explain how different identities intersect with each other. (1996)

We can see that the emphasis here shifted as a result of postmodern approaches, which asserted that identities could be fluid, shifting and plural. The idea of multiple or 'hybrid' identities has been particularly important in relation to the arguments within adoption, and specifically in the application of these ideas to 'mixed-parentage' identities (Tizard and Phoenix, 1994). This involves recognition that the child's identity will be multilayered, plural and complex rather than one-dimensional and reductionist. 'Race' is viewed here alongside other factors such as class, gender, religion, health, friends, school, neighbourhood, the child's and their family's wishes and so on. 'Race' and racism is not seen as the defining feature; instead a broader, more inclusive and representative view of identity is taken.

The two arguments need to be clearly distinguished because one, the New Right argument, seeks to individualize difference, whereas the other, the anti-essentialist critique, seeks to acknowledge diversity and difference but to resist the assumptions which sometimes follow on from that acknowledgement. Fiona Williams has commented that the notion of difference is under-explained in the former analysis (Williams, 1994). The arguments by Phillips could be viewed as one example of the individualization of difference. Here the child's individual needs are prioritized and 'race' as well as other forms of difference become visible.

A 1998 local authority circular on adoption reflects some of these changes in thinking and has advised that consideration be taken of all children's needs: 'simply identifying a child's ethnic background is not sufficient in itself'. Whilst still supporting the idea that a child's needs are most likely to be met by placement with a family of 'similar ethnic origin'. The government has 'made it clear that it is unaccept-able for a child to be denied loving adoptive parents solely on the grounds that the child and the adopters do not share the same racial or cultural background' (Department of Health, 1998: 3–4). It is debatable whether this circular, introduced by New Labour, is more a reflection of continuity with earlier New Right critiques of social work generally and anti-racist perspectives in particular, rather than being an approach which embraces the anti-essentialist arguments outlined above.

Anti-oppressive theory and practice in social work have a turbulent history and have been the site of intense struggle and contestation throughout the period since the 1960s. The brief account here of the issues surrounding trans-racial adoption illustrates this as well as any other area of practice. The issue raised, however, could be equally applied to other areas of social work policy, procedures, legislation and practice.

Future directions?

Social workers may be relatively powerless and have had their powers constrained within the past decade, but in relation to most service users social workers retain power as 'gatekeepers' to resources, information and support services, as well as holding statutory powers relating to legislation such as the Children Act 1989. Social workers who maintain a commitment to anti-oppressive social work practice will always look for specific ways in which to use legislation to support positive practice on issues of equality. Macdonald (1992) has argued that the pressures social workers are subjected to make it more challenging to maintain 'good practice'.

From the discussion above it is possible to trace the threads of the arguments and important contestations from the new social and welfare movements. Together these have helped to create the possibility for a renewed critical agenda within social work, which embraces 'the politics of representation' (Hall, 1988: 43 in Morley and Chen, 1996). The argument here is that the broader vision of anti-oppressive theory and practice, which links 'social exclusion' based on gender with that of 'race', disability, age, sexual orientation and class, still has a foothold in the future of social work itself. The tension remains around how to promote positive and sensitive practice, which opposes all forms of oppression while at the same time resisting essentialism and not homogenizing the needs and aspirations of service users. This is a debate which continues to be played out in the theories, legislation, policies, procedures and practices of social work.

References

Ahmed, S., Cheetham, J. and Small, J. (1986) *Social Work with Black Children and their Families*, London: Batsford.

Boushel, M. and Noakes, S. (1988) 'Islington Social Services: Developing a policy on child sexual abuse', *Feminist Review Special Issue. Family Secrets: Child Sexual Abuse*, 28 (Spring).

Brake, M. and Bailey, R. (1980) *Radical Social Work and Practice*, London: Edward Arnold.

Campbell, B. (1988) *Unofficial Secrets. Child Sexual Abuse: The Cleveland Case*. London: Virago Press.

CCETSW (1991a) *Paper 30, Rules and Requirements for the Diploma in Social Work*, London: CCETSW.

CCETSW (1991b) *One Small Step towards Racial Justice: the Teaching of Anti-racism in the Diploma in Social Work Programmes*, London: CCETSW.

Cheetham, J., James, W., Loney, M., Mayor, B. and Prescott, W. (eds) (1981) *Social and Community Work in a Multi-Racial Society*, London: Harper and Row.

Clarke, J. (ed.) (1993) *A Crisis in Care? Challenges to Social Work*, London: Sage/Open University.

Clarke, J. and Cochrane, A. (1998) 'The social construction of social problems', in Saraga (1998).

Coombe, V. and Little, A. (1986) *Race and Social Work. A Guide to Training*, London: Tavistock.

Corrigan, P. and Leonard, P. (1978) *Social Work Practice under Capitalism: A Marxist Approach*, London: Macmillan.

Department of Health (1998) *Adoption – Achieving the Right Balance*, LAC(98)20, London: DOH.

Dominelli, L. (1997) *Sociology for Social Work*, London: Macmillan.

Dominelli, L. and McLeod, E. (1989) *Feminist Social Work*, London: Macmillan.

Hall, S. (1988) 'New ethnicities', in Morley and Chen (1996).

Hanmer, J. and Statham, D. (1988) *Women and Social Work: Towards a Woman-Centred Practice*, London: Macmillan.

Hughes, G. (1998) 'A suitable case for treatment? Constructions of disability', in Saraga (1998).

Hughes, G. and Lewis, G. (eds) (1998) *Unsettling Welfare: The Reconstruction of Social Policy*, London: Routledge.

Katz, J. (1978) *White Awareness*, Norman, OK: University of Oklahoma Press.

Langan, M. and Day, L. (eds) (1992) *Women, Oppression and Social Work*, London: Routledge.

Lewis, G. (1998) 'Welfare and the social construction of "race"', in Saraga (1998).

Lewis, G. (1998a) 'Coming apart at the seams: the crisis of the welfare state', in Hughes and Lewis (1998).

Macdonald, S. (1992) *All Equal Under the Act? A Practical Guide to the Children Act 1989 for Social Workers*, Race Equality Unit, NISW.

Macey, M. (1995) 'Towards racial justice? A re-evaluation of anti-racism', *Critical Social Policy*, 44/45 (Autumn).

MacLeod, M. and Saraga, E. (1988) 'Challenging the orthodoxy: towards a feminist theory and practice', *Feminist Review Special Issue: Family Secrets: Child Sexual Abuse*, 28 (Spring).

Maxime, J.E. 'Some psychological models of black self-concept', in Ahmed et al. (1986).

Morley, D. and Chen, K.H. (eds) (1996) *Stuart Hall: Critical Dialogues in Cultural Studies*, London and New York: Routledge.

Oliver, M. (1990) *The Politics of Disablement*, Basingstoke: Macmillan.

Phillips, M. (1993) 'Oppressive urge to stop oppression', *Observer* 1 August.

Phoenix, A. and Owen, C. (1996) 'From miscegenation to hybridity', in B. Bernstein and J. Brannen (eds) *Children, Research and Policy*, London: Taylor and Francis.

Saraga, E. (ed.) (1998) *Embodying the Social: Constructions of Difference*, London: Routledge.

Secretary of State for Social Services (1988) *Report of the Inquiry into Child Abuse in Cleveland*, Cmnd 412. London: HMSO.

Small, J. (1986) 'Trans-racial placements: conflicts and contradictions', in Ahmed et al. (1986).

Tizard, B. and Phoenix, A (1994) 'Black identity and trans-racial adoption', in I. Gaber and J. Aldridge (eds) *In the Best Interests of the Child*, London: Free Association Books.

Williams, F. (1994) 'Social relations, welfare and the post-Fordism debate', in R. Burrows and B. Loader (eds) *Towards a Post-Fordist Welfare State?* London: Routledge.

Williams, F. (1992) 'Somewhere over the rainbow: university and diversity in social policy', in N. Manning and R. Page (eds) *Social Policy Review, 1991–1992*. Canterbury: Social Policy Association.

13

L. Culley

Working with Diversity: Beyond the Factfile

Culture, health and health care

In contemporary thinking about health and illness, the link between social deprivation and ill-health is largely uncontested. A much more controversial and uncertain issue, however, concerns the role of 'culture' in explaining patterns of health and illness. This is particularly evident in discussions of ethnic differences. Culturalist explanations for health inequalities between ethnic groups have been heavily criticized in recent years (Stubbs, 1993; Ahmad, 1996), yet the discourse of 'culture' remains the dominant discourse in the construction of ideologies of the health care needs of minority ethnic groups. Cultural differences are still called upon to 'explain' ethnic differences in health status and health behaviours and gaining appropriate knowledge about 'other' cultures is still regarded as the appropriate professional response to an ethnically diverse population. This is noticeable within nursing, where one of the major responses to 'meeting the needs of minority ethnic groups' has been the development of cultural factfiles and checklists which are said to aid the process of transcultural understanding and care. There are, however, many 'troubles with culture' (Ahmad, 1996).

Ahmad (1996) sees the dominance of a 'vehement culturalism' as one of the main obstacles to achieving improved health and health care for black people in Britain. It is certainly the case that the role of culture in explaining health differences is often over-emphasized (Sheldon and Parker, 1992) and it could be argued that cultural difference is conceived of in ways which limit rather than extend professional repertoires of interaction with minority ethnic groups. This chapter presents an outline of some of the major criticisms of a 'culturalist' approach. This is discussed first in relation to explanations of differences in health status between ethnic groups and secondly in relation to the delivery of health care to minority ethnic clients. The chapter goes on to discuss the concept of cultural safety, developed in the context of nursing practice in New Zealand, and concludes with a brief discussion of some of the challenges and dilemmas which face health care practitioners in developing strategies to manage cross-cultural encounters effectively.

Explaining ethnic differences in health: the role of culture

There is convincing research evidence to indicate the significance of socio-economic status for the health of minority ethnic groups. The nationally representative morbidity survey carried out by the Policy Studies Institute (PSI) (Nazroo, 1997) has provided detailed evidence of health status which allows comparisons across ethnic groups and which controls for socio-economic status, age and gender. Using a more sophisticated indicator of socio-economic status than most previous studies, the PSI report concludes that the relatively deprived socio-economic position of ethnic minority groups compared with whites contributes significantly to their poorer health and that controlling for standard of living gave a large improvement in the health of ethnic minority groups compared with whites. This does not, however, mean that ethnicity and 'race' can be reduced to class (Nazroo, 1998). As Smaje (1996) has argued, there is no theoretical basis for the position that the ethnic patterning of health can be explained purely on the grounds of socio-economic disadvantage and that ethnicity has no value as an analytical variable.

Yet research which invokes 'culture' as an explanatory category has typically deployed a very problematic concept of culture. The dominant approach has been to conceive of culture in an essentialist manner. Culture is seen as fixed in time, place and person and is seen to map on to ethnicity in an unproblematic way. Culture is constructed as a rigid and constraining concept which is seen to mechanistically determine people's behaviours (Ahmad, 1993, 1996; Sheldon and Parker, 1992; Culley, 1997). This can lead to a politics of 'victim blaming' in which minority communities are seen as dangerous to their own health. The alleged cultural attributes of minority ethnic groups are regarded not only as 'other' but as pathological (Pearson, 1986). Minority ethnic communities may be perceived as being problematic rather than the problem being located in inflexible, ethnocentric health services (Douglas, 1995) and ill-health perceived as emanating from primarily cultural attributes rather than structural issues of poverty, social exclusion and racism. This was apparent in the attempts to 'resocialize the culturally deviant' in campaigns such as Stop Rickets and the Asian Mother and Baby Campaign of the 1970s and 1980s (Rocheson, 1988) and has to some extent resurfaced in more recent debates about consanguinity and health problems in the Pakistani community (Ahmad, 1994). Healthy behaviours, healthy 'cultural' practices and the positive, supportive and protective aspects of cultural identity are invariably ignored (Smaje, 1995a).

An approach to ethnic inequalities in health which relies on a reified and deterministic view of culture, therefore, is very problematic. It tends to ignore racism and plays down the significance of wider social relations which place some minority ethnic communities in a position of socio-economic disadvantage. It tends to treat ethnic groups as homogeneous wholes and fails to recognize the significance of differences of socio-economic status, gender and age *within* broadly defined ethnic minority and majority groups, statuses which we know are likely to be extremely relevant to health (Nazroo, 1997). It assumes a linear link between cultural beliefs and behaviour which cannot be theoretically or empirically sustained and it fails to problematize the category 'white' which is implicitly or explicitly contrasted with the category 'other'. It is difficult to sustain the notion of an undifferentiated white 'British' culture. Not only are there enduring differences between social classes and between genders within the 'white' category, but the term also renders invisible groups such as the Irish (Greenslade et al., 1997). As Bradby (1995) has argued, being discriminated against is not dependent on being a member of a minority with a dark skin. It is necessary to develop an understanding of what the term 'white' conceals and what it means to be part of the majority ethnicity.

The oversimplistic concept of culture so characteristic of health research has been contrasted with a view of culture as a complex and dynamic *process* and ethnicity as one fluid and shifting aspect of identity (Hall, 1992; Rattansi, 1992; Nagel, 1994). Ethnicity cannot be treated as a fixed property of individuals, shaping behaviour in a deterministic way. 'We are all ethnic, yet our ethnicity does not define us. We all need our ethnic identity to be respected, yet we cannot be adequately understood solely in terms of our ethnicity' (Gerrish et al., 1996: 19). Ethnicity is situational, which means that it becomes relevant in particular contexts in particular ways (Wallman, 1986). Ethnic identity is overlaid with gender, age, socio-economic and professional identities, each of which may be more or less significant in any specific context, at any specific moment. Culture is constantly changing and evolving. As Ahmad (1996) has argued, 'Cultural norms themselves contested and changing, represent flexible guidelines within which behaviour is negotiated rather than an "independent variable" which is solely responsible for determining behaviour' (Ahmad, 1996: 215). As we shall see later, a failure to understand culture as a complex and dynamic process has led, in the nursing context, to an approach which may limit professional practice rather than liberate it from ethnocentricity.

While the traditional culturalist approach has many drawbacks, it is equally problematic to assume that culture has no role to play in explaining the ethnic patterning of health (Kelleher, 1996). Several more recent critics of culturalist approaches are also critical of crude anti-racist stances which often ignore cultural identities and resources, defining ethnic minority groups as the products of the racisms they experience and overlooking the small-scale developments and improvements which have taken place (Stubbs, 1993; Rattansi, 1992). As Smaje (1996) has argued, there is little to be gained from counterposing material and cultural explanations. We require analyses which build upon a more complex and dynamic concept of culture and its interaction with material factors and with racism. However, despite the recognition of the need for approaches which emphasize the importance of group affiliation and culture while acknowledging the contingent and contextual nature of ethnicity there has been very little empirical work of this kind undertaken to date (Nazroo, 1998).

Health professionals and minority ethnic users: cultural sensitivity and cultural factfiles

There is a growing body of research which suggests that health services are not adequately meeting the needs of minority ethnic groups (Smaje, 1995b). There is evidence of inaccessibility of maternity services (Phoenix, 1990); structural barriers to services for black elders (Cameron et al., 1989), black disabled people (Stuart, 1996), and those requiring palliative care (Hill and Penso, 1995); lack of provision of services for those who have sickle-cell and thalassemia (Anionwu, 1993); inadequacy of interpreting services (Gerrish et al., 1996) and misdiagnosis and differential treatment regimes in psychiatry (Fernando, 1991). In addition to structural barriers, health and social care professionals have been criticized for portraying negative attitudes and hostility to clients from minority ethnic groups across a range of provision. Despite some progress, some health professionals are failing to respond effectively and appropriately to clients from minority ethnic groups (Thomas and Dines, 1994; Rudat, 1994; Gerrish et al., 1996). Problems have been identified in GP services (Ahmad et al.,1991); community nursing services (Hek, 1991); maternity services (Bowler, 1993); mental health care (Fernando, 1995); health promotion (Douglas, 1995) and in a range of social services provision (Ahmad and Atkin, 1996).

Within nursing, midwifery and health care more generally, a lack of 'cultural' knowledge on the part of health professionals and the resultant cultural insensitivity of care is seen by many to be the major problem facing minority ethnic groups in the provision of health care. This construction of the problem is clearly signalled in the 'transcultural nursing' project initiated in the US by Madeleine

Leininger. According to Leininger, nurses need to provide 'culturally congruent care' (Leininger, 1978). Transcultural nursing, derived from cultural anthropology, develops cultural snapshots or databases of major 'cultures' and subcultures for nurses to draw upon in their encounter with patients. This approach has been dominant in nursing in particular (Baxter, 1997). Nurses see *themselves* as lacking 'cultural' knowledge, rendering them unable to communicate effectively with users (Murphy and Macleod Clark, 1993). Transcultural nursing theory is not without its critics, many of whom challenge its theoretical integrity and criticize its potentially negative impact when applied to nursing care (Bruni, 1988; Mulholland, 1995; Culley, 1996). One aspect of the latter can be seen in the difficulties which have been identified with the 'factfiles' approach to transcultural care.

The use of professional support resources such as ethnic or cultural 'factfiles' has become the health care strategy most commonly proposed as a means of overcoming the problem of cultural insensitivity. Minority groups are categorized according to religious or 'cultural' beliefs and practices – language, dietary norms, naming systems, personal hygiene norms, rituals surrounding birth and death and so on (Henley, 1987; Qureshi, 1989; Bal and Bal, 1995; Karmi, 1992).

The overall aim of such resources to assist practitioners to provide culturally sensitive care is a positive one, but in practice their use can be highly problematic. Although not wishing to dismiss the value of factfiles altogether, Gunaratnam (1997) provides an excellent critique of the effects of such resources on nursing practice. She is critical of the essentialism and reductionism of the concepts of culture and identity which are embedded in such resources. Not only do they portray one-dimensional snapshots of cultural practices, frozen in time and context, they suggest that it is possible to relate ethnic identities in a linear way to health care needs and behaviours. Gunaratnam argues that packaging cultural practices in this way can lead to the manufacturing of 'mythical stabilities' and turn the addressing of need into a 'task', rather than a process issue.

The resort to a factfile approach can lead practitioners to bypass the need to engage with the subjective experience and personal choice of users. She argues that a preoccupation with cultural identity can serve to limit professional intervention and make it more difficult for professionals to support the choices of individual users. Factfiles not only position ethnic minority users as 'exotic' and as 'Other'; the differentiations they construct actively work *against* developing the empathetic alignment which is often a key starting point for professional support. Factfiles, she argues,

> translate cultural and religious practices into a series of visible and objectified 'needs' which can be met through practical measures such as the provision of Kosher food for Jewish users or through the availability of the

Koran for Muslims. Multi-cultural practice can then be condensed into highly practical, task-based competencies which by-pass the need for professionals to engage with subjective experience and personal choice. Yet, by portraying cultural and religious needs as rigid and non-negotiable, factfiles can also threateningly concretise the possibilities of professionals 'getting it wrong'. So rather than allaying fears, reified information can paradoxically serve to heighten professional anxieties while also channelling practice into 'safe' and unimaginative areas. (Gunaratnam, 1997: 173)

Gunaratnam's critique is derived from extensive fieldwork in palliative care, where she observed the dilemmas created for staff when individuals make demands and choices which contradict the alleged cultural prescriptions and stereotypes.

A further major criticism of factfiles and their effects on practice concerns what they are silent about. Personal and institutional racism, relationships of power and wider organizational and political barriers to meeting the needs of minority ethnic users are ignored. This is not simply an academic issue which has no bearing on practice. As Gunaratnam argues, 'the distance between the "safe" and manageable multi-cultural territory of factfiles, and the reality of power-based and emotionally charged multi-culturalism in practice, can leave professionals stranded without guidance or reference points' (1997: 181). Gunaratnam observed instances of professional anxiety and fears about managing interpersonal issues – fear of confronting their own racism, fear of confronting racism in others, fear of being identified as racist, fear of confronting the anger of minority ethnic people. Factfiles and cultural knowledge can reduce the levels of professional threat, but they only scratch the surface of professional anxieties.

Gerrish et al. (1996: 20) agree with this general critique of cultural factfiles. 'There are very few "simple rules of thumb", basic Health Service Lonely Planet Guides to minority ethnic communities, which will furnish an adequate basis for meeting the individual needs of particular clients. The practitioner as tourist is not an attractive model for caring in a multi-ethnic context.' What then is the alternative? Recognizing, respecting and responding to the cultural needs of users is central to effective health care. This has been repeatedly expressed by minority ethnic users (Torkington, 1991; Atkin and Rollings, 1993; Rudat, 1994; Gerrish et al., 1996).

Cultural safety and nursing practice

The idea of cultural safety has emerged in New Zealand as an approach which overcomes some of the limitations of earlier approaches and has been contrasted quite explicitly with the 'transcultural' approach of Leininger (Cooney, 1994; Coup, 1996). Kawa Whakaruruhau or cultural safety, began with a challenge from Maori nurses and users. The starting point of cultural safety is that the health of indigenous people can be placed at risk by unaware nursing and midwifery practice (Ramsden, 1992). Consumers must feel safe in the nursing care they receive and their views must be seen as legitimate rather than lesser knowledge. But, proponents argue, cultural safety goes beyond the appearance of relationships in clinical contexts. Cultural safety demands that the taken for granted character of health care interactions be unveiled and the power dynamics within them be recognized (Kearns, 1997). There has been an insistence that it must include an analysis of the historical power relations within health care and the positioning of Maoris within processes of historical and social change which have subordinated their culture and materially disadvantaged them as a people. Cultural safety is about life *chances* (access to health services, education, housing) rather than *lifestyles* (Dyck and Kearns, 1995).

While factfiles have been politically uncontentious in the UK, cultural safety in New Zealand has been a very controversial issue. This must be seen in the unique context of racial politics in New Zealand, but there are many parallels with the challenge to anti-racism in social work education and practice in the UK (Pinkey, 1998; this volume). In 1992 the Nursing Council of New Zealand made cultural safety a requirement of registration for all nurses and midwives and the curriculum and state examination was changed to include a cultural safety component. Public debate in the media located these moves in terms of 'political correctness' and 'social engineering' and a select committee of the New Zealand Parliament commenced an inquiry into cultural safety and nursing education in 1995. Papps and Ramsden (1996) argue that to some extent 'cultural safety' became a political scapegoat for some of the problems brought about by radical changes in the health system not dissimilar to the post-1991 reforms in the UK. But cultural safety has survived and indeed the Nursing Council has extended its application to encompass other forms of exclusionary behaviour such as ageism, sexism and homophobia (Nursing Council of New Zealand, 1996).

While cultural safety represents a considerable advance in recognizing the wider context of nursing practice neglected in Leininger's transculturalism, it is not without its critics. There are those who argue that despite an insistence on the importance of the wider socio-political dimension, advocates of cultural safety are still concerned primarily with changing individual attitudes. The concept does not directly address issues such as institutional racism (Polaschek, 1998) and it therefore implies that 'attitudinal changes by nurses will, of themselves, positively alter the health care situation' (Polaschek, 1998: 454), a position not unlike the rationalist stance of multiculturalism (Culley, 1996). Polaschek (1998: 454) argues that effective change on a large scale cannot follow from purely personal changes in outlook. This needs to be 'complemented by attention to collective issues such as general nursing policies, the nursing settings in which care is provided, and the broader health care structures of which nursing is a part'.

Working with diversity: responding to difference

Gerrish et al. (1996) have made an important contribution to the debate about what is required of health professionals in working with ethnic diversity. The authors argue that cross-cultural nursing and midwifery contacts often are stressful experiences which constitute a challenge for both the carer and the client. Health professionals must work at overcoming such difficulties since racist strategies of retreat from or rejection of this challenge are ethically unacceptable. They argue that we must work towards developing strategies to manage cross-cultural encounters efficiently. Drawing on the work of Kim (1992) the authors suggest that there may be generic communicative skills which can be learned and which prepare individuals to be optimally flexible and adept at meeting the challenge of intercultural interactions, regardless of the specific cultures involved in the exchange. These skills are defined as 'intercultural communicative competence'. Adaptability (cognitive, affective and behavioural) is at the heart of this competence.

> It involves the acquisition of a cognitive style and an attitudinal stance towards 'the stranger' which prevents the practitioners from artificially and hastily reducing the ambiguity present in the encounter. It enables the practitioner to work with that ambiguity through an open and empathetic negotiation of the client's identity and needs. This competence must surely exist as a necessary range of abilities characteristic of any practitioner who claims to offer holistic care. (Gerrish et al., 1996: 29)

In addition, however, there is also the requirement for practitioners (from both minority and majority ethnic backgrounds) to familiarize themselves with the specific implications for practice of the client's ethnic identity.

The professional thus requires a repertoire of knowledge of cultural practices to draw upon (cultural communicative competence) and a repertoire of generic behavioural skills of intercultural communicative competence which together form what Gerrish et al. call 'transcultural communicative competence' (Gerrish et al., 1996). One could add here that an understanding of the complexity of ethnicity as structure and identity and an understanding of the historical positioning of minority ethnic communities in British society is also a crucial body of knowledge to contextualize the professional–user encounter (Culley, 1997). It is important that health professionals can situate users *and themselves* in the context of an ethnically diverse society in which minority ethnic communities have been marginalized and in which a variety of racisms operate.

Although most of the literature on transcultural nursing tends to assume the delivery of health care by 'white' professionals to minority groups, it is important to remember that around 8 per cent of nurses in the NHS are themselves from minority ethnic backgrounds. A recent survey of minority ethnic nurses found that racial abuse from patients and their families is commonplace. More than one third of respondents also said that they had been racially harassed by work colleagues (Beishon et al., 1995).

Whilst advocating the development of transcultural communicative competence, it is also important to recognize the challenges to which this inevitably gives rise. The complex and shifting character of ethnic identities presents the professional with a dilemma. Practitioners must avoid stereotypes, but must have sufficient prior knowledge to know what *might* be relevant to the caring encounter. The danger of stereotyping is real, yet professionals require the knowledge base to anticipate which particular beliefs, cultural prescriptions etc. *may* have relevance. Lack of such knowledge can not only lead to personal distress and offence but may have serious consequences for treatment.

As Gunaratnam (1997) has argued, professionals must be enabled to see that practice is not always harmonious and unproblematic. Providing intercultural care is complex and practitioners should not be compelled to see the issue in binary terms as 'getting it right' or 'getting it wrong'. Ambiguity should be recognized as a fundamental characteristic of intercultural work since changing experiences of ethnicity means that there are no certainties of practice – any such certainties may exist only temporarily and only in relation to a limited range of experiences.

In attempting to respond to difference in this way, individual practitioners need appropriate institutional support. Managers need to initiate and/or support the efforts of all health workers to practise effectively and policies must be in place to support minority ethnic staff who may face racist abuse. Those responsible for professional education and training need to review a curriculum which is currently failing to equip practitioners to provide appropriate care (Gerrish et al., 1996).

Conclusion

This chapter has examined some of the issues in the debate surrounding culture, health and health care. It has criticized the traditional culturalist approach to explaining ethnic patterns of health and the 'factfiles' approach to cultural sensitivity in health care delivery. Improvement in the relatively poor health status of some ethnic minority groups is very much dependent on wider challenges to social and economic deprivation and racist exclusions. In addition, health care itself is not just about the individual responsibilities of nurses but about health policy and the priorities invested in this. Nevertheless there *are* important issues which need to be addressed concerning the practice of health care professionals.

The ideas embedded in the movement for cultural safety and the concept of transcultural communicative competence have been introduced as alternative strategies to take health care practice forward. However, whilst stressing the importance of competent individual practice and institutional support for this, it is also necessary to make the point that transculturally competent practitioners are an essential but not a sufficient precondition of a more equitable health care system. As Gerrish et al. argue, the temptation to scapegoat health professionals must be avoided.

> Ensuring an effective and sensitive mode of interpersonal communication in practitioner–client interaction is rewarding for both participants; as well as being a professional necessity in ensuring good nursing and midwifery care. But it cannot be the practitioners alone who must demonstrate creative adaptability; the health care system must show an ability to respond flexibly to the health care needs of minority ethnic service users. (1996: 32)

References

Ahmad, W. (1993) 'Making black people sick: "race", ideology and health research', in W. Ahmad (ed.) *'Race' and Health in Contemporary Britain*, Open University Press: Buckingham.

Ahmad, W. (1994) 'Reflections on the consanguinity and birth outcome debate', *Journal of Public Health Medicine*, 16 (4): 423–8.

Ahmad, W. (1996) 'The trouble with culture', in D. Kelleher and S. Hillier (eds) *Researching Cultural Differences in Health*, Routledge: London.

Ahmad, W. and Atkin, K. (eds) (1996) *'Race' and Community Care*, Open University Press: Buckingham.

Ahmad, W., Baker, M. and Kernohan, E. (1991) 'General practitioners' perceptions of Asian and non-Asian patients', *Family Practice*, 8 (1): 52–6.

Anionwu, E. (1993) 'Sickle cell and thalassaemia: community experiences and official response', in W. Ahmad (ed.) *'Race' and Health in Contemporary Britain*, Open University Press: Buckingham.

Atkin, K. and Rollings, J. (1993) *Community Care in a Multi-Racial Britain: A Critical Review*, HMSO: London.

Bal, P. and Bal, G. (1995) *Health Care Needs of a Multi-Racial Society: A Practical Guide for Health Professionals*, Hawkar Publications: London.

Baxter, C. (1997) *Race Equality in Health Care and Education*, Harcourt Brace: London.

Beishon, S., Virdee, S. and Hagell, A. (1995) *Nursing in a Multi-Ethnic NHS*, Policy Studies Institute: London.

Bowler, I. (1993) '"They're not the same as us": midwives' stereotypes of South Asian descent maternity patients', *Sociology of Health and Illness*, 15 (2): 157–78.

Bradby, H. (1995) 'Ethnicity: not a black and white issue. A research note', *Sociology of Health and Illness*, 17 (3).

Bruni, N. (1988) 'A critical analysis of transcultural theory', *Australian Journal of Advanced Nursing*, 5(3): 26–32.

Cameron, E., Badger, F. and Evers, H. (1989) 'District nursing, the disabled and the elderly: who are the black patients?' *Journal of Advanced Nursing*, 14: 376–82.

Cooney, C. (1994) 'A comparative analysis of transcultural nursing and cultural safety', *Nursing Praxis*, 9 (1): 6–12.

Coup, A. (1996) 'Cultural safety and culturally congruent care. A comparative analysis of Irihapeti Ramsden's and Madeleine Leininger's educational projects for practice', *Nursing Praxis in New Zealand*, 11 (1).

Culley, L.A. (1996) 'A critique of multiculturalism in health care: the challenge for nurse education', *Journal of Advanced Nursing*, 23: 564–70.

Culley, L.A. (1997) 'Ethnicity, health and sociology in the nursing curriculum', *Social Sciences in Health*, 3 (1): 28–40.

Douglas, J. (1995) 'Developing anti-racist health promotion strategies', in R. Bunton, S. Nettleton and R. Burrows (eds) *The Sociology of Health Promotion*, Routledge: London. pp. 70–7.

Dyck, I. and Kearns, R. (1995) 'Transforming the relations of research: towards culturally safe geographies of health and healing', *Health and Place*, 1 (3): 137–47.

Fernando, S. (1991) *Mental Health, Race and Culture*, Macmillan: Basingstoke.

Fernando, S. (ed.) (1995) *Mental Health in a Multi-Ethnic Society*, Routledge: London.

Gerrish, K., Husband, C. and Mackenzie, J. (1996) *Nursing for a Multi-Ethnic Society*, Open University Press: Buckingham.

Greenslade, L., Madden, M. and Pearson, M. (1997) 'From visible to invisible: the "problem" of health of Irish people in Britain' in L. Marks and M. Worboys (eds) *Migrants, Minorities and Health*, Routledge: London.

Gunaratnam, Y. (1997) 'Culture is not enough: a critique of multi-culturalism in palliative care', in D. Field, J. Hockey and N. Small (eds) *Death, Gender and Ethnicity*, Routledge: London.

Hall, S. (1992) 'The new ethnicities', in J. Donald and A. Rattansi (eds) *'Race', Culture and Difference*, Sage: London.

Hek, G. (1991) 'Contact with Asian elders', *Journal of District Nursing*, December: 13–15.

Henley, A. (1987) *Caring in a Multiracial Society*, Bloomsbury Health Authority: London.

Hill, D. and Penso, D. (1995) *Opening Doors: Improving Access to Hospice and Specialist Palliative Care Services by Members of the Black and Ethnic Minority Communities*, National Council for Hospice and Specialist Palliative Care Services: London.

Karmi, G. (1992) *The Ethnic Factfile*, The Health and Ethnicity Programme, North East and North West Thames Regional Health Authorities: London.

Kearns, A. (1997) 'A place for cultural safety beyond nursing education?' *New Zealand Medical Journal*, 119 (1037), 14 February: 23–4.

Kelleher, D. (1996) 'A defence of the use of the terms "ethnicity" and "culture"', in D. Kelleher and S. Hillier (eds) *Researching Cultural Differences in Health*, Routledge: London. pp. 69–90.

Kim, Y. (1992) 'Intercultural communication competence: a systems-theoretic view', in W.B. Gudykunst and Y.Y. Kim (eds) *Readings on Communication with Strangers*, McGraw-Hill: New York.

Leininger, M. (1978) *Transcultural Nursing: Concepts, Theories and Practice*, John Wiley: New York.

142   *Connecting*

Mulholland, J. (1995) 'Nursing, humanism and transcultural theory: the "bracketing out" of reality', *Journal of Advanced Nursing*, 22: 442–9.

Murphy, K. and Macleod Clark, J. (1993) 'Nurses' experiences of caring for ethnic minority clients', *Journal of Advanced Nursing*, 18: 442–50.

Nagel, J. (1994) 'Constructing ethnicity: creating and recreating ethnic identity and culture', *Social Problems*, 41 (1): 152–76.

Nazroo, J.Y. (1997) *The Health of Britain's Ethnic Minorities*, Policy Studies Institute: London.

Nazroo, J.Y. (1998) 'Genetic, cultural or socio-economic vulnerability? Explaining ethnic inequalities in health', *Sociology of Health and Illness*, 20 (5): 710–30.

Nursing Council of New Zealand (1996) *Draft Guidelines for the Cultural Safety Component in Nursing and Midwifery*, Nursing Council of New Zealand: Wellington.

Papps, E. and Ramsden, I. (1996) 'Cultural safety in nursing: the New Zealand experience', *International Journal for Quality in Health Care*, 8 (5): 491–7.

Pearson, M. (1986) 'The politics of ethnic minority health studies', in R. Rathwell and D. Phillips (eds) *Health, Race and Ethnicity*, Croom Helm: London. pp. 100–16.

Phoenix, A. (1990) 'Black women and the maternity services', in J. Garcia, R. Kilpatrick and M. Richards (eds) *The Politics of Maternity Care*, Clarendon Press: Oxford.

Pinkey, S. (1998) 'The reshaping of social work and social care', in G. Hughes and G. Lewis (eds) *Unsettling Welfare: The Reconstruction of Social Policy*, Routledge: London.

Polaschek, N. (1998) 'Cultural safety: a new concept in nursing people of different ethnicities', *Journal of Advanced Nursing*, 27: 452–7.

Qureshi, B. (1989) *Transcultural Medicine*, Kluwer Academic Publishers: Dordrecht.

Ramsden, I. (1992) *Kawa Whakaruruhau: Guidelines for Nursing and Midwifery Education*, Nursing Council of New Zealand: Wellington.

Rattansi, A. (1992) 'Changing the subject? Racism, culture and education', in J. Donald and A. Rattansi (eds) *'Race', Culture and Difference*, Sage: London. pp. 11–48.

Rocheson, Y. (1988) 'The Asian mother and baby campaign: the construction of ethnic minorities' health needs', *Critical Social Policy*, 22 (4): 4–23.

Rudat, K. (1994) *Black and Ethnic Minority Groups in England: Health and Lifestyles*. Health Education Authority: London.

Sheldon, T. and Parker, H. (1992) '"Race" and ethnicity in health research', *Journal of Public Health Medicine*, 4 (2): 104–10.

Smaje, C. (1995a) 'Ethnic residential concentration and health: evidence for a positive effect?' *Policy and Politics*, 23 (3): 251–69.

Smaje, C. (1995b) *Health, 'Race' and Ethnicity: Making Sense of the Evidence*, King's Fund Institute: London.

Smaje, C. (1996) 'The ethnic patterning of health: new directions for theory and research', *Sociology of Health and Illness*, 18 (2): 139–71.

Stuart, O. (1996) '"Yes, we mean black disabled people too": thoughts on community care and disabled people from black and minority ethnic communities', in W. Ahmad and K. Atkin (eds) *'Race' and Community Care*, Open University Press: Buckingham. pp. 89–104.

Stubbs, P. (1993) '"Ethnically sensitive" or "anti-racist"? Models for health research and service delivery', in W. Ahmad (ed.) *'Race' and Health in Contemporary Britain*, Open University Press: Buckingham. pp. 34–47.

Thomas, V. and Dines, A. (1994) 'The health needs of ethnic minority groups: are nurses and individuals playing their part?' *Journal of Advanced Nursing*, 20: 802–8.

Torkington, P. (1991) *Black Health: A Political Issue*, Catholic Association for Racial Justice: London.

Wallman, S. (1986) 'Ethnicity and the boundary process in context', in J. Rex and D. Mason (eds) *Theories of Race and Ethnic Relations*, Cambridge University Press: Cambridge. pp. 226–45.

PART III

COLLABORATING: SHIFTING BOUNDARIES, CHANGING PRACTICE

Collaboration, co-ordination, partnership, teamwork. These are today's buzz words as policy makers, practitioners and consumer groups all call for a greater commitment to integrated care. This is not straightforward. Collaboration involves letting go of traditional professional boundaries, and listening to, and learning from, others – be they colleagues or service users. It involves dealing with conflict, seeking new ways of working – ways that deliberately empower others. At an organizational level, too, there are challenges. New mechanisms for joint decision making which reflect an anti-oppressive approach are needed.

These themes are explored in the opening piece of this part. Collaboration, argue Suzy Braye and Michael Preston-Shoot, involves working creatively across difference and a willingness to cede power to others, not just to share control. A genuine commitment to empower others will unlock benefits for workers, users and carers alike.

The next two chapters focus explicitly on teamwork. In the context of exhortations to work in teams, they draw attention to less positive aspects of teamwork, noting that operating in a team can be challenging and difficult. Idealistic assumptions about the team as a source of untrammelled, unqualified support can be contradicted by practice. Linda Finlay summarizes the findings of a qualitative research study which aimed to explore how professionals – in this case occupational therapists – experience working in multidisciplinary teams. The team emerges as an important source of identity and a place of refuge wherein therapists can heal, recover and develop away from everyday strains and stresses. But the team can involve destructive, defensive dynamics as individuals clash in their values, struggle to defend role boundaries and jostle for recognition. Researching perceptions of teamwork across a range of practitioners, Cheryl Cott argues that staff in different structural positions understand teamwork in very different ways. Nursing staff in the front line of care seem to see the team in more hierarchical terms, whilst higher-status professionals report more collaborative relationships. If lower-status staff see things this way, it can make them more difficult to control – a point which carries powerful implications as teams continue to diversify and 'cheaper'; subordinate staff are drafted in.

Accepting that problems and tensions arise in teams, what can be done? Kim Dent-Brown offers a thought-provoking account of how a psychotherapeutic approach can be used to examine the relationships between patients, treatment teams and their wider social context. Using the case example of a conflicted team who are 'split' over the treatment of a suicidal patient, he has a particularly interesting way of thinking about the dynamics of what may be occurring and why. He explains how the patient's experience of his own parents as being inconsistent, controlling and rejecting was mirrored in his relationships with the treatment team and reproduced in the team's response to their trust. Examining such patterns can reveal ways relationships in the present sometimes replicate those from the past. The first step towards avoiding such destructive games, Dent-Brown argues, is to see these patterns for what they are.

The final two chapters focus on collaborative relationships between practitioners and service users considering matters of organization structure and design. Mark Priestley argues that appropriate quality assurance systems must be designed with the full participation of service users. Too often, he believes, the design of quality assurance systems can seem to be a technical matter, something to be left to the experts, a set of requirements imposed from on high and of little relevance to day to day practice. Taking the case of disability, and working from a social model of disablement, he underlines the link between quality of service and quality of life and argues for more attention to the values that lie behind service delivery and more work to define user-relevant performance measures.

Agreeing that service users need to be actively involved in determining quality, Peter Beresford and his colleagues argue that schemes for user involvement have often become too bureaucratized and distanced from users' day to day experience of services. A number of obstacles are in play, among them basic communications difficulties arising from unequal roles, relationships and competing values (for instance between medical and social models of disability). The authors suggest that the active participation of service users is both a *route to*, and a *measure for*, quality. Participation and collaboration as an approach, in contrast to business or professional models, values personal autonomy and respect for individual choice.

All the pieces in this part, in their different ways, offer a similar message. Collaboration is an attitude, a way of being. Genuine collaboration involves a relationship between equals –one where others are respected and valued. Quality and equality should go hand in hand. In the context of exhortations to collaborate, we need to find ways of working across our differences to translate the rhetoric into action.

14

S. Braye and M. Preston-Shoot

Keys to Collaboration

. . . As the obstacles to collaboration occur both in relation to specific pieces of work and at the structural level of agency organization, so too must tools for managing the interprofessional system embrace both individual situations and arrangements for co-ordinating service programmes, professional networks involving several providers from one agency and those where different agencies are involved. These tools for action must be underpinned by eight keys to collaboration, to unlocking the potential benefits for workers, users and carers of interprofessional and inter-agency cooperation.

The first key is *vision*. This is not an apostolic calling to teamwork but an analytic stance of curiosity and questioning. Variously described as being multi-minded (Grimwood and Popplestone, 1993), adopting a wide angle (individuals in context) rather than telephoto (individual focus) or zoom (either individual or community) lens (Smale et al., 1993), or meta-perspective (Selvini Palazzoli et al., 1978), essentially it involves moving around the professional system from the perspective of those involved rather than maintaining one fixed perspective on problem definition and problem solving. It implies standing back to monitor processes and evaluate the work of the whole professional system, including oneself and one's own agency. The purpose is to reflect on how parties see and may be seen by the system in which they are working, and to understand the complex dynamics in which they might have become enmeshed. This can open up creative dialogue and possibilities, such as when agencies conduct a 'public perception' audit to consider policies and their delivery from the public's viewpoint (Mawhinney, 1993).

The second key is *power*. The imbalance of power between, say, purchasers and providers, social workers and domiciliary care workers, doctors and nurses, centred on images and perceptions of status, knowledge and training, and dimensions of race, gender and class between the individuals involved, all create unbalanced contributions, especially where these images and perceptions are internalized

First published in *Empowering Practice in Social Care* (Open University Press, 1995), pp. 154–61. Abridged.

by those occupying 'less powerful' positions and, in the form of internalized oppression, become beliefs about the hopelessness of speaking out and about inability to contribute anything of value. It is important to emphasize the centrality of power to questions of partnership and anti-oppressive practice, and the importance therefore of an open dialogue about power based on worker and agency recognition of power structures, worker and user perceptions of it, and how it may be used non-oppressively and anti-oppressively. Here the concern additionally is to effect change in and between organizations. For this workers and users must know where power is located and how to gain access to it. Thus, the questioning advocated as part of the first key to collaboration must include a focus on power and the extent to which the professional system is using its power, in the form of legal mandates, policy authority, resources and skills, for empowerment, for challenging oppression and for developing services *with*, not *for*, users. Decisions about provision must not be so rigid as to deny the power to develop services as needs evolve or become more clearly understood. . . .

Thus, if one collaborative endeavour is to manage power in a manner which empowers colleagues and users alike, another is to manage the transfer of power to alter power differentials. This requires a willingness to cede, not just to share control. It also requires an ability to assist users to identify, value and use their power and authority.

The third key is *the introduction of difference*. . . .

The recognition that welfare agencies can become part of the problem suggests that it is important to intervene in the professional system if the change effort with users or carers is not to be undermined (Dungworth and Reimers, 1984). This involves asking what makes it difficult for workers to abandon established ways of thinking and working, and to look anew at what services would meet users' needs. It involves keeping systems creative by introducing difference, and by creating channels for detoured conflict to be communicated and dealt with between those parts of the system where it properly resides. This commitment to 'something different' is necessary at personal, organizational and practice levels. At a personal level it is a process of unlearning and relearning, a critical scrutiny of value assumptions as a necessary foundation for considering the constructions which are placed on older age, health and (dis)ability and, therefore, the parameters which are built around social care. This 'pulling back' connects with the first key, stepping outside one's own position and viewing values, understandings and interactions between people from different perspectives.

At an organizational level it revolves around a dialogue about power, and particularly about the extent to which expert power can and should give way to learning with and facilitating users. The spotlight will be on oppressive systems, on the norms which agencies have represented. The objective will be using legislative mandates, underpinned by clear values, to inform and drive the work with and for users, rather than imposing these upon them. How do organizations perceive service users, their rights, needs and wants? What norms do standardized services express? What services would reflect an anti-oppressive approach?

At a practice level it involves promoting collective action by users, maximizing user control of processes of assessment and decision-making, and advocating clear rights for users within social care, such as resources to promote autonomy where competency is established and to promote safety for incremental risk-taking in less well-established areas, and resources to secure services which address needs as defined *by* users and which legitimize work on changing social attitudes and arrangements which restrict people's participation in society. Here the focus links with the fifth key, an emphasis on *structured* as well as personal change.

The fourth key is *creating a holding environment*. Empowering staff in the pursuit of effective anti-oppressive practice requires recognition of and dialogue about the tensions, practice dilemmas and conflicting imperatives in social care. If these are to be worked through rather than acted out, a safe and facilitating environment is required, one which encourages analysis, reflection and discussion rather than denial of complexity. If difficulties are to be resolved collaboratively, if organizations are seriously to encourage workers to discuss the impact of agency norms and processes on themselves and users, and if workers are to be supported effectively on the task, a culture must be created where workers feel sufficiently safe to acknowledge and articulate anxiety, discomfort and disagreement. Anti-oppressive practice requires workers to put race, gender, disability and other forms of oppression on the agenda, and to demonstrate how paternalism and Eurocentricity block the needs of disabled people (Barnes, 1992), women and black people. Since this may challenge one's own feelings, thoughts and actions, and will challenge established interests as encapsulated in agency policy and practice, a facilitating culture is central. Power and vision once again are keys to collaboration's potential to inspire change.

The fifth key is distinguishing between *first- and second-order change*. Traditionally social care law, policy guidance and practice have emphasized individualized problem-solving, leaving unchanged underlying relationships and power structures. Symptoms and tasks, rather than fundamental needs, processes and issues, are tackled. Issues which arise from the wider system are assumed to be located within individual, family or team systems and worked with as if there. When the symptoms return, or prove resistant to intervention, the system frequently responds with more of the same, for example refined procedural guidelines, rather than looking at the nature of relationships between those involved, the assumptions and norms on which these relationships are based and how intervention may have maintained or exacerbated the situation. Longer-term empowering and anti-oppressive solutions require second-order change too, based on the analysis of and intervention into the context, power, culture, organizational arrangements and structural relationships which impact upon individual users and workers. This takes workers and agencies into social and political action, challenging and enabling users to challenge how they and services 'for' them have been perceived. The focus is on transactions, patterns of relationships, problems and individuals in context, with everyone in the professional network included in both analysis of what is happening and promotion of change. Thus, training for the future . . . and the creation of new organizational and inter-agency arrangements should focus not only on the implementation of service changes and new systems to accommodate the new arrangements (first-order change – problem-solving), but also on a shifting of perspective as a basis for refocusing activity (second-order change – relationship change), for example towards partnership with users, carers and the voluntary and independent sectors.

The sixth key is *partnership*. All parts of the system must be engaged, respect must be shown for and use made of experiences, resources and contributions in individual cases and in policy formation and review. The choice of the word partnership is deliberate. It does not mean participation or consultation within pre-set local authority agendas, perhaps considering a draft community care plan or proposed care package. It does mean, first, all parties convening to agree how the professional system is to approach its legal and policy mandates, consulting on how to work in partnership in devising an overall framework for community care. Second, it implies joint planning, for example in matching the needs and expectations of purchasers and providers in relation to contracts for services. This approach promotes mutual learning and trust, shared ownership and service relevance. It clarifies and uses difference and, through enabling the development of inter-professional and inter-agency agreements about aims, principles and procedures (Hardy et al., 1993; Leedham and Wistow, 1993), it improves outcomes for users.

The seventh key is *visibility*. Developing joint mechanisms for achieving integrated care, and for monitoring and reviewing performance and outcome of objectives . . . requires commitment: to building new relationships and organizational structures, to dealing with disagreement and difference openly, to sharing information and professional territories. The creation and sustaining of this approach will be facilitated by its being visible (Ormiston and Haggard, 1993): in joint events, such as planning days to engage in or review joint work, or identify and use resources within the system; in action research; in training courses, linked to policy development, coordinated and planned by an inter-agency group; in publicity about achievements; in delegation to managers and workers of decision-making autonomy sufficient to progress work. The idea of a health and social care 'passport', a user-held record (Henwood, 1993), not only provides users with a greater sense of personal control, but also, in merging records of assessments, plans, actions by those involved and outcomes, demonstrates evidence of change from traditional practice to a shared philosophy and approach to collating information and enabling users to express their needs or exercise their rights in a coordinated service. Scepticism, resistance and cynicism about community care changes generally, and multidisciplinary collaboration, particularly, will not be overcome by encouragement alone. It requires managerial support and a clear demonstration of commitment and possibilities.

The final key to collaboration is *the distinction between task and process*. The erratic track record of multidisciplinary collaboration suggests some attention to processes to achieve the task. Guidance abounds:

- overarching values, to provide direction and standards, and to avoid stereotyping;
- clarity of purpose and structure (Onyett, 1992; Hardy et al., 1993), each informed by a comprehensive survey of needs;
- robust and coherent management arrangements (Hardy et al., 1993);
- defining the function of resources such as residential care (Neill, 1982) and focusing on objectives of resourcing rather than just on the resources available;
- team control over deployment of services and resources (Knapp et al., 1992; McGrath, 1993);
- team coordinators accepted by all the professions involved (McGrath, 1993);
- single transferable procedures for assessment, one entry point via different services (DoH, 1991);
- flexible service models, neither so loose as to be chaotic and unstructured, not so rigid as to restrict autonomy and workers' abilities to develop and implement expertise.

Within an overarching framework for the task, agencies must consider the collaborative structures and strategies needed to meet the legal mandate to coordinate services. This requires clarity about roles and responsibilities. Thus negotiation and agreement is required on:

- who will coordinate, at what organizational level, the interface with other agencies, monitoring individual cases, team functioning and services, with clarity about how this will inform planning, resourcing and objective setting;
- what type of teams or networks are required for policy planning and review, for service delivery to user groups. This relates to membership, supervision and management of teams, where different models (Øvretveit, 1986; Onyett, 1992) are possible;
- how workloads will be managed to avoid overload and to ensure effective targeting of services based on assessment of need and priority decisions (Orme and Glastonbury, 1993);
- what is profession-specific, on the basis of how each profession perceives and approaches its tasks, what overlaps different professions and may be undertaken variously, such as assessment, and what is common to different professions, i.e. not profession-specific (Øvretveit, 1986);
- communication based on need rather than position (Biggs, 1990);
- how roles will be allocated and disputes resolved.

Thus, when you are 'troubleshooting', teamwork problems may reside in the task: unrealistic goals; inadequate resources of time, services and/or skills available to team members; blocks in other systems. Equally, problems may arise from conflictual relationships, from doubts about investing in goals, from group processes.

This highlights the importance of maintenance work (Kitzinger et al., 1993) in negotiating and sustaining relationships, recognizing that team development is marked by stages (Preston-Shoot, 1987), with trust, experimentation with different ways of working, expression of difference and flexible working patterns requiring groupwork skills to develop.

Teamworking interventions

Several tools are useful for practitioners and teams seeking to implement the keys to collaboration and manage the obstacles in the interprofessional system. The first, *hypothesizing*, centres on key questions.

- What is the problem?
- Why is it a problem now?
- Where is the problem?
- What might be the meaning, function or purpose of the problem?

Where the 'stuckness' resides in the interaction between the professional system and the user/carer/family system, additional questions

(Dimmock and Dungworth, 1983; Dungworth and Reimers, 1984; Stratton et al., 1990) help to formulate an effective intervention.

- What role is being pressed on the team and why?
- Is this role appropriate to accept?
- With whom does the team need to clarify its role?
- How do people view the interactions, their position in this system and the position of others?
- Who believes there are (what) problems? Is there a problem definition which agencies are working on? Is this shared with the user/carer/family system?

Essentially, hypotheses are stories, meta-perspectives about processes and how these are enacted within and between systems. They help to clarify what is happening and thereby to give purpose and direction to the change effort. If unclear values are driving the work, questions of rights and risks may need to be debated. If misconceptions exist about what different professionals can and should do, stereotypical beliefs and models of understanding social care tasks may need to be shared. If the work is triggering anxiety and this is affecting decision-making, support may have to be sought.

The second tool is *naming*, setting out this understanding in a manner which values people's contribution where possible since they will find it more difficult to contemplate difference and change if they feel blamed. Positive reframes may then be followed with questions about what the system could do more effectively in this or similar situations. This requires a third tool, *convening the system*. This enables observation of how system members interact, the position people adopt. This can be useful in exploring the position of the referring person in the system referred (Selvini Palazzoli et al., 1980; Preston-Shoot and Agass, 1990), the nature of relationships and whether another agency or professional is being triangulated (Carl and Jurkovic, 1983) to resolve a problematic relationship. It may enable work done by one part of the professional system to be observed by others, thereby avoiding duplication or being drawn into problem sequences (Benbow et al., 1990; Bowman and Jeffcoat, 1990). Convening the system also helps to sustain working together, to share perspectives which help to define what intervention to make, and to explore openly differences in goals. The nature of relationships and communication can be illustrated by use of sculpting, geneograms and eco-maps (Stratton et al., 1990) to map significant strong, weak and/or conflictual relationships; significant events; how such relationships and events have been carried subsequently into organizational life; how structures and relationships may block or distort communication; boundaries, roles, feelings and the perceptions of system members about these.

Convening the system helps to avoid covert agendas and relates the worker–user encounter to the systems which underpin it. It engages the professional system in problem clarification and resolution, and reduces the likelihood of acting out disagreements, of splitting into 'good and bad' agencies, and enmeshment in one person's problem definition (Pottle, 1984; Dungworth, 1988; Stratton et al., 1990). The system to convene should depend on need, not position, and may include family, friends and local community figures who provide support (Pottle, 1984).

The fourth tool is *hunting the latitude* (Stratton et al., 1990), searching for those areas where system members have room for manoeuvre, alternative ways of understanding and tackling a problem. It involves acknowledging the common tendency to use favourite approaches, suspending 'bias' to ensure that possibilities are not neglected (Smale et al., 1993). One such latitude lies in reducing restraining forces rather than increasing driving forces, since the latter will increase anxiety and tension (De Board, 1978). Another is asking what decisions are non-negotiable, usual and possible, identifying which are least acceptable and why, and by a process of such elimination finding the decision people feel least anxious about (O'Brian and Bruggen, 1985). Negotiations can also be freed by recognizing that, while mutuality of complete agreement on objectives and methods of achieving them might be desirable, reciprocity, where exploration leads to narrowing differences and a balance of agreement which outweighs disagreement, might be a useful starting point, parties agreeing to work on each other's objectives. A consultant, someone outside the system, may provide a different perspective (Dare et al., 1990), expanding the team's imagination by generating fresh ideas about difficulties, the processes which maintain or aggravate them and the work required to overcome them. A consultant can help teams to track processes within the system, and between it and other systems, and how these processes might reflect the internal and interpersonal processes in the user/carer/family system (Preston-Shoot and Agass, 1990).

Conclusion

The inbuilt fragmentation between purchasing and providing, health and social care, local authorities and the independent and voluntary sectors makes a seamless service a difficult goal to achieve. The systems approach, on which this chapter is based, adds a useful dimension to understanding and intervening in interprofessional and inter-agency systems. It complements other essential competencies for multidisciplinary work in social care: identifying the parts of and relationships between agencies; understanding the different perspectives of other professionals, including the values, knowledge and skills each offers, being able to use knowledge from other professionals while being clear regarding one's own perspective (Biggs and Weinstein, 1991).

References

Barnes, C. (1992) 'Institutional discrimination against disabled people and the campaign for anti-discrimination legislation', *Critical Social Policy*, 34, 12 (1): 5–22.

Benbow, S., Egan, D., Marriott, A., Tregay, K., Walsh, S., Wells, J. and Wood, J. (1990) 'Using the family life cycle with later life families', *Journal of Family Therapy*, 12: 321–40.

Biggs, S. (1990) 'Consumers, case management and inspection: obscuring social deprivation and need?', *Critical Social Policy*, 10 (3): 23–38.

Biggs, S. and Weinstein, S. (1991) *Assessment, Care management and Inspection in Community Care*, London: CCETSW.

Bowman, G. and Jeffcoat, P. (1990) 'The application of systems ideas in a social services field-work team', *Journal of Family Therapy*, 12: 243–54.

Carl, D. and Jurkovic, G. (1983) 'Agency triangles: problems in agency–family relationships', *Family Process*, 22: 441–51.

Dare, J., Goldberg, D. and Walinets, R. (1990) 'What is the question you need to answer? How consultation can prevent professional systems immobilizing families', *Journal of Family Therapy*, 12: 355–69.

De Board, R. (1978) *The Psychoanalysis of Organisations*, London: Tavistock.

Dimmock, B. and Dungworth, D. (1983) 'Creating manoeuvrability for family/systems therapists in social services departments', *Journal of Family Therapy*, 5 (1): 53–69.

DoH (1991) *Getting the Message Across. A Guide to Developing and Communicating Policies, Principles and Procedures on Assessment*, London: HMSO.

Dungworth, D. (1988) 'Context and the construction of family therapy practice', in E. Street and W. Dryden (eds) *Family Therapy in Britain*, Milton Keynes: Open University Press.

Dungworth, D. and Reimers, S. (1984) 'Family therapy in social services departments', in A. Treacher and J. Carpenter (eds) *Using Family Therapy*, Oxford: Basil Blackwell.

Grimwood, C. and Popplestone, R. (1993) *Women, Management and Care*, London: Macmillan.

Hardy, B., Wistow, G., Turrell, A. and Webb, A. (1993) 'Collaboration and cost effectiveness', in D. Robbins (ed.) *Community Care, Findings from Department of Health Funded Research, 1988–1992*, London: HMSO.

Henwood, M. (1993) 'Smart thinking', *Social Work Today*, 14 January: 18.

Kitzinger, J., Green, J. and Coupland, V. (1993) 'Labour relations: midwives and doctors on the labour ward', in J. Walmsley, J. Reynolds, P. Shakespeare and R. Woolfe (eds) *Health, Welfare and Practice. Reflecting on Roles and Relationships*, London: Sage/The Open University.

Knapp, M., Cambridge, P., Thomason, C., Beecham, J., Allen, C. and Darton, R. (1992) *Care in the Community: Challenge and Demonstration*, Aldershot: PSSRU/Ashgate.

Leedham, I. and Wistow, G. (1993) 'Just what the doctor ordered', *Community Care*, 7 January: 22–3.

McGrath, M. (1993) 'Policy implementation studies – the all-Wales mental handicap strategy', in D. Robbins (ed.) *Community Care. Findings from Department of Health Funded Research, 1988–1992*, London: HMSO.

Mawhinney, B. (1993) 'Check against delivery', Closing address to the Social Services Conference', 29 October, Solihull.

Neill, J. (1982) 'Some variations in policy and procedure relating to Part 3 applications in the GLC area', *British Journal of Social Work*, 12 (3): 229–45.

O'Brian, C. and Bruggen, P. (1985) 'Our personal and professional lives: learning positive connotation and circular questioning', *Family Process*, 24: 311–22.

Onyett, S. (1992) *Case Management in Mental Health*, London: Chapman and Hall.

Orme, J. and Glastonbury, B. (1993) *Care management*, London: Macmillan.

Ormiston, H. and Haggard, L. (1993) 'A long road ahead', *Community Care*, 17 June: 16–17.

Øvretveit, J. (1986) *Organisation of Multidisciplinary Community Teams*, Uxbridge: Brunel University Institute of Organisation and Social Studies.

Pottle, S. (1984) 'Developing a network-oriented service for elderly people and their carers', in A. Treacher and J. Carpenter (eds) *Using Family Therapy*. Oxford: Basil Blackwell.

Preston-Shoot, M. (1987) *Effective Groupwork*, London: Macmillan.

Preston-Shoot, M. and Agass, D. (1990) *Making Sense of Social Work: Psychodynamics, Systems and Practice*, London: Macmillan.

Selvini Palazzoli, M., Boscolo, L., Cecchin, G. and Prata G. (1978) *Paradox and Counterparadox*, New York: Jason Aronson.

Selvini Palazzoli, M., Boscolo, L., Cecchin, G. and Prata, G. 91980) 'The problem of the referring person', *Journal of Marital and Family Therapy*, 6: 3–9.

Smale, G. and Tuson, G. with Biehal, N. and Marsh, P. (1993) *Empowerment, Assessment, Care Management and the Skilled Worker*, London: NISW/HMSO.

Stratton, P., Preston-Shoot, M. and Hanks, H. (1990) *Family Therapy Training and Practice*, Birmingham: Venture Press.

15

L. Finlay

Safe Haven and Battleground: Collaboration and Conflict within the Treatment Team

The multidisciplinary treatment team is often perceived as an important source of mutual support, identity and esteem, as team members collaborate in therapy and decision-making. In reference to occupational therapists, Sweeney et al. (1993) suggest that work stress is considerably lessened through team support and interaction, while Leonard and Corr (1998), among others, have demonstrated the importance of supervision and support from other team members.

But within teams, as within families, relationships vary and experiences can be mixed. Team relationships can involve destructive or defensive dynamics as individuals clash in terms of values and levels of understanding. McNeely (1994) found that, for nurses, communication with colleagues, doctors and departments was a major source of stress. Adamson et al. (1995) reported that nurses were dissatisfied with their status and the power differentials built into their relationships with doctors; these acted as a barrier to collegial relationships. Toulouse and Williams (1984) uncovered poor liaison with other professions as a key area of dissatisfaction for newly qualified therapists. Hopkinson et al. (1998) found that community workers experienced much role uncertainty, with misunderstandings about boundaries constituting a considerable source of stress. Øvretveit (1997) suggested that the erosion of clear professional roles was a particular source of tension in a community mental health team whose members felt that others were encroaching on valued areas of work.

How do practitioners actually experience their team work? What do they identify as sources of support or zones of conflict? How do they manage tensions within the team? This chapter summarizes the findings of a qualitative study which set out to answer these questions by exploring how one group of professionals (occupational therapists) experienced their team relationships.

Method

The study focused on 12 occupational therapists drawn from a range of health care contexts: physical and psychiatric hospitals, social services and community mental health. Qualitative methodology was employed in the form of in-depth, non-directive interviews and participant observation carried out by the author, herself an occupational therapist. This methodology was chosen as it was suited to capture the subjective experiences of each individual and the meanings derived from these experiences. A phenomenological approach was adopted to describe the individual's life world rather than seek to explain how or why particular meanings had arisen.

After analysing each interview and drawing observations, the researcher sought to identify common themes and meanings. This involved repeated and systematic reading of the transcripts, in line with the analytical method suggested by Wertz (1983) and Giorgi (1975). After first 'dwelling' on the phenomenon (through empathetic immersion and reflection), the psychological structures involved were then described by identifying constituents and recurrent themes.

Findings

While the study uncovered considerable variation in what the team meant to individual therapists, certain common experiences emerged. These experiences can be understood in terms of four key themes: caring for one another; 'good' colleagues versus 'bad' colleagues; 'sibling rivalry'; and ideal images versus tough reality. These themes are discussed below, in part drawing on the voices of the individual therapists (whose names have been changed to preserve anonymity).

Caring for one another

The team is experienced by the therapists as a source of identity and support. They feel positive about the process of sharing and co-operating in decision-making. Mary, for instance, identifies strongly with her community mental health team. The weekly team meeting, at which the process of assigning clients to practitioners is negotiated, structures her schedule. She particularly enjoys the sense that she and her fellow team members are aware of one another's skills and expertise. As she puts it,

> I work in a multidisciplinary team with community psychiatric nurses and social workers and there's also medical input and a psychologist as well. Basically the way we work here is we have a meeting each week and

anybody can pick up any referral. . . . I think it's nice because although we all do similar sort of work, each profession has its own sort of speciality. . . . So there's that recognition, which is good.

In the interviews, the practitioners reveal the importance they attach to collaborating on treatment planning. Fellow professionals, they report, inspire confidence as well as ideas; it comes as a relief to share with others, and collaboration means safe practice, even survival. For Stephen, such team liaison is vital. Accustomed to working alongside others, he consults his colleagues on his treatment interventions. Recalling one occasion when he experienced near panic ('My immediate reaction was "Oh, my God, what are we going to do here?"'), he found that, aided by the social worker he was with at the time, he was able to talk the situation through and come up with a plan.

For Jenny, too, team collaboration is vital. In the special unit she works in, physical survival can depend on the support team members offer each other. The staff function as a coalition to control the patients; they watch over each other and intervene to keep each other safe. She needs, and expects, the team to back her. As she says, when 'people are aware that there is a potential problem . . . I expect staff to jump in.'

The team is experienced not only as a refuge and zone of safety but also as an ongoing source of support, supervision and advice. Practitioners find the sense of sharing with others who 'really understand' beneficial. They express the relief of being with team members with whom it is unnecessary to justify or defend one's professional identity. Susan, who receives regular supervision from another occupational therapist, values the relationship for the nurturing it offers alongside general professional development. Supervision is her space to 'off-load', be herself, heal and learn; she can, she feels, be totally honest in this non-threatening environment in which she will not be judged negatively or called upon to justify her practice. For Jane, the team helps counteract the intense isolation of being alone on the road all day: 'We've always got each other. If any of us has got a problem we can always go back to the office and say, "Look at this" or "Would you come out? I'm really stuck here."'

'Good' colleagues versus 'bad' colleagues

Within teams, however, levels of trust, respect and appreciation vary considerably. Some team members are experienced as supportive, 'good' colleagues, others as 'bad' colleagues who seem dismissive, disrespectful and rejecting.

Good colleagues are the ones with whom the therapists are able to collaborate, for instance in the running of treatment sessions or in co-leading therapy groups. As an example, Karen allies herself firmly with the physiotherapists:

We're fortunate in sessions in that we would have joint sessions. So in the kitchen we would actually have both of us working together with the client. So the physio would be looking at the side-stepping, the standing and posture, and we would be looking at actually doing the functional tasks in the kitchen.

While collaboration comes easily with certain team members, relations with others are tense, distant or even conflictual. Cathy, for instance, struggles with some of her relationships, particularly with certain consultants who are not interested in, and do not appreciate, what she does. Julie, for her part, has laboured to be valued as a skilled and legitimate team member. She has found it personally painful not to be given that status and has had to fight to prove herself:

It got very personal. People would tell me, 'for my own good', that I shouldn't be doing the sort of things I was doing because that wasn't an OT's job . . . I started running relaxation groups and a stress management group, and I had it fed back to me by a community nurse that he had heard that people were very unhappy about it, and really I wasn't qualified to do that sort of work.

Sibling rivalry

Despite its many positive aspects, the team can also be a place of strife in which members compete over territory and vie for recognition. The occupational therapists sometimes find themselves struggling to make their voices heard, to assert their presence. Cathy, for one, sometimes finds herself working up the courage to do so. She dislikes being ignored and feels she has to 'shout' to get others to give her attention and respect. A particular problem, in her experience as an occupational therapist, is being outnumbered by community psychiatric nurses (CPNs) which results in her expertise as an occupational therapist (OT) being overlooked:

I was in a meeting the other day, a training session, and we were talking about community teams referring to the CPN. And they kept saying, 'CPN, CPN', so in the end I had to say, 'Excuse me, but I work on a community mental health team and I'm an OT'! And these are colleagues that I work with! It does become annoying to feel that you've got to justify and keep shouting out 'OT! We're OT!'

Stresses emerge, too, when one team member seeks to usurp the professional role of another. Cathy expresses the resulting competition in terms of 'guarding her back'. She feels she is in a battle for territory; if others are out to take over her role, she in her turn can encroach on that of others. As she says: 'a little bit of antagonism is set up and it's sort of covering your own back and saying, "Well the physio hasn't passed any exams in mental health . . . what are they doing here . . . or, if you teach me how to give injections then I can do the same as a CPN."' Julie, too, has had a battle on her hands: to gain access to her clients' medical and nursing notes against the blocking efforts of an autocratic and old-fashioned consultant and some of the nurses on her team.

For her part, Jenny feels constantly engaged in small role battles with other professionals, trying to defend or carve out territory. Tired of endlessly fighting the same battles, she sees team collaboration and interdisciplinary working as the way forward:

> Why do I have to do this again? I'm tired of doing this . . . we're not always asking nurses why they're doing what they're doing . . . there are really big barriers to break down. They're enormous barriers . . . it feels very much like collaborative working is the way forward . . . that's the vision that I want to see.

Sometimes jostling for status extends to vying for patients' approval and co-operation. Mary, for one, struggles to value herself, and to be valued, as a fully legitimate therapist. She was particularly upset on one occasion when a neighbour of one of her clients, who was a nurse, denied she was a 'proper therapist'. That accusation stung as it may have destroyed the trust she had so painstakingly built up with her client and she had assumed that, among professionals at least, there would be greater mutual respect.

Ideal images versus tough reality

The team can also be experienced negatively when harsh reality seems to mock idealistic expectations. Team members may find it hard to hold on to positive images of the team when it is passing through divisive, damaging or destructive times. Jenny, describing her many battles to defend her staff from macho-management and her patients from incompetent staff, views the staff team as potentially very difficult, possibly because of the closed environment. She believes one of her main values is being able to do battle, but she also knows that sometimes the battles can backfire. 'Sometimes you feel you're walking on eggshells,' she reports. 'If you upset somebody that can actually interrupt your treatment . . . you have to be careful.'

When a team is passing through a particularly stressful or problematic period, it is important to be vigilant and to seek ways to minimize the damage. Julie, recognizing the need for patience, emphasizes that problems do not sort themselves out overnight. And sometimes it may prove to be a 'no win' situation. In her interview, she recalls how student nursing placements within her occupational therapy unit created so many strains and tensions that team members indulged in 'sabotage' and the placements had to be ended.

In some instances, practitioners may feel betrayed by the realities of team practice. There is a sense, for example, that Mary is experiencing a sudden 'tear' in her feeling of connectedness to others in the team; she has come to realize the support she had previously taken for granted simply was not there. She had thought the team members would protect each other in the face of abusive, damaging clients. Now she feels can no longer trust other members not to set her up and deliberately place her in the firing line. She feels alone in her struggle – a struggle with both difficult clients and difficult staff.

Discussion

These findings demonstrate that the relationship with the multi-disciplinary team plays a powerful role in the therapist's life world. However, this picture is complex as the team means different things and is perceived ambivalently in both positive and negative terms. The therapists engage in multiple relationships at various levels – both close and distant – with different team members. Further, any discussion of how teams are experienced must also recognize that therapists are often involved with more than one team – for instance, each of the therapists interviewed belong to at least two teams: a multidisciplinary team and an occupational therapy team. For these therapists, the profession-specific team was often viewed in especially positive terms as it offered supervision and the therapists did not feel under pressure to justify their role. Thus, the team means something different, at different times, and in different contexts.

In general, both the occupational therapy and the multidisciplinary treatment team would appear to be an important source of identity, meaning and social interaction for the therapists. Team relationships are also a prime source of support, helping to relieve stress. Therapists see themselves as working collaboratively and sharing in team decision-making. This vision of the team as a positive force is reflected in much literature (e.g. Sweeney et al., 1993; Hopkinson et al., 1998; Leonard and Corr, 1998; Robertson and Cummings, 1991).

However, the team can at the same time be viewed in terms of problems and conflict. Over and above ideological divisions such as those between bio-medical models of disability and models with a stronger social dimension, team members may find themselves drawn into a range of conflicts. Therapists seem to compete with others (often nurses) over territory and vie for recognition within the hierarchy. Interactions with other team members can be experienced as stressful and disempowering (Sweeney et al., 1993; Toulouse and Williams, 1984; Hopkinson et al., 1998). Within this battleground, the team is experienced in terms of power struggles in which therapists have to fight to be valued and respected (Hugman, 1991).

Explaining why team problems and conflicts arise in any depth is beyond the scope of this chapter. However, some explanations can be suggested through using three levels of analysis:

1 At a **group level** of analysis, it may be relevant to consider unconscious group dynamics and how a team may put up psychological defences to combat anxiety. Following Menzies Lyth (1988), Loxley suggests that 'suspicion, avoidance, scapegoating, stereotyping, denial, blaming, self-idealisation are all common defence mechanisms in the interchange between professions involved in individual or social distress' (1997: 57).

2 At an **organizational level** of analysis, the team may not have systems in place which can clarify the division of labour in terms of roles, responsibilities and how clinical decisions are made (Øvretveit, 1997).

3 At a **society level** of analysis, the team can be understood to reflect wider social divisions in society (class, race, gender and age). The fact of working in a hierarchy where practitioners have different levels of status, power, pay and experience is a potential source of tension (Kenny and Adamson, 1992; Adamson et al., 1995). Further, in the context of marketization (Jones, 1998), the fact of competition between team members for their very jobs also underlies some team conflict.

Several of the therapists in the research admitted feeling hurt and surprised when first confronted with team conflict. They seemed to be inadequately prepared to deal with the problem. Further research on the challenge of team work, the causes of problems and possible strategies for overcoming these, seems called for – particularly in the current context of evolving practice and the emergence of a new, collaborative professionalism (Davies, 1998).

Conclusion

The findings presented here indicate something of the complexity of the experience of working in a multidisciplinary team. For the occupational therapists interviewed, this experience has many positive features. The team emerges as an important source of identity, support and esteem. It offers opportunities for collaboration and participation in decision-making. It stands as a haven and place of refuge wherein therapists can heal, recover and develop away from everyday strains and stresses.

But the team is also a source of tension, conflict and negative feelings. In a real sense, it can be experienced as a battleground. Team members may perceive themselves in competition with others. They may jostle for recognition or struggle to defend role boundaries. In their different ways, the therapists seem caught up in a never-ending battle to be respected and valued by the other members of their team.

Operating in a team, is often challenging and difficult. Easy, idealistic assumptions about the team as a source of untrammelled, unqualified support seem likely to be contradicted in practice. Professionals working within a multidisciplinary team need to learn how to live with, and handle, a much more complex reality.

References

Adamson, B.J., Kenny, D.T. and Wilson-Barnett, J. (1995) 'The impact of perceived medical dominance on the workplace satisfaction of Australian and British nurses', *Journal of Advanced Nursing*, 21: 172–83.

Davies, C. (1998) 'The cloak of professionalism', in M. Robb and M. Allott (eds) *Understanding Health and Social Care: an Introductory Reader*, London: Sage Publications.

Giorgi, A. (1975) 'An application of phenomenological method in psychology', in A. Giorgi, C. Fischer and R. van Eckartsberg (eds) *Duquesne Studies in Phenomenological Psychology*, Vols I and II, Pittsburgh: Duquesne University Press.

Hopkinson, P.J., Carson, J., Brown, D., Fagin, L., Bartlett, H. and Leary, J. (1998) 'Occupational stress and community mental health nursing: what CPNs really said', *Journal of Advanced Nursing*, 27: 707–12.

Hugman, R. (1991) *Power in Caring Professions*, Basingstoke: Macmillan Press.

Jones, L.J. (1998) 'Changing health care', in A. Brechin, J. Walmsley, J. Katz and S. Peace (eds) *Care Matters: Concepts, Practice and Research in Health and Social Care*, London: Sage Publications.

Kenny, D.T. and Adamson, B.J. (1992) 'Medicine and the health professions: Issues of dominance, autonomy and authority', *Australian Health Review*, 15: 319–35.

Leonard, C. and Corr, S. (1998) 'Sources of stress and coping strategies in basic grade occupational therapists', *British Journal of Occupational Therapy*, 61 (6): 257–62.

Loxley, A. (1997) *Collaboration in Health and Welfare: Working with Difference*, London: Jessica Kingsley.

McNeely, S. (1994) 'Communication: another source of stress among nurses?', *The Occupational Psychologist*, 25: 5–7.

Øvretveit, J. (1997) 'Evaluating interprofessional working – a case example of a community mental health team', in J. Øvretveit, P. Mathias and T. Thompson (eds) *Interprofessional Working for Health and Social Care*, Basingstoke and London: Macmillan.

Robertson, J. and Cummings, C. (1991) 'What makes long term care nursing attractive?', *American Journal of Nursing*, 91 (11): 41–6.

Sweeney, G.M., Nicholls, K.A. and Kline, P. (1993) 'Job stress in occupational therapy: an examination of causative factors', *British Journal of Occupational Therapy*, 56 (3): 89–93.

Toulouse, J. and Williams, S. (1984) 'First appointments: a survey of influencing factors', *British Journal of Occupational Therapy*, 47 (4): 111–13.

Wertz, F.J. (1983) 'From everyday to psychological description: analyzing the moments of a qualitative data analysis', *Journal of Phenomenological Psychology*, 14 (2): 197–241.

16

C. Cott

Structure and Meaning in Multidisciplinary Teamwork

The purpose of this study was to examine the relationship between structure and meaning in multidisciplinary long-term care teams. In-depth semi-structured interviews were conducted with 26 staff working on five multidisciplinary teams in the same long-term care facility in Metropolitan Toronto. Staff in different structural locations have differing meanings of work and teamwork. Direct caregiving nursing staff have simple role-sets, minimal involvement in team decision-making and ritualistic orientations towards their work and teamwork. Multidisciplinary professionals have complex role-sets, greater involvement in team decision-making and organic orientations towards their work and teamwork. Supervisory nurses are in a contradictory structural location and shared aspects of both orientations to teamwork. The lack of shared meanings results in alienation from work and teamwork for staff in lower structural positions which, in turn, has considerable implications for team functioning. . . .

Findings

As the study progressed, it became apparent that although all the staff members valued teamwork, staff in different structural positions held different perceptions of meanings of teamwork because they were engaged in different kinds of teamwork. The structure of the team is essentially alienating for staff in lower structural positions with the result that they do not share the same meanings of teamwork as staff in higher structural positions. These differing meanings of teamwork have considerable implications for the way the team functions. . . .

First published in *Sociology of Health and Illness*, 20: 848–73 (Blackwell, 1998). Abridged.

The main theme: getting the work done

The main theme underlying all the respondents' comments about teamwork was how being part of the team helped them to do their job, usually in the context of sharing knowledge and information or work tasks. Sharing work tasks with other team members helped alleviate the difficulty of working with multi-problem frail institutionalized elders. For example, one respondent said: 'Because by teamwork . . . it's much easier for everybody . . . if you work together it's much, much easier.'

'Getting the work done' was the main underlying theme common to all respondents and was an important foundation for whether staff valued teamwork. Also, whomever staff defined as helping to 'get the work done' was defined as being part of the team. Depending on their structural position, staff differed on how they defined the team and their perceptions of the meaning of teamwork.

The structure of the teams

It is largely supposed, in the literature, that the 'team' is the multi-disciplinary group of professional health care providers working together for the well-being of the patients. In this study, the team was defined very broadly to include all health care providers on a particular unit who provided direct care to patients. As the interviews progressed, it became increasingly clear that there were two sub-groups within the larger team. The differentiation between 'nursing' and the 'multidisciplinary team' was commonly made by all respondents.

These two sub-groups were quite different in their structure (Cott, 1997). The multidisciplinary sub-group consisted mainly of non-nursing professionals such as physicians, therapists and social workers. It was non-hierarchical. These health care professionals had no supervisory capacity over each other, and proceeded with their work tasks autonomously and independently. They met regularly for team meetings which were attended only by other multidisciplinary professionals and supervisory nurses (head nurses and team leaders). The direct caregiving nursing staff, which included mainly registered nurses (RNs) and health care assistants (HCAs), rarely, if ever, attended multidisciplinary rounds. The multidisciplinary professionals interacted mainly with each other and with the supervisory nurses. They had little contact with the direct caregiving nursing staff, particularly those nursing staff working the evening or night shift.

The nursing sub-group consisted of RNs, RPNs and HCAs on the day, evening, and night shifts. In contrast to the multiprofessional sub-group, it was very hierarchical. . . .

This common team structure reflects social class distinctions within society (Navarro, 1976) with higher-educated, higher-status professions assuming responsibility and control of the team and lower-educated, lower-status, workers carrying out tasks delegated to them from above. It represents the 'we decide, you carry it out' division of labour in health care (Cott, 1997) in which one group of professionals decides on a course of action that another group of health workers is expected to carry out.

As the analysis progressed, it became increasingly clear that the team to which respondents were referring differed depending on their structural position. When staff were referring to the 'team' they were referring to those staff who helped them to get their work done. However, the nature of the work that staff in different structural positions were trying to 'get done' differed, and influenced the type of teamwork in which they were involved, resulting in differing perceptions of the team and teamwork.

Direct caregiving nursing staff

. . . The direct caregiving staff were involved in teamwork that involved helping each other complete work tasks. For them the team consisted of those nursing staff who were on duty together and who provided assistance and support for one another in the fulfilment of their tasks of providing for the basic care needs of the patients. As one RPN said:

> You get them [patients] washed and dressed and then you get somebody to help you with a transfer or a lift. If I'm on medication that day, somebody else has to feed them, so then you have to ask them, 'Did they eat everything, and what did they eat?' You have to put them back to bed after lunch too.

The lack of engagement of these direct caregiving staff in their work was also reflected in the way they talked about teamwork. For the most part, they did not talk about how teamwork improved the quality of the work done, only how it made it easier. A few who were more engaged in their work did talk about how being part of a team improved the work. However, even these more engaged nurses were only talking about nursing. They did not feel engaged with the multidisciplinary professionals, nor did they consider themselves part of a larger multiprofessional team. They talked about nursing as 'we', but referred to the multidisciplinary professionals as 'they'.

Most of the direct caregiving nursing staff were quite ambivalent when they talked about the multidisciplinary team. As one said, 'So, I guess having a [multidisciplinary] team does work sometimes'. These nurses saw the multidisciplinary professionals as separate from themselves and not essential to helping them complete their work tasks. The direct caregiving staff's ambivalence about the multidisciplinary professionals reflected the low levels of interaction between the two groups. Coser (1991) also found that low frequency of interaction among health professionals was associated with weakness of interpersonal sentiments resulting in little motivation to work collaboratively with one another. . . .

These nursing staff had a ritualistic notion about teamwork just as they had a ritualistic notion about their work. The structure of the team placed little onus on them for decision-making. They rarely attended multidisciplinary team rounds, nor were they expected to be part of team decision-making. These limited expectations were incorporated into their attitudes towards their work and teamwork. . . .

The multidisciplinary professionals

. . . When discussing the team, the multidisciplinary professionals differentiated between themselves and nursing, but they tended not to differentiate between the direct caregiving nursing staff and supervisory nurses, usually referring to nursing as a whole. Like the direct caregiving nursing staff, whoever helped to get the work done was the criterion for who the multidisciplinary professionals defined as part of the team. However, they defined the team quite broadly because, due to the nature of their work, they needed the input and cooperation of many others. They had complex role-sets. They were linked to individuals who were different from themselves in that they belonged to different professional groups, and, in the case of the peripheral professionals, might work with a number of different teams. They had more extensive responsibilities *vis-à-vis* the organization, plus complex work tasks that required more integration and planning and therefore input from a variety of other health professionals. In addition, they needed nursing to fulfil their work requirements. For example, if the dietitian had the responsibility of ensuring that a patient was adequately nourished, she needed the skills and cooperation of others to do her work. She might need a complete medical workup to plan the appropriate diet, she might need assistance from speech-language pathology, occupational therapy and physiotherapy to assess swallowing difficulties, and she would need the nursing staff to ensure that the patient took in the food that was provided. She defined the team extensively to include all the multidisciplinary professionals and the nursing staff because she needed all these staff to help her to get her work done.

The core multidisciplinary professionals felt very much a part of the team. Even the physicians who had little interaction with the others on a day-to-day basis felt part of a team because they attended and usually chaired team rounds. This sense of belonging was an important aspect of teamwork for the core professionals and was incorporated into their social identity. One said, 'It's just easier being part of a team, you're not alone . . .'. These multidisciplinary professionals had an organic conceptualization of teamwork. For example, one said:

> I think that being part of the team enables me to share my expertise and knowledge with them and the knowledge and expertise of the other disciplines, especially nursing, medicine and recreation. That certainly makes it easier and more effective when you're dealing with impaired residents and the family.

. . .

The supervisory nurses

The supervisory nurses were in an interesting structural position in that they were the link between the direct caregiving nursing staff and the multidisciplinary professionals. They were the conduit through which information was passed between the two other groups. This intermediary position was reflected in their orientation to their work and to teamwork. . . .

These supervisory nurses saw themselves as somewhat apart from both the direct caregiving nursing staff and the multidisciplinary professionals. They referred both to the direct caregiving nursing staff and the multidisciplinary professionals as 'they', although they used 'we' when referring to nursing overall. This terminology reflects their paradoxical structural position in the team. On the one hand, they were at the top of the nursing hierarchy; on the other hand, they were interacting with the less hierarchical multidisciplinary professionals. They were engaged in two different kinds of teamwork, depending upon with whom they were interacting.

This separation of the supervisory nurses from both the direct caregiving nursing staff and the multidisciplinary professionals reflects their linking position in the structure of the team. It is similar to contradictory class locations within a mode of production in which professionals are simultaneously in two different classes (Parkin, 1979; Wright et al., 1982). The supervisory nurses shared some characteristics with the multidisciplinary professionals and direct caregiving nursing staff but they were not distinctly part of either group. They were in a contradictory structural location which was reflected in the way they talked about teamwork.

When talking about teamwork with the multidisciplinary professionals, the supervisory nurses reflected some of the ideology about collaborative teamwork and how being part of a team improved the way they did their work:

> . . . and sometimes you're right and sometimes you're not right, so you try to work together the best way because who is going to benefit in the long run? It's the patient who you are working for – it's not for you.

However, when they were talking about teamwork with the direct caregiving nurses, they usually referred to how it helped to get the work done, with little reference to improving the quality of the work.

Unlike the direct caregiving nursing staff, the supervisory nurses were not alienated from the larger multiprofessional team by the structure of the team. They were included in team decision-making and had a more organic conceptualization of their relationship to the team. . . .

Meaning, structure and team function

Differences in meaning of teamwork for staff in different structural positions are reflected in how the team functions and perpetuate the 'we decide, you carry it out' division of labour within the teams. The notion of teamwork is important to maintaining this social order, but is limited in this function by the differing meanings of teamwork held by staff. . . .

The orientation to teamwork held by the multidisciplinary professionals and, to a certain extent, by the supervisory nurses reflects the ideals of collaborative teamwork, as espoused in the literature, that are key to promoting cooperation amongst disparate groups of health professionals who are working together without clear lines of authority over each other. It is a means of social control. The rubric of teamwork provides the justification and rationale for staff cooperating with other disciplines. Because they feel that they are part of a team, the multidisciplinary professionals and supervisory nurses feel obliged to try and work things out with other disciplines instead of proceeding independently. As a supervisory nurse said:

> Sometimes you agree and [sometimes you] disagree, but you have to take into consideration it's the welfare of the patient and so you can't be dogmatic and say this is what I think, I'm not going to change. . . . We have to work together.

The ideology of collaborative teamwork works as a social control for the multidisciplinary professionals and supervisory nurses because they share aspects of an organic orientation to teamwork. The structure of the team, when they are interacting with each other, reflects the ideology of collaborative teamwork. However, interaction becomes more problematic when it involves the direct caregiving nursing staff.

The meaning of teamwork shared by the multidisciplinary professionals and supervisory nurses has little meaning for the direct caregiving nursing staff because the overall structure of the team does not reflect the ideology of teamwork – egalitarian, cooperative decision-making. The multidisciplinary professionals' roles may be to make decisions and recommendations about care and treatment plans, but their job is not complete until these decisions or plans are implemented. Invariably, implementation of their patient-related

recommendations involved the direct caregiving nursing staff. As one of the multidisciplinary professionals said: 'I use the nursing team to input my recommendations and that's probably the hardest part of my job – just getting my recommendation implemented.'
. . .

Despite their subordinate position in the hierarchy, the direct caregiving nursing staff were able to exert some control over their conditions of work. Simply giving orders and expecting them to be carried out did not work for the multidisciplinary professionals because they had no authority over the nursing staff, and even if they had, the nursing staff had ways of undermining what orders they received. As one therapist commented: 'they [the nursing staff] can really sabotage what you're doing [she laughs] if they don't understand why the specific diet's recommended'.

Even the supervisory nurses, who do have legitimate power through their supervisory authority over the direct caregiving nursing staff, found that giving direct orders was not always sufficient to gain cooperation. All of them described instances in which they had had difficulty obtaining the cooperation of the direct caregiving nursing staff.

The implications of these negotiations within the 'we decide, you carry it out' chain of command are fragmented patient care and problematic interactions with patients and families. Because their authority was not sufficient to ensure cooperation, the supervisory nurses had tried to use teamwork to ensure that they got the cooperation they needed to get their work done. They were sometimes successful in their attempts to promote teamwork with the direct caregiving nursing staff because they were able to help the direct caregiving nurses with their work tasks. . . .

The paradox is that while the integration of the direct caregiving nursing staff is important for their cooperation, the structure of the team works against this happening by excluding the lower-status staff from any formal participation or membership in the team. Because the direct caregiving nursing staff are alienated from the larger multiprofessional team and have a ritualistic understanding of teamwork, the multidisciplinary professionals have to spend much of their time trying to counteract the effects of the structure as they try to gain the cooperation of the direct caregiving nursing staff.

Discussion and conclusions

. . . The unanticipated consequence of teamwork is that, if the structure of the team does not reflect the ideology of egalitarian, cooperative teamwork, it can promote alienation from teamwork in lower-level staff who are key to the implementation of the decisions made by the higher-status professionals. Just as medicine supported the notion of teamwork in order to ensure the cooperation of subordinate professions, now these professionals find themselves having to promote more collaborative teamwork for the lower-status staff with whom they interact in order to accomplish their goals. However, in order to achieve the kind of teamwork that the higher-status professionals profess to desire, the structure of the team would have to change to allow for more equitable or meaningful participation in decision-making for all staff, and therefore a more similar orientation to teamwork for all team members.

Do definitions of health care teamwork espoused in the literature reflect the day-to-day interactions in multidisciplinary long-term care teams? The answer is equivocal. Not all staff are included in the type of egalitarian, cooperative teamwork described in those definitions. For those who are, the ideology of teamwork for the benefit of the patient prevents the potential splintering, factioning and lack of cooperation that could occur among the disparate professionals. However, the ideology of teamwork is not always successful in this function because it is not always reflected in the structure of teamwork. The findings of this study provide further evidence that not only do team members not share understandings of roles, norms and values, they do not share similar meanings of teamwork. Although professional affiliation may provide part of the explanation for these differing meanings of teamwork, structural position, particularly when resulting from differential involvement in different types of teamwork, is an important consideration. As multidisciplinary health care teams continue to diversify, and as more layers of 'cheaper' subordinate staff are brought in to perform tasks traditionally performed by higher-status professionals, it will be increasingly important to consider whether the structure of health care teams is appropriate and supports their supposed functions. . . .

Acknowledgements

The author would like to acknowledge the financial support of the Ontario Ministry of Health through Health Research Personnel Development Fellowship # 04224, and the comments from Dr Susan Rappolt and two anonymous reviewers on previous drafts of this manuscript.

References

Coser, R. (1991) *In Defense of Modernity: Role Complexity and Individual Autonomy*, Stanford: Stanford University Press.

Cott, C. (1997) 'We decide, you carry it out: a social network analysis of multidisciplinary long-term care teams', *Social Science and Medicine*, 45 (9): 1411–21.

Navarro, V. (1976) *Medicine under Capitalism*, New York: Prodist.

Parkin, F. (1979) *Marxism and Class Theory: a Bourgeois Critique*, New York: Columbia University Press.

Wright, E.O., Hachen, D., Costello, C. and Sprague, J. (1982) 'The American class structure', *American Sociological Review*, 47: 709–26.

17

K. Dent-Brown

A Split in the Mirror: Using psychotherapeutic concepts to understand team conflict

This chapter will describe how the work of mental health teams with certain divided, conflicted individuals can have the effect of opening up divisions and generating conflict in those teams. It will show how concepts from psychotherapeutic theory and practice can be helpful in understanding how best to help the individual patient,[1] as well as in understanding what is going on in the team as a whole. The case study is derived from actual clinical experience, but has been considerably altered to preserve anonymity.

The patient group

Staff in NHS community mental health teams (CMHTs) and in-patient units find themselves dealing with a clearly identifiable sub-group of patients who present them with particular problems. These patients often present in some kind of crisis, frequently involving self-harm by overdosing or cutting themselves. They can challenge staff and services with chaotic behaviour which cannot be ignored; one patient progressively broke all the windows in her housing association flat, then took outside and burned all her furniture. Another left hospital, took a large drug overdose then returned to hospital to be found unconscious and near death by nursing staff. They will often complain (with some justification) that the NHS and other services are slow to react and offer little practical or useful help in times of crisis.

And yet when they are offered something, this group of patients will frequently reject it. Someone who begs for admission to a ward may stay for two days then go absent and refuse to return, citing a petty ward rule as their reason for leaving. Or someone who rings a CMHT in crisis and is offered regular sessions with a community psychiatric nurse may never keep their appointment, only reappearing after a visit to casualty. This group seems, anecdotally, to make a large number of formal complaints to the NHS, and even go to the extent of suing their health authority or trust. Indeed, one of the labels this group attracts is 'help rejecting complainers'.

Casenotes on this patient group are often several inches thick. Individuals will often have attracted several different diagnoses – depressed, schizophrenic, anxious, personality disordered – and several different forms of treatment, none of which seems to have made much difference. Their notes (particularly, but not exclusively, the older entries) will contain words like 'manipulative', 'acting out', 'attention seeking', and 'behavioural'. They do not appear to conform to the diagnostic categories of mental illness that doctors and nurses are trained to recognize and treat – indeed they may sometimes be described as 'not mentally ill' or having 'no treatable mental illness'.

Effects on the staff group

Staff report feeling many contradictory feelings in response to these patients. Some of the more critical and judgemental reactions have already been noted. But along with dismissive and even punitive impulses come reactions of sadness, hopelessness, empathy with the suffering being described and a desire to make things better. A hard-headed decision that this patient is a manipulative attention seeker cannot always be maintained when faced with a patient who is so obviously sad, desperate and in trouble. So individuals can be aware of contradictory feelings within themselves, and similar contradictions can run through the teams as a whole.

The effects of working with this patient group can be summarized under intra-personal effects (i.e. those affecting individual functioning) and inter-personal effects (i.e. those affecting team functioning.)

Intra-personal effects:

- feeling deskilled, thinking 'If only I knew more . . .';
- feeling abused, criticized and overwhelmed by the patient, colleagues, managers and the whole system;
- forgetting or not applying core professional skills;
- calling in sick;
- having to be inauthentic with the patient (e.g. smiling calmly while feeling violently angry);
- having intrusive recollections of traumatic incidents (e.g. dealing with suicide attempts);
- feeling angry with the patient, blaming them for their situation;
- feeling guilty or angry with oneself for having any or all of the above reactions.

Inter-personal effects:

- feeling the team as a whole has no model/skills/facilities for this patient;
- calling in 'experts', feeling deskilled by them and then let down when they cannot help;
- discriminating against this patient because every interaction is interpreted suspiciously;
- spending fruitless time discussing this patient to the exclusion of others;
- feeling angry with the admitting, absent consultant;
- feeling angry with management 'who leave us to get on but will be down like a ton of bricks if there's a problem';
- being overtly or covertly critical of or sabotaging colleagues' work;
- dividing into two or more camps with diametrically opposing views of the patient and no mechanism for resolution.

Staff often refer to there being two camps in respect of these patients. (This is frequently the case in in-patient units, where the care is shared by a number of staff rather than being provided by one or two staff members as in a community mental health team.) These camps could be characterized as having the following differences:

	THE HARD NUTS	THE SOFT CENTRES
How they see the patient	A time-waster, manipulating others to get what they want. Unwilling to take responsibility for themselves.	Genuine, needing to be looked after in times of crisis, needing others to step in and take responsibility.
How they see themselves	Professional, able to maintain boundaries, willing and able to make tough decisions in the best interests of others.	Caring, empathic, non-judgemental, able to see through the chaos to the real person underneath.
How they see the other group	Over-involved, unable to be objective, taken in by the patient, unprofessional.	Defensive, frightened of their own and others' strong feelings, hiding behind procedures, uncaring.
What unspoken model of treatment they adhere to	The 'tough love' model – refusing to bow to demands because this will only lead to further demands.	The 'empty tank' model – just provide enough input to the patient and eventually we'll fill up their emptiness.

It is as if there are only two mutually exclusive explanations for the patient's condition, and staff members must eventually align themselves with one or the other. This is further given as evidence about how the patient 'plays staff off against one another' and the blame for the split is often laid at the patient's door. But splitting can work two ways. Is the patient splitting the team or is the team splitting the patient? Teams complain that the patient acts inconsistently, singles out some team members and acts differently towards them. They may not see the possibility that the team as a whole is acting inconsistently when individual members adopt different attitudes and behaviour towards the same patient. Perhaps the team's inconsistent position is reinforcing – or even causing – the patient's inconsistency?

This divergence happens so frequently and in so many teams that it is probably familiar, in some guise, to practitioners who work in mental health services. It is a divergence that may not be tested too far with most patients, so that a team will function well enough. Indeed, there may be times when having a range of positions is useful, in order to allocate as key worker to any one patient a member of one or the other camp. But there will be times – particularly with the patient group we are discussing – when the divergence stops being a healthy, continuous spectrum of opinion and becomes a thorough-going, reciprocal split. At this point the team is no longer able to respond flexibly to changing patient need but is being driven more by the need to oppose those team members who hold an opposing view; the team is no longer functioning effectively.

Concepts of splitting in psychotherapy

The concept of splitting into polar opposites is one which psycho-analyst Melanie Klein (1975) described in her work in the first half of this century. She saw it as a primitive defence mechanism used by the infant in the first months of life. The infant is confronted with dichotomous, contradictory elements of mother – the 'all-good' mother who provides food and warmth and the 'all-bad' mother who sometimes leaves him/her unsatisfied, or does not come when the child calls. Klein hypothesized that these two concepts are so incompatible that the infant sees his/her mother not as one, integrated figure but as two separate objects.

In the healthy child, whose environment is consistent and whose carers are relatively predictable, this dichotomous, black-and-white, 'either-or' style of thinking disappears by the age of three or so. The thinking style has become more 'both-and', with ambivalence possible and shades of grey tolerable; mother is sometimes good and sometimes bad but she is always the same mother. The philosopher Hegel would have recognized this as a shift towards dialectical thinking; he suggested that the best way to struggle towards truth was through the presentation of one argument (thesis), the countering of this with an opposite view (antithesis) and the integration of these into a single new view (synthesis). The new view incorporates elements from both thesis and antithesis, and as such is integrative, tolerant of ambivalence and more robust than either original argument. Just like the developing infant!

Institutions, organizations and teams can sometimes be described in the same way as individuals and it is possible to see that some teams, for example, might be more integrative and tolerant of ambivalence than others. Less psychologically mature teams will want black-and-white answers to questions, will be anxious with uncertainty or ambivalence and will tend to veer between mutually exclusive and contradictory attitudes towards the same issue from time to time.

Clinical example

John has been admitted again to the 12-bedded community in-patient unit. As usual, the admission came after a visit to casualty. Casualty staff had asked a duty psychiatrist to see him, and he had admitted John because of his description of suicidal thoughts.

Staff on the unit were unhappy with the admission because they had no part in its planning and the admitting psychiatrist had no part in John's treatment after admission. Staff felt that they had been handed a problem and then abandoned. Many people's instinct was to discharge him, but his notes reported suicidal feelings. What if he was discharged and then killed himself? They felt they had to go through a risk assessment process in order to be seen to have followed procedures, even though many were sceptical about the efficacy of the process.

For example, in John's case, in looking at his early life it was clear that his parents treated him inconsistently; sometimes they were over-controlling, punitive and rigid – at others they were *laissez-faire*, unconcerned and even abandoning. He would respond differently to their differing treatment in the reciprocal ways shown in Figure 17.1.

In adult life, it was as if these roles were duplicated with other people at other times. For example, in an admission to hospital (a year before the incident we are now examining) John's thinking had become very disordered, he was very scared and felt he could trust no one. He had been admitted compulsorily to hospital and treated with medication which he did not want. In response to what he saw as controlling and punishing behaviour from the health service he

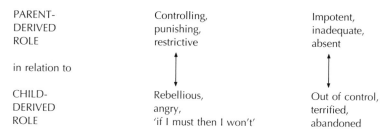

Figure 17.1

became violent, threatening and abusive towards staff. In response to this staff did not know what to do, backed away from him and in the end he was discharged. He felt abandoned and terrified once more.

Here the reciprocal roles were perhaps being repeated, in an interlocking fashion, with the NHS system taking the roles that had been occupied by John's parents in his childhood (Figure 17.2).

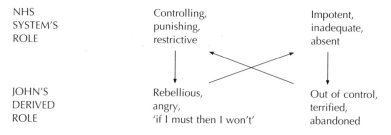

Figure 17.2

Here is where the Kleinian notion of splitting can help us to see what is happening. John himself was subjected as a child to parenting which was not consistent enough to allow him to move from dichotomous thinking to dialectical thinking. He could not arrive at a synthesized, coherent view of his world because his world was not coherent, predictable or stable enough for him to do this.

Unfortunately for John, the team he was now working with was also at this primitive dichotomous level. Having worked for years in a large, Victorian, edge-of-town psychiatric hospital the team was now in a new, small, unit. Set in the middle of the town it was closer to the community it served but much further from the other small units dotted around the town. Some staff saw this as a step forward, others as the wanton destruction of a caring institution. New procedures, new managers, the change from health authorities to an NHS internal market, a radical change in the role, expectations and training of student nurses all provided a rich fund of possible fault lines along which splits could occur. Everybody sought certainty and did so by sticking rigidly to their own thesis, rather than by the more anxiety-provoking process of accommodating other people's antitheses and arriving at a synthesis. For example, younger nurses, with better academic training but less experience, felt angry but impotent at the attitudes of older staff, perceiving them as stuck in the past. The more experienced staff in turn felt threatened by the more highly qualified newcomers and tended to belittle the qualifications as 'no substitute for experience'. Each side felt as though to value what the other was bringing might diminish their own contribution.

It should not be thought that this team were alone in their primitive, dichotomous thinking; the split played out between John and the team was also perhaps being played out between the team and the senior management of the trust. In the team's perception, trust management were of no practical help, and would only get involved if there was a problem when their attitude would be one of imposing procedures, rules or even disciplining staff (Figure 17.3).

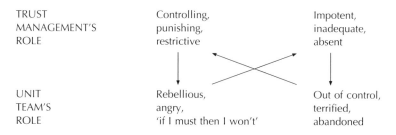

| TRUST MANAGEMENT'S ROLE | Controlling, punishing, restrictive | Impotent, inadequate, absent |
| UNIT TEAM'S ROLE | Rebellious, angry, 'if I must then I won't' | Out of control, terrified, abandoned |

Figure 17.3

The team now find themselves in the same reciprocal role with their higher management that John found himself in with them. It is easy to see that if we expanded the field of view even wider (to include the Department of Health, for example) trust management might find themselves relegated to the underdog roles. And so, like reflections in mirrors facing each other, the game of top dog/underdog gets played out to infinity.

What else could be done? Can the game be avoided somehow? It can if it is possible to get out from between the two mirrors and look, not at the images they generate but the system which they form. Rather than looking *in* the mirrors at the apparent content of the situation we need to stand outside them and look *at* them and perceive the process of the system as a whole. This distinction between process and content is one where psychotherapy can make a contribution to mental health practice —not necessarily by direct therapy with patients but by offering a way of thinking about process, about reciprocal roles and repeating patterns which reveals the way relationships in the present may sometimes replicate those from the past. Dunn and Parry (1997) describe one way this can be done; a short, focused series of assessment sessions from an experienced psychotherapist to determine what reciprocal roles are being played out and by whom.

When this was done in John's case two things happened. First, he himself was given some feedback about how his ways of thinking, feeling and acting might be based on old patterns of relating and might not always be helpful to him now. Second, both he and the team he was working with were given a bird's eye view of themselves sitting, as it were, between the mirrors. None of this was done with any imputation of blame – thus hopefully avoiding the tendency to react by feeling punished, rebellious, impotent or abandoned. Both John and the staff team were able to move towards a Hegelian synthesis of their own positions; the staff became less restrictive and punitive while not throwing up their hands and abandoning John. He in turn was able to take more control over his own actions while not feeling this meant he was being left to his own devices. At the next level up, the fact that this kind of consultancy was available made the team start to think differently about the management of the trust; after all, senior managers had found the resources to make such psychotherapy consultancy available, and were perhaps not entirely punitive or abandoning.

Once the system of mirrors is seen for what it is, the illusion can never be recaptured, and the ever-receding images will never look the same again.

Note

1 The term 'patient' is used throughout this chapter. Recent work in the author's NHS trust appears to show that people who use the NHS mental health services prefer this term to others such as 'user', 'client' or even 'customer'.

References

Dunn, M. and Parry, G. (1997) 'A formulated care plan approach to caring for people with borderline personality disorder in a community mental health service setting', *Clinical Psychology Forum*, 104: 19–22.
Klein, M. (1975) *Envy and Gratitude and Other Works, 1946–63*, New York: Delacote Press.

Recommended reading

Hegel's works are required reading for philosophers but can be hard work for those of other disciplines. The following work gives a good lay person's introduction to Western philosophy: J. Gaarder (1995) *Sophie's World*, London: Phoenix House.

Melanie Klein's writing can be very impenetrable even to specialists in psychotherapy. A good general outline of her work is H. Segal (1978) *Klein*, Glasgow: Fontana/Collins.

Further information about personality disorder and the use of reciprocal role theory is contained in A. Ryle (1997) *Cognitive Analytic Therapy and Borderline Personality Disorder*, Chichester: John Wiley.

18

M. Priestley

Dropping 'E's: the Missing Link in Quality Assurance for Disabled People

... In the current climate of consumerism and user participation, it is useful to consider how the theoretical and practical contributions of organizations controlled by disabled people can be better incorporated in the evaluation of contemporary social policy. The current preoccupation with 'quality' as a policy evaluation tool provides an important opportunity to address this issue.

It is important at the outset to distinguish between two distinct but related aspects of quality – 'quality of service' and 'quality of life'. The linking factor between the two is the formation, implementation and evaluation of social policy. Both the definition of quality and the evaluation of disablement services are inherently value led. They are also interdependent, since services of high quality will be those whose outcomes, structures and processes impact positively on disabled people's quality of life. However, this relationship is in no way simplistic. While there are definite links between quality of life and quality of service, there can be no obvious causal connection – for example, a person may get a poor service but experience a better quality of life due to other contributory factors (and vice versa).

The following discussion deals first with the issues of defining and measuring quality of life. These issues are then related to the definition and measurement of service quality. Specific attention is paid to the design of appropriate quality assurance systems. The discussion concludes with a critical examination of the relationship between 'quality' and 'equality' for disabled people in Britain.

Defining quality of life

It is immediately apparent that the literature on quality of life is characterized by conceptual dichotomy. For example, Rescher (1972) writes of 'artistic' and 'hedonistic' domains while George and Bearon

First published in *Critical Social Policy*, 44/45, 15(2/3): 9–21 (Sage, Autumn 1995). Abridged.

(1980) consider the 'conditions' and 'experiences' of life. Robertson (1985) uses the terms 'welfare' and 'happiness'. Osborne (1992) reviews existing dichotomies in the quality of life literature and attempts to characterize them under the headings 'welfare' and 'well-being', noting that the former has traditionally been associated with objective criteria and the latter with subjective ones.

Quality of life may be defined in terms of physical, cognitive, material and social well-being (e.g. Blunden, 1988) or equated solely with health status (Kaplan, 1985; Williams, 1987) or physical function (Katz et al., 1963). It may be related to the experience of material consumption (Gillingham and Reece, 1979; Ackoff, 1976) or considered in more existential terms – such as the ability to engage in rational and virtuous action (Megone, 1990). It may be measured across whole communities or as an idiosyncratic property of the individual (Brown, 1988).

These differing definitions of life quality give rise to differing conceptual frameworks which, in turn, influence the selection of the evaluation criteria and measurement tools employed in social policy analysis. Ultimately, the value-base used to define 'quality' may be seen to shape the form and content of disablement services. It is a central feature of the argument presented here that definitions of quality (used to judge both disabled people's quality of life and the quality of the services available to them) are derived from, and determined by, a variety of dominant and oppressive social values about the role of disabled people in society (Ritchie, 1994). Thus, Hirst (1990: 72) asserts that the way in which disablement is depicted has implications for social policy because the value judgements used in decision-making are not only technical but also political. In this way, the social construction of 'quality' is inextricably bound up with the social construction of 'disablement'.

The quality standards used to judge disablement services are thus not immutable but dynamic, arising from an ongoing dialectic in which public opinion, political ideology, bureaucratic imperatives, theory, practice, research activity and social movements all make a contribution. Within the current state of this dialectic, the pursuit of greater quality of life and quality of service for disabled people often conflicts with dominant social values. Thus, Richie and Ash (1990: 21) argue of their work on quality that:

> Services which seek to promote valued lives for people with learning disabilities are working against the grain of major economic and social trends. They are working within resource constraints against long-established patterns of service designed to achieve the exact opposite.

Bradley and Bersani (1990) suggest that generally held values about quality of life for non-disabled people may sometimes run counter to the values and life expectations imposed on disabled people as service users. For example, quality of life in a general sense might be said to include the ability to exercise a preference for interdependence over independence (French, 1991), choice over productivity or private over integration. . . .

Quality of service

. . . Increasingly, quality definitions have been imported into the welfare services from industry, a trend which is consistent with policy evaluation approaches based on a production of welfare model (Osborne, 1992) and with the developing marketization of welfare. However, the industrial analogy has its limitations. Nelson (1970), for example, notes that quality information about social care products is generally only available *after* consumption (while industrial products can often be quality measured before purchase). Richie and Ash (1990) draw a clear distinction between industrial and human service processes and suggest that a lack of clarity about the exact identity of the latter's 'products' and 'customers' has resulted in a tendency to define service quality only in relation to inputs (such as the amount of resources available, staffing ratios, etc). The discussion here seeks also to recognize the role of outcomes, processes and service delivery structures.

Outcome-oriented approaches

Bradley and Bersani (1990) argue that the measurement of service quality provides service managers with a means of demonstrating to policy-makers the value of a service in terms of its impact on service users' quality of life. In this respect, they assert that the measurement of service quality should have a particular focus on service outcomes. Conroy and Feinstein (1990) also adopt an outcome-oriented approach to the measurement of service quality. They argue that services should be judged primarily from the disabled person's viewpoint as consumer.

To be consistent with a social model of disablement, outcome measures of service provision should focus on the impact which those services have on the life quality of disabled people. Specifically, they would need to evaluate service delivery outcomes against measures of their success in removing oppressive physical and social barriers from a person's life. Such an approach to service evaluation would thus be in stark contrast to many existing service outcome measures which focus on the disabled person's level of functioning rather than on their disabling environment.

Process-oriented approaches

Ackoff (1976) suggests that traditional approaches to service quality measurement, based on the expected value of outcomes, have failed to recognize the importance of aesthetic factors in service delivery (particularly the 'style' of delivery and the pursuit of ideas). For Ackoff, people have preferences and ascribe value to means as well as ends. Parmenter is concerned that traditional approaches to outcome-oriented studies have been dominated by empiricism rather than theory. Thus 'we have tended to emphasise regular features or structures to the neglect of processes in our study of disability, possibly because it is easier to measure static structures more reliably' (1988: 9). Culyer (1990) points out that demand for a service may often be confused with demand for the *characteristics* of that service. It might be argued, for example, that it is not 'personal assistance' or 'benefits' that many disabled people want, but the greater 'independence' or 'freedom of choice' which they feel such services might bring. Thus, Culyer is concerned that while users may appear to value a service it may well be the characteristics of that service which they value. In this case it is equally possible that such characteristics might be available in a different mode of service delivery. An alternative to the preoccupation with outcome and process measurement is to consider whether there are identifiable attributes of a service delivery structure which lend it added quality – by facilitating positive outcomes and processes. It is argued here that the degree of service user participation and control may constitute a useful quality measure in this respect. (Bornat et al., 1985, use the term 'participation standards' in relation to services for older people.)

There is, it would seem, a fundamental flaw in the preoccupation of service purchasers, providers and policy-makers with the measurement of life quality for disabled people. Ackoff (1976: 299) argues that the policy problem should not be how to improve other people's quality of life but *'how to enable them to improve their own quality of life'*. It is significant that this reformulated problem does not require life quality measures for its solution. Thus 'the key to improved quality of life is not planning for or measurement of others, but enabling them to plan and measure for themselves' (p. 303). In a similar way, O'Brien (1990: 20) argues that 'human services organisations cannot manufacture better lives. People weave better lives from the resources afforded by individual effort, personal relationships, available opportunities, and help from services'.

It is thus possible to envisage an approach to service quality measurement which takes into account not only the established criteria of outcomes and process but also the service delivery structure, in terms of the degree to which that structure facilitates and empowers disabled people. The recognition that service structures which empower users to improve their own quality of life may have intrinsic value is of paramount importance in considering the potential role of organizations controlled by disabled people as potential providers of community care services, since such organizations are most likely to be able to demonstrate genuinely participative service delivery structures.

Designing a quality assurance system

Having reviewed differing approaches to the measurement of service quality it is important to consider the mechanisms by which that quality might be assured. Specifically, it is relevant to consider how quality assurance (QA) systems might incorporate the ideals, processes and structures required by a social model of disablement.

Firstly, it is likely that service providers will bear the primary responsibility of quality assurance. Common and Flynn (1992: 26) argue that it is logical that service providers rather than purchasers should have the central role in developing QA systems, since 'it is they who deal with the client and have to implement appropriate procedures'. . . .

In the light of the initial discussion on the value-led nature of quality measurement, it is important to note that different service provider organizations will tend to generate different QA systems which reflect their organizational values and goals. Quality measurement which operates within a social model of disablement will thus require service provider organizations committed to the social emancipation of disabled people. It is arguable that organizations within the disabled people's movement are uniquely placed to fulfil this requirement.

Secondly, the values and goals on which a service is based would need to be explored and made overt within the provider organization. Both Bradley and Bersani (1990) and Richie and Ash (1990) express concern that many existing QA systems are aimed at maintaining a 'lowest common denominator' of minimum standards rather than providing 'benchmarks' to inspire service providers towards outstanding performance. In line with arguments presented earlier, O'Brien (1990) emphasizes the central role of 'vision' and 'organisational purpose' in developing high-quality disability services, Rhodes (1987) and Richie and Ash (1990) note that strong organizational values are also a key element of quality assurance systems imported from industry. Thus, O'Brien recommends that a successful QA system should strive to be visionary by incorporating the ongoing discussion, articulation, clarification and sharing of ideals relating to a better future for disabled people. Such a process should seek to identify tensions between the existing situation and the service ideal; it should wherever possible seek out opportunities to act consistently with the vision.

Thirdly, a successful quality assurance system would need to operate within a participative structure. Bradley and Bersani (1990) suggest that as disabled people become more integrated ('invisible') in society, the need for effective monitoring becomes ever greater, yet 'real' homes should be free from the bureaucratic scrutiny often associated with quality assurance. In this context, they suggest that disabled people themselves can make an important contribution to an unobtrusive and successful monitoring process: 'using other people with disabilities to serve as independent monitors can assist in maintaining the integrity of consumers and their living and working arrangements' (1990: 347). Again it is tempting to note that organizations controlled by disabled people are particularly well placed to design and implement quality assurance systems within this model.

Conclusions: quality and equality

This discussion began by seeking to review critically traditional approaches to quality and quality measurement within the context of a social model of disablement. Aggregate measurements of life quality for whole communities (such as social indicators research and large-scale psychological studies) have tended to contribute to the oppression of disabled people by obscuring both their presence and their needs. Life quality measures targeted specifically at disabled populations have sustained that oppression by medicalizing the state of disablement. Existing service quality measures have valued functional outcomes and administrative hegemony over participative processes and structures.

It is important at this stage to reconsider the points made at the outset about the relationship between quality of life and quality of service. While there is (or should be) a clear link between the two, there can be no necessary causal association. More to the point, it can be argued that assuring service quality *alone* can never be a sufficient condition for improving disabled people's quality of life (although it may be a necessary one). There is a danger in becoming preoccupied with the technicalities of quality assurance systems in the delivery of services at the expense of considering life quality issues which are beyond the reach and scope of 'services' (see Oliver, 1991). Specifically, there is a danger of employing 'quality' as an inadequate conceptual substitute for the notion of 'equality'. . . .

The Local Government Management Board (1991) make an explicit link between the notions of quality and equality, linking recent work on quality by local authorities with simultaneous advances in local equal opportunities policies. The two themes are related through the overarching concept of 'service to the whole community'. Thus 'the phrase "service to the whole community" describes an approach which integrates quality and equality, a way of working which sees these two themes as interrelated and interdependent rather than separate' (1991: 1).

It is inherent within this approach to quality that the service provider (and local authority purchaser) is required not only to treat each person as an individual customer but also to recognize that person's identity as a member of a particular group within the community. If applied to the present context, such an integrated approach requires authorities to recognize and respond to disabled people both as customers with *individual needs* for services and also as members of an oppressed group in the community with *collective needs* for equal civil rights.

The argument presented here suggests that organizations controlled by disabled people have a unique contribution to make in the pursuit of quality. They are well placed to act both as providers of participative community care services to individuals and as the collective representatives of disabled people's needs for civil rights. . . .

References

Ackoff, R. (1976) 'Does quality of life have to be quantified?', *Operational Research Quarterly*, 27: 289–303.

Blunden, R. (1988) 'Quality of life in persons with disabilities: issues in the development of services' in R. Brown (ed.) *Quality of Life for Handicapped People*, London: Croom Helm.

Bornat, J. et al. (1985) *A Manifesto for Old Age*, London: Pluto.

Bradley, V. and Bersani, H. (1990) 'The future of quality assurance: it's everybody's business', in V. Bradley and H. Bersani (eds) *Quality Assurance for Individuals with Developmental Disabilities*, Paul H. Brookes.

Brown, R. (ed.) (1988) *Quality of Life for Handicapped People*, London: Croom Helm.

Common, R. and Flynn, N. (1992) *Contracting for Care*, York: Joseph Rowntree Foundation.

Conroy, J. and Feinstein, C. (1990) 'A new way of thinking about quality', in V. Bradley and H. Bersani (eds) *Quality Assurance for Individuals with Developmental Disabilities*, Paul H. Brookes.

Culyer, A. (1990) 'Commodities, characteristics of commodities, characteristics of people, utilities, and the quality of life', in S. Baldwin et al. (eds) *Quality of Life: Perspectives and Policies*, London: Routledge.

French, S. (1991) 'What's so great about independence?', *New Beacon*, April: 2–3.

George, L. and Bearon, L. (1980) *Quality of Life in Older Persons*, Human Sciences Press.

Gillingham, R. and Reece, W. (1979) 'A new approach to quality of life measurement', *Urban Studies*, 16: 329–32.

Hirst, M. (1990) 'Multidimensional representations of disablement: a qualitative approach', in S. Baldwin et al. (eds) *Quality of Life: Perspectives and Policies*. London: Routledge.

Kaplan, R. (1985) 'Quality of life measurement', in P. Koroly (ed.) *Measurement Strategies in Health Psychology*, Chichester: Wiley.

Katz, S. et al. (1963) 'Studies of illness in the aged: the index of ADL', *Journal of the American Association*, 185: 914–19.

Local Government Management Board (1991) *Quality and Equality: Services to the Whole Community*, Birmingham University/LGMB.

Megone, C. (1990) 'The quality of life: starting from Aristotle', in S. Baldwin et al (eds) *Quality of Life: Perspectives and Policies*, London: Routledge.

Nelson, P. (1970) 'Information and consumers behaviour', *Journal of Political Economy*, 78: 311–29.

O'Brien, J. (1990) 'Developing high quality services for people with developmental disabilities', in V. Bradley and H. Bersani (eds) *Quality Assurance for Individuals with Developmental Disabilities*, Paul H. Brookes.

Oliver, M. (1991) 'Speaking out: disabled people and the welfare state', in G. Dalley (ed.) *Disability and Social Policy*, London: Policy Studies Institute.

Osborne, S.P. (1992) 'The quality dimension: evaluating quality of service and quality of life in human services', *British Journal of Social Work*, 22: 437–53.

Parmenter, T. (1988) 'An analysis of the dimensions of quality of life for people with physical disabilities', in R. Brown (ed.) *Quality of Life for Handicapped People*, London: Routledge.

Rescher, (1972) *Welfare: Social Issues in Philosophical Perspective*, Pittsburgh: Pittsburgh University Press.

Richie, P. and Ash, A. (1990) 'Quality in action: improving services through quality action groups', in T. Booth (ed.) *Better Lives: Changing Services for People with Learning Difficulties*, Joint Unit for Social Services Research, Sheffield University.

Ritchie, P. (1994) 'The process of quality assurance', in R. Davidson and S. Hunter (eds) *Community Care in Practice*, London: Batsford.

Robertson, A. (1985) 'Social Services planning and the quality of life', in A. Robertson and A. Osborn (eds) *Planning to Care*, Aldershot: Gower.

Williams, A. (1987) 'Measuring quality of life', in G. Teeling Smith (ed.) *Health Economics: Prospects for the Future*, London: Croom Helm.

19

P. Beresford, S. Croft, C. Evans and T. Harding

Quality in Personal Social Services: The Developing Role of User Involvement in the UK

. . .

The growth of the user perspective

The shift towards a market ideology coincides with the emergence of increasingly vocal, well-organized and effective independent service users' organizations and movements. This emergence is a worldwide as well as European development, with growing movements of disabled people, people with learning difficulties, older people, psychiatric system survivors and people living with HIV/AIDS in many different countries.

While progress is sometimes slow and often uneven, the disability and service user movements in the UK have scored some notable achievements. The Disability Discrimination Act is now on the statute book (though a much weaker version than had been hoped for); and legislation to give people the option to receive cash to arrange their own support in lieu of services arranged by the local authority care manager is now in place. This legislation (the Community Care [Direct Payments] Act 1996) has been fought for by disabled people, psychiatric system survivors and people with learning difficulties to enable them to have control over the nature, purpose and quality of the assistance they receive, and it is a notable achievement that it has reached the statute book in a recognizable form, in spite of its (in the UK welfare system) revolutionary nature. If service users are to be seen as consumers, there could not be clearer evidence that existing social service provision was failing to deliver what at least some consumers wanted; they have taken steps

First published in A. Ever, R. Haverinen, K. Leichsenring and G. Wistow (eds) *Developing Quality in Personal Social Services: Concepts, Cases and Comments* (European Centre Visuals, 1977), pp. 63–80. Abridged.

to ensure that they themselves will in future do the purchasing, instead of the local authority. They will be true consumers, with real purchasing power. (However, it seems likely at present that only a minority of service users will opt for direct payments, not least because of restrictions on eligibility.)

At the local level, organizations run by service users themselves have in places developed their own independent living schemes and other direct services, and all over the country, disabled people and other service users have formed groups to work together and exert greater influence over the environments and conditions which affect their lives.

Most local authorities and managers responsible for planning and providing services now recognize, at least in principle, that it is important to consult and involve service users in the decisions that affect their lives. The values of social justice and respect for individuals that lie behind that message accord with those of many social service professionals (Morris, 1994), and strong encouragement from the Department of Health in its guidance documents and progress reports has given weight and legitimacy to those principles. It is rare these days for social service professionals not to acknowledge the importance of consulting and involving service users in all aspects of service planning and development.

So a key feature of the community care reforms has been to emphasize the centrality of the service user in policy and practice. Both service user organizations and service agencies have been concerned to ensure service users a more active role in decisions affecting them and in the organizations responsible for taking those decisions. The 1990s have seen a considerable growth of initiatives for 'user involvement' in the planning and development of services, and a plethora of consultations, market research exercises, participative forums, committees and groups, set up by health and welfare agencies, at local, regional and sometimes national level.

However, such involvement has not always been effective. While much has been learned, many initiatives are now being re-evaluated by service users' organizations and independent researchers, both of whom highlight their limited impact and effectiveness and the significant costs, both personal and in terms of resources, to service users.

At the root of the problem, it seems that both the idea of user involvement and schemes for user involvement have frequently become distanced from service users' actual experience of and preferences for services. They have been too removed from reality, too distant from the coal face to have an impact on the day-to-day experience of service users.

User involvement has largely focused on consultation about the drawing up of annual community care plans by local social services departments, which is a requirement of the legislation. Such plans, which are more often descriptive than prescriptive, have only a distant relationship with day-to-day service delivery, and it is hard for those who have been involved and consulted to see the impact of their work. User involvement in this context tends to become 'bureaucratized'.

Less attention has been paid by service agencies to how service users can play a more central role in influencing the nature and quality of the services and support they receive as individuals. But it is this that is likely to be the priority for most service users and is the underlying rationale behind the idea of user involvement. Service users' organizations themselves are increasingly measuring the value of their involvement in terms of the degree of control individuals can gain as a result, over their own lives and over the interventions of the agencies, services and practitioners which affect them, which entails both individual and collective action. Many attempts at user involvement to date have missed the mark because they have failed to address the issues of purpose and quality most central to users' concerns.

Bringing service users more fully into the debate about what constitutes quality would, then, more closely reflect their concerns and priorities and give greater purpose to their role.

Obstacles to user involvement in the quality debate

What then are the obstacles to user involvement in the debate about the quality of services, and how can these be overcome? We suggest that there are three key kinds of obstacle which inhibit full effectiveness: the communication difficulties to be overcome before service users and providers can engage with each other on a basis of equality; the nature of the competing discourses; and the values which each party brings to the debate.

Communication difficulties to be overcome

All attempts at user involvement face certain basic difficulties due to the unequal roles and relationships involved.

Firstly, service users themselves are disempowered. It is not easy to participate on a basis of equality with powerful professionals, when people have spent a considerable period – sometimes a lifetime – without control over the decisions which affect their lives and unable to exercise much autonomy. It takes time and resources, as well as determination, for service users to build confidence, decide what they want and make themselves heard. The source of such confidence is usually other service users; the role of independent service user organizations is therefore crucial, and this takes time and resources to develop. Until service users have a sense of and confidence in the validity of the contribution they have to make, it will be difficult to establish relationships of trust with professionals and to work together on a basis of mutual respect.

Secondly, the agenda for such involvement is usually set by the professionals involved; not only does that create instant inequality, but the agenda itself and the whole style of working, the way meetings are conducted, the language used, appear obscure and alienating.

Thirdly, amongst both service users and service providers, there are real obstacles to open dialogue, due to fears and anxieties on both sides. The views of service users are often a real challenge to the received wisdom of many professionals. Service users often fear the power professionals have to influence their lives. These fears are deep-seated and genuine and can readily become real obstacles to communication.

Fourthly, it is often difficult for service users to see that their involvement has any effect. It is only by seeing results that service users can have confidence that they are influencing services and creating change. If there is no change, or no feedback about changes that have occurred, then motivation is quickly lost.

Finally there are numerous competing agendas and priorities to that of user involvement; the prevailing culture within local authorities is one in which professional concerns and managerial resource control are the overwhelming priorities. User involvement is set against a background of turbulent organizational change, as social services departments separate their 'purchasing' and 'providing' roles, local government undergoes a massive redrawing of geographical boundaries, and the interface between health and local authority responsibilities shifts significantly, putting additional pressures on social services. Service agencies are bombarded by challenges on many fronts. Unless user involvement is an integral part of all aspects of service development, it is very easy for it to be relegated to a side issue, where it fails to have a significant impact.

Competing discourses

When it comes to the debate about quality, it quickly becomes apparent from the UK experience (and this does not seem to be isolated) that there is not so much one set of discussions going on, as several, including academic, professional, managerial and political debates. While these are overlapping and to some extent interchangeable, a more fundamental distinction can be drawn between personal social services agencies' and service users' discussions or discourses.

The discourses from these two constituencies are fundamentally different in nature, and they do not sit comfortably together. The terms of the debate are significantly and qualitatively different in their objectives, philosophy, concerns, forms and process.

Service agency discourse, not surprisingly, is primarily concerned with policy and services; with service organization, management, efficiency, effectiveness and economy. The involvement of service users in this context is primarily as a source of data to help manage restricted resources, to inform rationing and targeting decisions and to set priorities. The focus has been on refining and adjusting services, not on substantive change. Decision-making has remained with the agencies.

Service users' discourse is concerned much more explicitly and specifically with people's lives; with managing their lives, dealing with difficulties, securing suitable support to live as they want to, maintaining or increasing choices and opportunities and challenging restrictions and obstructions which they face. This discourse is not concerned narrowly with specialist or dedicated health and welfare support and service systems, but also with access to the mainstream: to employment, education, training, public transport and recreation.

The central concern of service users' organizations is to increase people's control over their lives and over the way agencies intervene in them. They place particular priority on ideas and objectives of participation, inclusion, equality, autonomy and rights, stressing the achievement of their civil and human rights, rather than just welfare rights (Croft and Beresford, 1995).

> It is important to us that our involvement is based on our terms and within a background of rights: the rights that we have as citizens like any others – the democratic right to participate in society and to have choice and control over our lives – which must mean that we have as much choice and control as we can over the services we receive. (Evans, 1995)

Service agencies' and service users' discourses therefore reflect totally different starting points, different value bases and different purposes. They have significantly different personal, professional, political and organizational concerns. Under those circumstances, a dialogue is not going to be easy; assumptions have to be questioned and some hard listening done on both sides if people are to understand each other's concerns.

Different values

One of the clearest expressions of the different ideologies and value bases of service users' organizations on the one hand and of service agencies and professionals on the other, consists of the models and theories developed by service users. A key example is the social model of disability developed by members of the disabled people's movement.

Thanks to this new thinking, there are now competing models of what disability is and how it is perceived. These have been labelled as the 'medical' and 'social' models of disability, although Oliver, the disability activist and academic, prefers a slightly different distinction:

> In short for me, there is no such thing as the medical model of disability, there is instead, an individual model of disability of which medicalization is one significant component. . . . The individual model 'locates the problem' of disability within the individual . . . it sees the causes of this problem as stemming from the functional limitations or psychological losses which are assumed to arise from disability.
>
> Disability, according to the social model, is all the things that impose restrictions on disabled people; ranging from individual prejudice to institutional discrimination, from inaccessible public buildings to unusable public transport systems, from segregated education to excluding work arrangements, and so on. Further, the consequences of this failure do not simply and randomly fall on individuals, but systematically upon disabled people as a group who experience this failure as discrimination institutionalized throughout society. (Oliver, 1996: 31–3)

By drawing the distinction between individual impairment and social disablement, the social model of disability enables disabled people to locate the restrictions and problems they experience and make sense of their social relations. Similar developments have taken place among the movements of people with learning difficulties, older people, psychiatric system survivors and people living with AIDS, and these have similarly made it possible for people to reassess the roles and identity attached to them, the oppression they experience and ways in which their rights and needs are or, more often, are not met.

Where the way one sees and interprets the world and its impact on the individual is so fundamentally at variance between two parties to a discussion, it is going to require a great deal of goodwill and a lot of patience to reach understanding. Furthermore, there is an imbalance of power and resources between the two perspectives, which makes such a dialogue even harder to achieve. Disabled people's and other service users' organizations have less funding, less credibility, less support and less access to the mainstream. They cannot assume that their agendas and proposals will be readily accepted either by the service system or by broader society. Instead they see struggling for the acceptance of their goals as an inherent part of what they must do.

Definitions of quality, of course, are based on and emerge from values, whether these are explicit or implicit. Writing about quality assurance for disabled people, Priestley argues that the definition of service quality is value-led and that dominant ideologies have contributed to the continued oppression of disabled people:

Definitions of quality (used to judge both disabled people's quality of life and the quality of the services available to them) are derived from and determined by a variety of dominant and oppressive social values about the role of disabled people in society. . . . In this way, the social construction of 'quality' is inextricably bound up with the social constriction of 'disablement'. (Priestley, 1995: 7, 10, 11; see also Priestley, this volume)

Where service users dispute the dominant values, they are also likely to dispute the quality of services framed within those values. For example, psychiatric system survivors who reject a psychiatric model of 'mental illness' are likely to be equally critical of 'treatments' based on a medical model, whether or not those meet other criteria for quality. People with learning difficulties who challenge measures of intellectual or 'mental' age attached to them, which equate them with children, are similarly likely to be unsympathetic to quality measures built on such (implicit) assumptions about their abilities and emotional development. A segregating institutional service for service users who want to take part in mainstream recreational and occupational activities is likely to fail their quality test, even if it has very high material standards, offers sensitive and appropriate personal support and ensures good accessibility within its premises.

Agencies might develop quality measures for their provision and services based on ideas of ensuring 'quality of life', physical conditions and personal rights within them consistent with broader dominant standards; but if such provision and services are not consistent with service users' *own* priorities for their inclusion, participation, autonomy and civil rights, then their movements would be unlikely to accept them as satisfactory.

These three kinds of obstacle to the involvement of service users in defining quality present a somewhat formidable barrier. But there is already a growing body of experience and confidence that such barriers can be overcome, given the will to do so. If quality standards are to reflect the values and choices of service users, service users need to be brought into the centre of the debate about quality. . . .

Conclusion

Service users are judging the quality of services in two ways: they are concerned that services will help them achieve the outcomes they aspire to; and they are concerned that services are delivered in ways which empower rather than disempower them and their peers as individuals. The motivation for getting involved with service agencies is primarily to achieve these two objectives. User involvement is not an end in itself, but a means of effecting change both in the outcome of services and in the behaviour of workers.

> We are very proactive in seeking opportunities for user involvement. . . .
> The aim is not participation for the sake of it . . . it is actually to bring
> about change. Users in the network say 'What is the point of me going and
> being involved, what effect will it have?' and they will not go and
> participate unless they know that they are going to be able to have an
> effect by giving their perspective as service users. (Evans, 1995)

It is encouraging that in the UK currently there is a new focus on the
outcome of services – not on organizational structure or efficient
systems alone, but on the basic purpose of services and what they are
there for.

As with the debate about quality, there is an ever-present risk that
it is service providers alone who will set the parameters by which
outcomes are defined and specified. But a new project, funded by the
Department of Health, is setting out to enable service users to
develop their own definitions of outcomes: to create the space and the
opportunity for people from service user organizations to define
desired outcomes from the point of view of their own values, their
own priorities and their own form of discourse.

It seems likely that service users will want to avoid coming up with
any predetermined set of quality standards. Rather they are more
likely to see quality as the extent to which services enable individuals
to meet their own aspirations, which will vary from person to person;
and as the extent to which they enable people to enhance control over
their own lives.

In this context, the participation of service users can be seen as
both a route to quality and a measure or criterion of it.

It offers a route to quality in the sense that service users are fully
involved in defining, developing, monitoring and evaluating quality
according to their own values. Participation is also a criterion of
quality since a key objective is that service users have more say and
control over their lives and over decision-making about the specific
service or arrangements for support.

This approach begins to offer a new paradigm for assessing quality
in the personal social services, based neither on a business nor a
professional model but rather on a model of personal autonomy and
respect for individual choice.

References

Croft, S. and Beresford, P. (1995) 'Whose empowerment? Equalising the competing
    discourses in community care', in R. Jack (ed.) *Empowerment in Community Care*,
    London: Chapman and Hall. pp. 59–76.
Evans, C. (1995) 'Disability, discrimination and local authority social services – users'
    perspectives', in G. Zarb (ed.) *Removing Disabling Barriers*, London: Policy Studies
    Institute.
Morris, J. (1994) *The Shape of Things to Come? User-led Social Services*, London: Social
    Services Policy Forum, National Institute for Social Work.

Oliver, M. (1996) *Understanding Disability: From Theory to Practice*, Basingstoke: Macmillan.

Priestley, M. (1995) 'Dropping "E's": the missing link in quality assurance for disabled people', *Critical Social Policy*, 44/45: 7–21.

PART IV

COPING: CHALLENGES AND CONSTRAINTS

What are the conditions that enable practitioners in health and social care not just to cope but to cope constructively with the diversity of challenges that others bring? Some of the answers can be found in Part III of the present book. What helps, however, when practice is severely constrained by factors which individuals and immediate work groups cannot easily address or control? Part IV deals with a range of these.

David Thompson and his colleagues, in what is still an all too rare account of the dilemmas of gender in daily practice, focus on a setting in which the behaviour of men with learning difficulties, in day care regimes that have become more sexually liberal, poses dilemmas for women staff. Defining just what behaviour is unacceptable and abusive – both towards female staff and towards clients – can be particularly difficult. Treading a line between conforming to gendered assumptions about being caring yet keeping a distance is shown to be a real dilemma. Clear acknowledgement of the issue by co-workers and well-developed management guidance, the authors suggest, are needed if staff are not themselves to be abused and are to cope more positively. Writing in a more abstract way, Pam Smith and Ellen Agard show that gender poses dilemmas for staff in nursing more generally. Nursing work is classically coping work – picking up the tasks that others have left, doing whatever is needed in the interests of the patient. But an ethos of committed caring that owes so much to implicit ideas about women, they argue, has restricted practice and devalued nursing. And in times when managers challenge costs, more explicit arguments about the value of the work are needed. Without these, it can be particularly hard to describe and defend the use of skilled nurses to provide care.

This brings us to the matter of giving an account of your practice to significant and possibly threatening others – be those others clients or managers, members of elected and appointed boards or representatives of external regulatory bodies. Employing an unusual technique of three 'staged' dialogues, Steven Shardlow teases out issues of accountability and confidentiality for the front-line social worker. His fictional client asks just what a social worker keeps confidential and how a client might check up on this. The conversations reveal what a fine line there is to be drawn between statutory obligations, duties to the employer and responsibilities to a client. Accountability and confidentiality, the writer concludes, can come into collision. Putting abstract concepts into practice in a way clients can accept is also no easy matter.

Two linked chapters then follow. Nick Black and Elizabeth Thompson interviewed doctors in the early days of medical audit after the 1990 NHS and Community Care Act. They vividly reveal the mix of emotions and the strategies to embrace or evade these new demands which were being employed by members of a profession until then quite unused to any questioning of its performance. Today, with clinical governance on the cards for all clinicians and new forms of inspection both in the NHS and in local government, it is important to ask how far structures for monitoring and review take account of human dimensions and histories. Monitoring cannot succeed unless the monitored respect the monitors. Those being monitored also need a chance to influence the monitoring tools that are in use and to feel that they have not just the one opportunity but a series of opportunities to put things right, to learn from the process and to demonstrate progressive improvements. Ellie Scrivens's chapter is a rare account of what it feels like to be on the receiving end of a process of inspecting and judging standards of work in a hospital setting. The importance of good preparation of staff, the significance of the stance of those visiting on the day, the quality of report preparation and the extent of follow-up, were all important factors in the perceived usefulness of the process. These factors offer clues to answering the question with which the introduction to this part of the book opened.

Chris Corkish and Bob Heyman bring the focus back to learning disability. The resettlement of residents of long-stay institutions into small homes in the community, alongside commitments to respecting user needs and preferences, raises questions of safety, protection and risk. These authors hold out the alarming prospect of environments being impoverished and options being closed down as reactions to one unfortunate incident after another result in the withdrawal of freedoms and opportunities from clients on the grounds of their safety and protection. How much better, they argue, if risk appraisals can be shown to have been regularly and proactively carried out for individual clients.

The final two chapters shift the angle of vision to demands being made on those working in health and social care to adjust to new contexts and to maintain their essential values and commitments in a new and often much changed climate. Margaret Harris gives a vivid account of the way that demands on voluntary organizations to be direct service providers have brought new kinds of people into their management. A loss of founders' values and visions can ensue. Diana Leat and Elizabeth Perkins deal with the dilemmas of social workers who in recent years have found themselves in care manager roles. Once again, there is the difficulty of remaining true to values while working with new demands. What unites these voluntary sector providers and care managers with others discussed in this section is their shared need to cope with change, to acknowledge that situations carry risks and may not be the ideal ones in which they would like to work. Such situations, nevertheless, may still provide opportunities for responsive and sensitive practice that is capable of further improvement.

The real key, perhaps, to coping with the challenges of others is a proactive working through of policies, a realistic attitude to constraints, a confidence in current practice and a willingness to countenance, indeed welcome, the possibility of change. Practice will not always be perfect, but it does need to be defensible, rather than defensive.

20

D. Thompson, I. Clare and H. Brown

Not Such an 'Ordinary' Relationship: the Role of Women Support Staff in Relation to Men with Learning Disabilities Who Have Difficult Sexual Behaviour

. . . This chapter shows how acutely aware some women staff are of the contradictions within their role so that they are put in a double bind when it comes to performing their caring responsibilities without compounding the risk of sexual harassment from their male clients. The pilot study which we describe seeks to identify how this dilemma is managed. It shows how women staff set boundaries in their practice with men with learning disabilities and seek to clarify the nature of the relationship between them. The fact that women have to make isolated, individual responses to protect themselves from abuse indicates how learning disability services fall into the trap of locating responsibility for abuse with the person who is a 'victim' rather than identifying the behaviour of men with learning disabilities as a concern for the whole agency and taking appropriate collective action.

As part of a wider study of men with learning disabilities with unacceptable/abusive sexual behaviour, focus groups were set up to ascertain staff perceptions about men who use their services. Aside from their potential to provide 'believable' qualitative data (Kruger, 1994: 8), it was believed that the process would usefully mirror the discussions within staff teams and case conferences. Four groups were run to explore the kinds of problems which service workers face with respect to the sexual behaviour of male service users; to avoid prejudicing the enquiry participants were asked to explore what they actually experience as 'difficult' rather than to limit themselves to a preset definition of unacceptable or abusive behaviour. . . .

First published in *Disability and Society*, 12(4): 573–92 (Carfax Publishing, 1997). Abridged.

Prior to any discussion, participants were asked to complete information sheets with descriptions of the 'difficult' sexual behaviour of up to three men with learning disabilities with whom they had some current contact: some participants did not fill out any forms because they were not aware of men who fulfilled the criteria. The aims of this were to provide data about the range of sexual behaviour which is defined by service workers as difficult or challenging, but also to provide a pool of potential case studies. A procedure for confidentiality was agreed with the host districts which allowed, at this stage, for details of men's behaviour to be available to the research team without any personal identifiable information. This procedure supplemented research ethics committee approval for the study from the relevant health agencies in both districts. . . .

Historically, people with learning disabilities have been subjected to the blanket repression of their sexual options, a legacy of which is that for many services any sexual behaviour is framed as difficult; however, an examination of the information sheets showed that the participants had been discerning in the behaviour they had described. We categorized the behaviour under the following headings:

- unconsented sexual behaviour, that is with a partner who has not consented, could not consent or was being unduly pressured into consenting;
- behaviour where consent was questionable;
- concern about masturbation;
- behaviour which, though not intrinsically abusive, was difficult because staff had to witness it;
- frustration and perceived unmet sexual desires;
- conflicting sexual values between family, staff and the man himself;
- experience of being sexually abused, as opposed to sexually abusing.

. . . Sometimes it was not obvious why a particular behaviour was deemed to be a problem; for example, 'cross-dressing' and spending 'considerable time in bed masturbating' were cited, but it is unclear whether staff found these a problem because of their own embarrassment or because they impinged unfairly on other users or were seen to cause problems for the men themselves in terms of exclusion from more valued activities or social stigma.

Table 20.2 shows that of the total of 32 men, 23 had been identified as instigating some form of sexual behaviour towards an unconsenting person. In nine instances there were concerns about the man's masturbation: these included potential harm to himself, the use of inappropriate places, lack of success and suggestions that it was being done too much. For two men it appeared that other people's

Table 20.2 *'Difficult' behaviour patterns*

Category	Example	No.
Unconsented sexual behaviour, i.e. sexual abuse/sexual harassment	'Continually touching other people's genitals' 'Verbal threats to others of aggressive sexual acts'	23
Behaviour where consent was questioned	'. . . He has been found in toilets in day centre with men. It is difficult to be clear whether these men are consenting'	1
Concern about masturbation	'Anal masturbation difficult because of health issues to himself . . .' 'Continued masturbation to the point of penis bleeding'	9
Witness of non-abusive sexual behaviour	'Sexual activity with (willing) women but in inappropriate places' 'Cross dressing'	2
Frustration and perceived unmet sexual desires	e.g. 'He is aware of his needs but unable to fulfil'	2
Conflicting sexual values	'Is confused on conflict between family education and emotional physical needs'	1
Inappropriate attachments	i.e. 'Forms strong inappropriate attachments to a female'	1
Experience of having been sexually abused	i.e. 'Sexually abused by a group (2)–(3) of other men in his residential home'	1

awareness of the sexual behaviour was the problem rather than the behaviour *per se*. Only one case was cited in which the task of establishing the consent of participating individuals was difficult. One participant identified two men whose 'needs' they considered were being 'unfulfilled'. The same person also identified that one of these men was experiencing conflict between his family's religious perspective on sexuality and the liberal views of his service. One case was reported of a man forming inappropriate attachments to women staff and another was described as presenting difficulties to staff as a result of being sexually abused.[1] Added to this list is the risk of HIV to men with learning disabilities having sex with men, which was identified by one participant at the start of the focus group. . . .

The discussions within the focus groups provide a more detailed picture of the ways these men's behaviour had been construed and responded to within their services. In other areas of sexual abuse research the choice of terminology is thought to be an indicator of how seriously the behaviour is regarded. More commonly, the men were said to have 'inappropriate sexual behaviour', a term which masks the impact of this behaviour for any victim: participants avoided terms such as sexual abuse or sexual assault even though these offer more valid descriptions of much of the men's behaviour. Although the behaviour was not named as sexual assault or harassment, it was evident that for staff, particularly women, the men's behaviour presented not just a management issue, but was experienced as an intrusion, as these examples illustrate:

> . . . whilst working with a female member of staff on his own, he actually got them into a grip and that person felt they couldn't get away.

> . . . he actually comments quite a lot on your physical, you know appearance.

Women described how the job they were employed to do exposed them to situations that were very uncomfortable and for which they had little training or forewarning. For example, there seemed no limits for women offering personal support:

> [When we go] in to help with this hygiene, he plays with his penis every morning.

> She still found it a real shock to take the men to the loo. . . . She had never seen naked men before.

One focus group participant noted that it was not only staff who were in this predicament, family members also had to witness men's sexual behaviour during the provision of intimate support. Furthermore, it was clearly a difficult subject for support staff to acknowledge and one mother had confided that

> what she really found dreadful to speak about was that when she was bathing her son he was masturbating and this was something she couldn't share with other people.

In addition to the women's forced observation of the men's behaviour, they described how at times they felt lured into the men's sexual world:

> . . . if he has an enormous erection on and he doesn't want you to leave, it feels like you are being drawn into somebody else's personal space.

> You are drawn into some sexual fantasy without your consent.

Because being touched by men with learning disabilities was accepted by women staff in some situations they were left in a vulnerable position when individual men overstepped the boundary by initiating intimate sexual contact.

Although participants displayed little doubt when people without learning disabilities, including themselves, had been sexually violated they found it more difficult to 'draw the line' between acceptable and unacceptable behaviour where service users were on the receiving end. Examples of such dilemmas were:

> He would encourage our users into the toilets . . . but quite vulnerable people were involved.

> . . . there was some sexual activity going on and it was seen by a member of staff and because this woman can't communicate through speech it was

automatically assumed that the man was the one who was leading the situation. But on further observation it was thought that this may not be the situation, although we couldn't be sure.

These statements show that staff have moved away from the historical prohibition of sex for people with learning disabilities to a position where they are concerned about consent. The transcripts further show that at least some staff are taking a holistic interpretation of consent, being aware of the potential for barriers and inequality to invalidate supposedly free choices (see Brown and Turk, 1992). They had perhaps occasionally bent over backwards to put a positive slant on some relationships, perhaps unaware of the growing evidence of research such as that of Michelle McCarthy (1993) which shows that for many women with learning disabilities who do nominally consent, sex is still perfunctory, unpleasurable or painful. . . .

However, participants also noted the inevitability that sex would be an issue in day centres given the prohibition which often exists within client's homes coupled with the difficulties of meeting fellow service users without the means of independent travel.

Lastly, the focus groups agreed that it was reasonable to give exclusive attention to the difficult sexual behaviour of men as opposed to women service users, acknowledging its greater incidence, but there was some dissent:

> We do have, I suppose, inappropriate sexual behaviour that does occur at the centre but it is no more men than women.

A few women with learning disabilities had also been identified as displaying difficult sexual behaviours. This included 'promiscuity' which was not mentioned for the men, demonstrating the persistence of sexist beliefs and double standards. On balance it was suggested that men's sexual behaviour was more offensive than that displayed by women, which was described as being less aggressive. . . .

Sexual abuse of women staff

Considerable allowances were made for the men's unacceptable/ abusive behaviour towards staff. The primary justification offered for this was the very unusual relationship that exists between staff and men with learning disabilities: one person described it as 'a very strange job'. Staff described how the ambiguity of the relationship and the lack of normal 'analogue' made it very difficult for the men to understand the boundaries:

> We have so many different sorts of relationship on different levels with them that it must be quite difficult for them to hold on to what you are.

> Misread overtures of friendship.

One woman commented – she would not be as *nice* to any other man unless she *was* intending to have a sexual relationship with him. When men were thought to have overstepped the boundary, a common response was for staff to 'stand back' in the relationship and/or to redefine the relationship by stressing the existence of their own partner or husband. The men's behaviour could not always be explained as confusion over the 'caring nature' of the relationship as it was noted that some men would discuss sex very differently with women and male workers and that new women staff were particularly vulnerable to harassment.

So the women, whilst facing a significant barrage of sexual harassment, are also burdened with, and maybe paralysed by, concern for the men who they see as being deprived of normal sexual opportunities, and on the receiving end of complicated and ambivalent sexual messages, without parallels or clear markers. The men have not so much 'misread' the signals as been placed in a position in which the signals simply don't add up, but the women themselves, although seen as powerful by the men they support, are hardly in a position to influence the process. They are caught between contradictory expectations: by conforming to gendered assumptions about 'caring' they are led to being warm and giving, and yet as professionals they are supposed to 'keep their distance'.

Responses to the men's behaviour

Although less time was spent on recording responses to the men's difficult sexual behaviour, some common themes emerged. First, responses were often dependent on who was on the receiving end of the men's behaviour; this tended to mean that nothing would be done unless members of the general public were involved. Moreover, where abuse was internal – being directed at other service users or staff – management was portrayed as unsympathetic:

> A lot of the time the managers don't always do their job because staff are looking for advice, someone to turn to and they have a manager who is portraying this sort of 'ignore it' attitude – brushing it under the carpet.

Some participants also identified how easily they themselves came to tolerate some of the men's behaviour:

> You can become complacent with it though – can't you? But once you become familiar with this it doesn't become threatening verbally.

A number of suggestions were made to improve the management of men with learning disabilities who have difficult sexual behaviour. One solution canvassed was the greater availability of male staff, although where they were in post they were not always sympathetic to the experience of their women colleagues. In one case where a man always masturbated when being given intimate support by women, but not by men staff, having men give him this support would have seemed an obvious solution. However, men were seen to be often unwilling to take on the intimate support needs of other men: 'The male staff won't deal with him all the time.' . . .

Boundary issues

The pervasiveness of unacceptable/abusive sexual behaviour directed at women staff requires further examination. It is clearly a commonplace occurrence for there to be either a lack of, or breach of, boundaries between male client and women staff members. To explore this in more depth a pilot study was undertaken with five women workers. During structured interviews they were asked to explore how they determined what touch was appropriate with male clients and how they saw their 'role'. . . .

Touch which was potentially 'allowed' included kissing, holding hands, hugging and sitting on laps, though this varied for individual men and different settings. For example, there was a reduced concern about touch with less able men. Contact with men who were seen as either too young or too old to be regarded as potential sexual partners for the women were also seen as less threatening. Here, staff seem to be making a judgement about which men are potentially sexual: by regarding some of the men they work with as being asexual (for example, severely disabled men), women staff are able to tolerate more physical contact. Conversely, men whom they identify as being like other men are kept more at arm's length. Prior knowledge of male clients also emerged as a factor in the drawing of boundaries. In particular, where they were aware of men with previous histories of inappropriate/abusive sexual behaviour they were much more guarded about any physical contact. Although the women were not specifically asked to compare their attitudes towards touch with women clients as opposed to men, there was some evidence of greater caution in relation to touching men and one reason given for this was the way the contact would be perceived by others. For individual men, touching which would be tolerated would extend to special occasions such as bereavement, being upset and marking the end of a piece of work. . . .

These women were fairly clear that their role with men with learning disabilities was a professional one: in practice, this meant adhering to 'codes of contact', 'keeping a distance' and being 'objective'. At times, this was thought to be 'too clinical' but no more informal analogue could be agreed upon. Mothering was rejected as a role because it was suggested that this patronized people with learning disabilities. However, there was some feeling that where clients did not have a mother, women staff in some way could act as a surrogate. The roles of 'daughter' or 'sister' were also rejected, but one woman said she did draw parallels between her experience of being a sister and her work: in both, she recognized herself as 'protective, a bit domineering, a bit knowing and giving companionship'.

Opinions about whether the women saw themselves as a 'friend' to the men they worked with were more diverse. The women found it most relevant, as an analogue, defining friendship as encompassing: 'giving companionship, sharing experiences, wanting to know and understand what's happening'. However, one woman noted that the friendships were not proper ones since clients are 'dropped' when staff move on. Tension between being a professional and being a friend was clear, with one woman saying it was very difficult to maintain a boundary when people were lonely or the work takes place in the client's home. Another view was that being friendly – 'pally' – was a tool that the women used to facilitate their work so that men with learning disabilities might 'relax', as part of 'relationship building'. One woman said that she measured how friendly she was with men according to the likelihood of men misconstruing it. None of the women wanted to be perceived as the girlfriend of the men with whom they worked. One made it clear that she tried to give out signals that this was not the case, although they are recognized that this did not always get across to some of the men with learning disabilities, who at times may hope for this relationship or believe it exists.

All the participants described informal ways in which they attempted to limit or redefine their relationships with men with learning disabilities. A fundamental boundary concerned access to the women's homes: the women were very resistant to giving men their home address or phone number and were cautious about taking clients to their homes. One woman said that she was even wary of letting clients know the area she lived in. Other strategies were not giving birthday cards and avoiding attending social functions with clients. The way these boundaries were described suggested that these were personal choices made by the women, rather than policies advocated by their agencies. They do however indicate a conflict of interests inherent in 'ordinary life' services which envisaged service workers integrating service users into their own networks (see, for example, Brown and Brown, 1989). . . .

A very public responsibility

. . . The pilot study indicates that even for those women whose role has clear 'professional' boundaries and markers, and who are not heavily involved in giving intimate support, setting and maintaining an appropriate sexual boundary is problematical. Although addressing sexual issues is not an officially sanctioned or legitimized part of the work of support staff, they cannot avoid being faced with dilemmas and sexual behaviours as part of their employment obligations. Normative boundaries are inevitably broken, taking with them the fiction that caring is just an 'ordinary' relationship. Furthermore, the issue is not being addressed by *all* staff as part of a coherent programme of staff training or service development. Keeping the lid on sexuality remains women's work within services as it is within the family.

In raising these issues, there are echoes of the way sexual harassment and sexuality are discounted within the workforce at large. . . . The role of women staff in containing sexual abuse by service users mirrors the extent to which women are forced to collude in containing men's sexual, and sometimes violent, behaviour within their homes and workplaces, and the pressures upon them to ensure that these are kept within the private domain. Unless and until sexuality and sexual abuse become part of the publicly acknowledged agenda for service agencies, people with learning disabilities and the women who care for them are at risk of having their experiences of abuse ignored.

The agenda for services

Hence, we see that as a first step the abuse of staff by men with learning disabilities must be named and taken seriously. We respect and endorse the commitment for this to be done in a way which does not disregard the men's disadvantages in their personal and sexual lives. However, we believe that women staff have rights as employees as do other service users, and that these can only be upheld by prompt intervention and problem-solving. Just as service users and their advocates are beginning to take a more serious litigious view of abuse which is allowed to persist through negligence, we believe that the conditions under which many women currently work may be illegal, as well as unsafe.

A training agenda must reframe this as an issue for everyone, not just as a women's issue. For men, in their roles as colleagues and managers, talking with women about these issues is an important competence and one which will require sensitivity given the unequal positions of men and women within the gendered hierarchies of service organizations. Certainly, women should be given support as they consider how to maintain some distance in their role with men who use services, but it is for managers to develop and communicate clear expectations about the limits of the caring role and the legitimate boundaries which women staff can put around their work. They must be clear that a gender-blind approach is not appropriate in situations where women are bearing the brunt of sexual harassment and abuse. Above all, they must take this issue back on to the public agenda of the service and not allow it to burden women workers in private.

Acknowledgements

The main study reported here is supported by funding from the Mental Health Foundation. We are also grateful to the staff and agencies who participated.

Note

1 It is important not to assume that this is the extent of known abuse *of* men in the two districts because participants were directed to think about aspects of the men's sexual behaviour which might be abusive to others, not to catalogue their experiences of being victimized.

References

Brown, H. and Brown, V. (1989) *Building Social Networks: Bringing People Back Home* (series of video-assisted training packages), Bexhill: SETRHA.

Brown, H. and Turk, V. (1992) 'Defining sexual abuse as it affects adults with learning disabilities', *Mental Handicap*, 20 (2): 44–55.

Kruger, R.A. (1994) *Focus Groups: A Practical Guide for Applied Research*, London: Sage.

McCarthy, M. (1993) 'Sexual experiences of women with learning disabilities in long stay hospitals', *Sexuality and Disability*, 11: 277–86.

21

P. Smith and E. Agard

Care Costs: towards a Critical Understanding of Care

. . . In both the USA and UK, the delivery of health care is being restructured. Although the health-care systems are very different, both are faced with the need to contain costs, to deliver services more efficiently, and to reduce waste. Nurses in both health-care systems are experiencing similar stresses as the conditions of their work change. In this chapter we reflect on these changes, situating them in their social and economic context and exploring their significance. . . .

In recent decades a rich body of nursing scholarship has been devoted to describing, analysing and validating the practice of nursing. In this literature, the language of care is so pervasive, and the association between nursing work and caring attitudes and actions so explicit, that even a brief excursion into the nursing literature yields a wealth of information about care and its distinctive place in nursing. This literature views care as a basic human need and capacity, and as a system of learned skills and practices. Underlying these aspects of care is an understanding of care as a relationship and moral commitment. Nursing responds to basic human needs for care in a skilled manner, but ideally this response is guided by a caring attitude. . . .

These efforts to define nursing work contribute to our understanding of what caring work entails. Caring work involves both tasks and emotional style – tasks performed with an attitude of care, and an attitude of care expressed in some form of caring activity. In an attempt to define and validate what nurses do, the nursing profession claims this blend of action and attitude as their distinctive territory. However, despite considerable efforts to identify what is unique about nursing practice, the nursing profession has been unable to claim a territory which belongs to nursing alone. Instead, the scope of nursing practice, and therefore the work that nurses do, expands and contracts in response to external demands. In order to

First published in G. Brykczynska (ed.) *Caring: the Compassion and Wisdom of Nursing* (Arnold, Hodder Headline, 1997) Abridged.

reduce the costs of providing health care, more highly skilled tasks commonly performed by junior physicians or therapists can be passed on to nurses, and the less skilled tasks commonly performed by nurses can be passed on to less highly skilled personnel, or to relatives.[1] We are left with an understanding of nursing work which remains vulnerable to exploitation as nursing labour, which we shall examine in the next section.

Care as labour

Nursing work is a product which can be sold and exploited, that is, wages can be set according to economic forces rather than according to the full value of the work or the cost to the person performing it. As nursing labour, the services which nurses perform are shaped by changes in the social and economic context within which nursing work is performed.

We suggest that, since emotions, feelings, communication and relationships are so central to nursing discourse, the notion of emotional labour provides one way of understanding what nurses provide that is not fully recognized or fully compensated.

Our concept of emotional labour is drawn from Hochschild's study of flight attendants, within which she developed the idea of emotional labour as 'the induction or suppression of feeling in order to sustain in others a sense of being cared for in a convivial safe place' (Hochschild, 1983: 7). Emotional labour is sold for a wage and has exchange value.

Smith (1992) describes the emotional work nurses do in helping patients to cope with illness and hospitalization, explores how that work can be done or not done according to its context, and raises issues about the gendered nature of nursing work. Smith found that care included the emotional labour involved in setting a caring attitude or caring atmosphere created by the ward sister (head nurse).

Emotional labour as a component of care is gendered. At the time of Hochschild's study in the early 1980s, she estimated that over half of all working women had jobs that call for emotional labour. . . .

In nursing during this time period the nursing process was introduced as a philosophy and work method which raised the profile of emotional care by emphasizing people and communication, rather than tasks. However, unlike the airline industry, which paid flight attendants for their emotional labour, the emotional rewards of nursing are still seen as supplementing the financial ones. A 1990 national recruitment advertisement in the UK reassured prospective nurses that, although they are unlikely to be attracted to the job for financial reasons, they will be well paid for their skills. The predominant message is clearly that nursing, as one of the 'most emotionally satisfying professions', offers more than financial rewards. This message does not differ substantially from that in an early edition of the *American Journal of Nursing* (Turkoski, 1992), which suggests that women should never expect the same wages as men because providing a service is more important than remuneration.

In the case of nursing, these skills are blended with technical expertise and a psychosocial, emotional, ethical and moral commitment to care. According to Ray (1987), this unique blend of skills was apparent in critical-care nursing, which 'displayed both human and technocratic aspects and was seen as an ethical and moral process' (Ray, 1987: 167). However, Hart (1991) saw nurses' multiple skills and their ability to cover for domestic and medical shortages as both their strength and their undoing. Their adaptability to changing situations was their strength, but in management terms this was also their undoing since it proved that nursing skills were 'unspecialized, interchangeable and easily transferable' (James, 1991, cited in Hart, 1991). . . . Just as women's management of complex domestic situations is neither visible nor valued by society (Hochschild, 1989), the adaptability of nurses is not seen as a skill.

According to Gordon (1991b), the consequences of women's work being invisible and undervalued are twofold. In addition to economic effects, women also suffer psychologically from lowered self-esteem and lack of self-confidence as a result of performing public and private tasks that at best are seen as inferior, and at worst are neither recognized nor rewarded.

An adequate account of care-giving must therefore include an analysis of both care as work and care as labour. It must also explain its gendered and marginalized nature.

Care and gender

. . . In recent years, a number of sociological and feminist theories have been postulated to explain and analyse the gendered nature of women's domestic and paid work (Finch and Groves, 1983; Glazer, 1993). While a full exploration and assessment of these theories is beyond the scope of this chapter, they effectively challenge some of the stereotypes and assumptions surrounding women as 'natural' care-givers.

First, the division of roles and responsibilities by gender, and the perception that women's care-giving and emotion management are an expression of their nature, is associated with an imbalance of power. Historically, men have had greater access to the public sphere, greater social and economic rewards and greater power than women.[2] The effects of this imbalance of power may not be felt by individuals or groups, but it affects the structure of society in ways which oppress women (Dahlerup, 1987).[3] Important indicators of structural oppression include segregation of work between the sexes (Dahlerup, 1987) and, citing Hartmann (1979), the servicing of men by women.

Secondly, the division between a domestic and a public sphere has been challenged; we cannot obtain a full account of women's oppression until we understand how their work in the domestic sphere and their paid employment in the public sphere are intimately and structurally related (Dahlerup, 1987). The oppression of women has roots in their confinement to the activities and responsibilities of the domestic sphere, but we need an account of women's work which recognizes not only their exclusion from the public sphere, but also the ways in which their participation in the public sphere is shaped and restricted by gender. The public sphere expands or contracts according to economics, and women take up the slack as both paid and unpaid care providers.[4]

Thus nursing work, a particular set of knowledge and skills, and nursing labour, a product sold for a wage, are shaped by women's social location and by the gender division of labour in health care. Both the scope of nursing practice and the value set on their work are largely outside their control. . . .

Role of nurses in health-care delivery

. . . Perspectives on social values, the common good, and individual and collective responsibilities vary widely. Historically, the UK has been more willing than the USA to subsidize social services with public funds; the differences in social-care arrangements in the USA and the UK reflect the underlying social values of each country. However, there is a shift in the UK towards emphasis on individual rather than state responsibility for the provision of welfare or care, and an associated shift from a service to a market ethos (Smith, 1996). In the USA, health-care restructuring indicates a commitment to competitive health care, with little attention being paid to the implications of this approach for health-care delivery. . . .

In the 1990s, health care, whether publicly or privately funded, is about reducing costs. Inevitably, nurses as the largest occupational group are used in a variety of ways to save money. . . .

Until the current crisis in health-care costs, nurses were used in the US health-care industry to attract patients to their hospitals (compare the example of flight attendants cited earlier). For example, during the 1980s, the 'Magnet' hospitals cited as representing some of the top management practices amongst US industry promoted primary nursing (one-to-one patient care from admission to discharge) as a means of improving nurse recruitment and patient satisfaction.

Evidence suggested that patients chose those hospitals because of the quality of nursing offered (Kramer and Schmalenberg, 1988).

In the UK's relatively small but expanding private sector, the nurse has been used as an advertising image to encourage prospective patients to take out private health insurance. One leading company with its own network of private hospitals projects the following image. The smiling, uniformed nurse in pleasant hospital surroundings holds the patient's hand and joins in cheerful conversation with her family. The caption reads: 'Feel confident that when you or a member of your family need hospital treatment, you'll enjoy comfort, privacy and individual attention.' The language appears to be directed to a middle-class, elite clientele. . . .

In summary, nurses as the largest occupational group within health care are used by both public and private systems to promote a caring image which can help profits in good times and save costs during economic cut-backs. In the case of state provision they are used . . . to meet the needs of complex groups who would otherwise fall through the net of diminishing resources. . . .

Impact of market forces on women's participation in the workforce

. . . In this context, the ideology of altruism becomes a powerful mechanism of social and economic control over those who perform service work. In order to promote the image of nursing in the USA in the early part of this century, nursing leaders promoted the ideals of altruism and service. This contributes to the economic devaluation of nursing labour, and its susceptibility to market forces. . . .

Thus in the shift from private duty to hospital nursing which took place when private individuals could no longer afford to hire nursing services during the Great Depression, and as the federal government began to support the development of hospitals and the health-care industry, nursing leaders persuaded the nursing rank and file to accept wages and working conditions from hospitals which were not economically too exacting. Instead, the ideals of vocation and service attracted women into socially acceptable nursing work (Turkoski, 1992). . . .

Nurses have been among the first casualties of . . . economic stringencies. As a group, they are expensive, accounting for half the workforce and a quarter of the NHS budget (Buchan, 1992). In the USA, nurses account for 28 per cent of total hospital costs (Gordon, 1995). Under cost constraints, US employers attempt to reduce the costs of nursing labour by making each nurse carry a greater workload, taking on additional duties and additional patients (Gordon, 1991b), and/or by replacing registered nurses with cheaper, less skilled personnel (Gray, 1993: Scott, 1993). In the UK, many nursing skills are seen by managers and policy-makers as 'unspecialized, interchangeable and therefore easily transferable' (James, 1991, cited in Hart, 1991). . . .

The move towards advanced practices roles, while encouraged in both the USA and the UK as part of health-care reforms, may offer nurses new challenges but also expose their vulnerability to market forces. By developing alternative models of professional caring practice, they may find themselves being used as cost-cutting devices and cheaper alternatives to physicians. The caring aspects of the job may remain unrecognized as nurses develop ways of giving quality care at lower costs than medically dominated or delivered services. . . .

In the UK, Hart (1991) describes a situation in which the 'managerial-medical' model of health care may mean that the 'nursing skills are devalued and down-graded, or up-graded and valued only to the extent that nurses take over the low status and routine technical work of junior doctors'. She sees this model as an attractive one for managers who need to cut their unit costs in order to compete in the emerging health-care market.

Evidence from the UK suggests that the implementation of the market, the breakup of the National Health Service into semi-autonomous trusts, and the purchaser/provider divide have indeed driven a rift between those who give care and those who are responsible for managing its organization and finance.[5] A study of morale among community nurses and health visitors in three first-wave English trusts during the first three years of health-care reforms revealed that front-line staff experienced a conflict of values between finance-oriented managers and their own commitment to care. The following quote represents a prevailing view among nurses in this study: 'Money has replaced the patient in our focus of care. We need to resist this insidious erosion to our commitment to people' (Traynor and Wade, 1994: 43).

On the other hand, managers in this study were found to believe that a 'business ethos' was highly compatible with the principles of good health care. Surveys in the USA revealed similar findings, with many changes being made in hospitals by administrators with a 'we know best' attitude who did not value 'hands-on care' (Noble, 1993).

A significant effect of the market on nursing in the UK is to attempt to reduce operating costs by reducing nurses' pay. Formerly paid according to a national pay scale, nurses now see their pay as being set by trusts that are in competition with each other. . . . The introduction of the internal market is being blamed for increased workloads, particularly paperwork, and threats to quality of patient care. In short, nurses feel that they are being expected to do more for less. . . .

Whether trust managers, like governments and private health-care corporations, are concerned about retaining qualified nurses or paying them adequately depends on whether they regard them as having unique rather than interchangeable skills. One approach to convincing them that the former is the case is to accumulate evidence that skilled nursing matters.

Value skilled nursing

. . . In the UK in 1991, the Audit Commission, the public finance watchdog, reported that one of the biggest problems facing health care in the UK was the 'undervaluing of nursing and nurses', which in turn prevented the efficient use of ward nursing resources (Audit Commission, 1991).

A US survey has revealed that three out of five nurses believed that cost containment had a detrimental effect on quality of care in their hospitals (Collins, 1988). Nearly 75 per cent of respondents felt that cost containment left 'no time for a caring attitude'. The little things, defined as 'psychological support, teaching, frequent turning and positioning', were the first items to go because nurses felt pressured to perform the visible 'high-tech' routines. The false economy of reducing skilled nursing is illustrated by the example of pressure sores, which may develop as a result of inadequate nursing care and which cost more to treat than to prevent (McSweeney, 1994). A federally funded study further confirmed the negative effect of cost containment on quality of care, suggesting higher death rates in hospitals facing stiff competition and stringent state regulation (cited in Collins, 1988). . . .

There is growing evidence for a direct correlation between qualified staff, good standards of care and positive patient outcomes (Scott, 1993). But as a leading US nurse states:

> The value of nursing derives from the content of its work. Nurses care for those who cannot care for themselves; such compassion is a hallmark of a civilized society. . . . Whether this care is supplied through the public sector or, as is much more common, through the private sector, there is a consensus that care should be given when it is needed. But we hate to pay for it. (Lynaugh, 1988: VII–2)

We return full circle to the question which we posed earlier, namely how to get at this complex phenomenon called care in order to make it visible and valued in a market-oriented society committed to costs. . . .

Towards a critical understanding of care

. . . Many studies of nurses take a phenomenological perspective. We find this perspective limited because it emphasizes individual experiences and interpretations. Critical theory demands that we situate phenomena within their historical and social context, and it asks not only what is happening, but why, and whose interests are being served. . . .

In carving out an area of practice, nursing has laid claim to a distinctive combination of attitude and skill. This commitment to care and expertise in care-giving is indeed a distinctive feature of nursing practice. However, the skills and effort involved in caring work are too easily obscured by the image of calling or vocation. The commitment of nurses to care is claimed as a practical and moral imperative and as a moral covenant (Bishop and Scudder, 1990). This moral language builds a self-image and public image of nurses as selfless and devoted, motivated by vocation and feeling rather than by material concerns, but it does not serve the profession well in holding its position within the health-care system.

Nursing has adopted the language and ethos of care without sufficient critical examination of where this ethos comes from and whose interests it represents. In nursing, the ethos of care contributes heavily to the gender division of labour and the subordination of nurses. When nurses present themselves as uniquely committed to care, it is very difficult for them to argue about the terms and conditions under which they perform their caring work and sell their caring labour. . . .

Condon (1992) suggests that caring provides a new and authentic metaphor for nursing, grounded in women's direct experience as mothers, nurses and care-givers. Freely chosen, the metaphor of care can point the way to a personal and social ethic; nursing is a 'space' in which this can happen. From the perspective of critical theory, however, nursing cannot establish a space unconnected with the values and structures of society. Even if the nurse chooses this space and his or her activities within it, the space itself and his or her choices and actions are shaped by the external context. In our view, we cannot understand nursing fully without understanding how attitudes, behaviours and opportunities in our society are shaped by gender, and how they operate in all spheres to diminish the economic value placed on women's work.

Feminist theory brings us to the paradox of care (Gordon, 1991a) – can we continue to value care without perpetuating the structures of subordination and exploitation within which the work and labour of care have traditionally been situated? According to Gordon, some feminists say that this cannot be done, and therefore measure women's progress by how far and how effectively we are able to distance ourselves from care-giving. However, we share with Gordon the hope that we can 'keep the market-place in its place' and organize care-giving in ways that reaffirm this basic human capacity. . . .

Central to our discussion is our concern with both individual and social responses to the human need for care. We suggest that neither the work of care-giving nor the moral commitment to care can be abandoned, but that we must examine critically the social arrangements which determine who provides care and the terms and conditions under which they do so. Far more than individual vocation or moral commitment, these social arrangements inhibit or sustain our capacity to care.

Notes

1 Levi (1980: 336) refers to the 'functional redundancy' or nursing: nursing has developed in such a way that substitutions for what nurses do can be made from both above and below; thus nursing cannot maintain a firm hold on its own scope of practice and professional territory.

2 We refer here to the notion of patriarchy as stated by Rosaldo and Lamphere (1974) and cited by Dahlerup: 'Everywhere we find that women are excluded from certain economic or political activities, that their roles as wives and mothers are associated with fewer powers and prerogatives than are the roles of men. It seems fair to say, then, that all contemporary societies are to some extent male dominated, and although the degree and expression of female subordination vary greatly, sexual asymmetry is presently a universal fact of human life' (Dahlerup, 1987: 3). Dahlerup (1987) notes that common to all definitions of patriarchy is the focus on men's power, authority or dominance over women, particularly over women's sexuality and labour.

3 Shue (1980) makes a useful distinction between systemic oppression, in which arrangements that exploit some members of society to the advantage of others are built into the structure of society and widely taken for granted, and systematic oppression, in which deliberate attempts are made, through legislation, segregation or coercive force, to oppress individuals or groups.

4 For an excellent discussion of the limitations of the public/private split, see Juteau and Laurin (1989). In a rigorous review of the feminist literature, and a specific study of Quebecoise nuns, Juteau and Laurin argue that (1) gender relations function as do class relations, to equate the interests of the dominant group(s) with the collective or general interest, and (2) that this results in both private and collective appropriation of women's labour in 'a diversity of sites, places, relations and institutions'.

5 Although the factors contributing to cost containment and competition in the US health-care market differ from those in the UK, the effects are similar (Smith, 1996).

References

Audit Commission (1991) *The Virtue of Patients*, HMSO: London.

Bishop, A. and Scudder, J. (1990) *The Practical, Moral, and Personal Sense of Nursing*, State University Press of New York: Albany, NY.

Buchan, J. (1992) *Flexibility or Fragmentation? Trends and Prospects in Nurse Pay*, King's Fund Institute: London.

Collins, H.L. (1988) 'When the profit motive threatens patient care', *Registered Nurse*, 19 (8): 74–83.

Condon, E.H. (1992) 'Nursing and the caring metaphor: gender and political influences on an ethics of care', *Nursing Outlook*, 40: 14–19.

Dahlerup, D. (1987) 'Confusing concepts – confusing reality: a theoretical discussion of the patriarchal state', in Sassoon, A. Showstack (ed.) *Women and the State*, Routledge: London. pp. 93–127.

Finch, J. and Groves, D. (1983) *A Labour of Love: Women, Work and Caring*, Routledge and Kegan Paul: London.

Glazer, N. (1993) *Women's Paid and Unpaid Labor*, Temple University Press: Philadelphia.

Gordon, S. (1991a) 'Fear of caring: the feminist paradox', *American Journal of Nursing*, 91: 48.

Gordon, S. (1991b) *Prisoners of Men's Dreams*, Little, Brown: Boston.

Gordon, S. (1995) 'Is there a nurse in the house?' *The Nation*, 13 February: 199.

Gray, B. (1993) 'RN job market shifts as health system evolves', *Nurse Week*, 6 (24): 1–23.

Hart, E. (1991) 'Ghost in the machine', *Health Service Journal*, 101: 20–2.

Hartmann, H. (1979) 'Capitalism, patriarchy and job segregation', in Z. Eisenstein (ed.) *Capitalism, Patriarchy and the Case for Socialist Feminism*, Monthly Review Press: New York.

Hochschild, A.R. (1983) *The Managed Heart: Commercialization of Human Feeling*, University of California Press: Berkeley.

Hochschild, A.R. (1989) *The Second Shift – Working Parents and the Revolution at Home*, Viking/London; Piatkus Press: New York.

James, V. (1991) *Changing Babies*, unpublished report, Department of Nursing Studies, Nottingham University.

Juteau, D. and Laurin, N. (1989) 'From nuns to surrogate mothers: evolution of the forms of the appropriation of women', *Feminist Issues*, 9: 13–40.

Kramer, M. and Schmalenberg, C. (1988) 'Magnet hospitals: Part I. Institutions of excellence', *Journal of Nursing Administration*, 18: 13–24.

Levi, M. (1980) 'Functional redundancy and the process of professionalization: the case of registered nurses in the United States', *Journal of Health Policy, Politics and Law*, 5: 333–53.

Lynaugh, J. (1988) *Twice as Many and Still Not Enough*, US Commission on Nursing, US Department of Health and Human Services: Washington.

McSweeney, P. (1994) 'Assessing the cost of pressure sores', *Nursing Standard*, 8: 25–6.

Noble, B.P. (1993) 'Pushing nurses to a breaking point', *New York Times*, 10 January.

Ray, M.A. (1987) 'Technological caring: a new model in critical care', *Dimensions of Critical Care in Nursing*, 6: 166–73.

Rosaldo, M.Z. and Lamphere, L. (1974) *Women, Culture and Society*, Stanford University Press: Stanford, CA.

Scott, K. (1993) 'RN layoffs of growing concern to ANA', *The American Nurse*, 25 (3): 14.

Shue, H. (1980) *Basic Rights*, Princeton University Press: Princeton, NJ.

Smith, P. (1992) *The Emotional Labour of Nursing*, Macmillan Press: Basingstoke.

Smith, P. (1996) 'Health care reform in Britain and the United States – public or market-led? – a review', *International Journal of Public Administration*.

Traynor, M. and Wade, B. (1994) *The Morale of Nurses Working in the Community: A Study of Three NHS Trusts: Year 3*, Daphne Heald Research Unit, Royal College of Nursing: London.

Turkoski, B.B. (1992) 'A critical analysis of professionalism in nursing', in J.L. Thompson, D.G. Allen and L. Rodrigues-Fisher (eds) *Critique, Resistance and Action: Working Papers on the Politics of Nursing*, National League for Nursing: New York. pp. 149–65.

22

S. Shardlow

Confidentiality, Accountability and the Boundaries of Client–Worker Relationships

. . . There is a broad range of concepts in the social work firmament that serve to delineate and define the nature and quality of aspects of relationships between social workers and clients. Two concepts, confidentiality and accountability, will be examined here. . . . How these two concepts are expressed can tell much about acceptable and unacceptable relationships between social workers and clients. . . .

To examine and reveal some of the tensions in the interaction of confidentiality and accountability a rather unusual methodology is adopted: three fictional dialogues between a client and a social worker discussing aspects of confidentiality and accountability in practice. . . .

Confidentiality

When applied to social work practice, confidentiality may be taken as an exhortation to social workers to keep secret both written and verbal communications from clients. Social workers are given information by clients in the full expectation that this will be kept secret by the social worker. . . . As a requirement it can be grounded in one of three ways: prudentially, we tend to keep the confidences of those who we think will keep our trust; technically, because not keeping some information confidential will generate problems in providing social services to the public; morally, because to treat confidential information as being available to others would be an act of discourtesy and demonstrate that the individual was seen as having little moral worth (Timms, 1983). Timms also suggests that confidentiality may be in either a weak or a strong form. In the strong form all information obtained by virtue of being in a particular role (e.g. being a social worker) should be treated as confidential. In the

First published in R. Hugman and D. Smith (eds) *Ethical Issues in Social Work* (Routledge, 1995), pp. 66–82. Abridged.

weak form only information specifically identified as confidential should be treated as such.

> *Confidentiality* is then a system of rules and norms applied to information given by clients to social workers: it is expected that social workers will not divulge this information to others except in certain specified circumstances.

Accountability

As for confidentiality, a working definition of accountability appears to be fairly simple and straightforward: to be accountable is to be in a position to give an explanation for one's actions – with reasons and justifications. Clark states that in conventional usage the terms *accountability* and *responsibility* are synonymous – with the require-ment that somebody has to be responsible to someone else for some-thing (Clark with Asquith, 1985: 41). It is in deciding what social workers are responsible for, and to whom, that the problems arise – the practical problems deriving from the principle. However, Coulshed, following Wareham, distinguishes between accountability and responsibility: the former is organizational and derives from the position held, while the latter is personal and derives from being a citizen and human being and therefore responsible for one's actions (Coulshed, 1990).

> *Accountability* is where social workers give an explanation and justification of their actions to somebody else who might reasonably expect to be given such an explanation.

Confidentiality and accountability: three dialogues

There are three dialogues between an imaginary social worker (*SW*) and an imaginary client (*C*). Both have been stripped of the usual attributes of human identity: they have no gender, race or age. Nor does the social worker represent any particular form of social work practice. . . . The questions put do not relate to any particular social work agency. The dialogues can be extended by giving the parti-cipants particular identities and asking questions based on their personae. The dialogues serve to illustrate various difficulties in realizing notions of confidentiality and accountability.

The first dialogue

C: Do you mind if I ask you some questions about things that have been on my mind?

SW: No, go ahead.

C: Suppose I tell you about myself, my innermost thoughts, can I be sure that you will keep them to yourself?

SW: Yes, of course I will.

C: Would it matter what I told you? I used to go to the priest, he never told anybody, you could rely on the priest to keep things secret . . . some of the things he must have heard in his time. . . . He always said it was between him and God . . . telling him was just telling God.

SW: Well it couldn't be quite like the priest, you know.

C: Well could it be like with my solicitor? She told me that whatever I told her was absolutely private – no court in the land could make her tell. She told me that anything I said to her was 'privileged' or something like that.

SW: No, I'm afraid it wouldn't be quite like that either.

C: Why not? Tell me why it would be different.

SW: You see, a lawyer belongs to a recognized profession with special rights which are guaranteed by law. Social work isn't quite like that.

C: You mean it's not a profession?

SW: Possibly it is . . . possibly it isn't. . . .

C: . . . That's not much of an answer!

SW: The real point is that social workers are not recognized in the way that lawyers are. If a court asked me what you had told me, I would have to tell them. I would protest of course, and say that it was unfair, but in the end I would either have to tell the court or go to prison. It would be different if we lived in New York in the United States. They have a law which makes social workers and lawyers equal in this respect. Whatever is said to a social worker is treated in the same way as what is said to a lawyer.

C: But that isn't really much of a problem, I shall just have to be careful about not telling you anything that I don't want the court to hear! I can't imagine that most of what I want to tell you would be of any interest to the courts. So that's it then! Whatever I told you, you would keep secret unless for some reason you had to tell a court? I suppose that's fair enough.

SW: I still couldn't absolutely guarantee that *everything* you told me could be kept secret.

C: Why not?

SW: If you told me about a crime that had been committed I might have to report it to the police.

C: Would that be only if *I* had committed the crime?

SW: No, if you told me about a friend or someone in your family I might still have to report it.

C: What sort of a crime would it have to be?

SW: If you told me you had murdered someone, or stolen a large amount of money, then I would have no choice.

C: Do you mean that there is a law that makes you do this?

SW: No, I just think it would be my professional duty.

C: But why? A priest or even a doctor might just tell me that it was my responsibility to report the matter to the police, if and when I chose. I can see that in a very serious case it would be difficult.

SW: Yes, even a doctor would have little choice if they thought that somebody else was in danger; this is the duty to warn. Suppose a doctor knew in confidence from conversations with a patient that the same patient harboured murderous desires towards another person – say it was a social worker! Then the doctor would, if he or she believed the threat to be genuine, have the responsibility to inform the social worker and the police.

C: That seems fair enough, if somebody presents a real danger to others then I can see that it is reasonable to break a confidence. That is not bothering me so much as . . . as the kind of crime. What if it wasn't as serious as murder? What would happen if I told you I was growing some cannabis plants for my own use? That doesn't really affect anybody else.

SW: That is a more difficult question, I'm not sure what I would do. I know some of my colleagues who disapprove of illegal drugs would feel obliged to report this to the police; others . . . they might, as the saying goes, 'turn a blind eye'.

C: That's not fair, it depends on who you have as your social worker, whether or not you are reported to the police.

SW: Yes I suppose you are right, but there is no law or code of practice to tell social workers what to do.

C: So how do you decide in these cases?

SW: I use my discretion.

C: What's that? I'm not sure I have any discretion.

SW: It means that I take account of all of my training and experience to help me decide what to do. I might talk to other social workers, but I would certainly do a lot of thinking about social work knowledge, skills and values.

C: So in the end it would be your decision – based upon your views – what you would do with information about me that I had told you. Would you even ask me what I thought?

SW: Yes, I would ask, some social workers might not – but the final decision would have to be mine.

C: You would exercise your power to decide. It seems as if you would not be on my side but would be working for somebody else. Who is that? Yourself, your loyalty to your employer, or to a romanticized ideal of what a professional does?

SW: No, it's not like that.

C: It seems to me that you are more accountable to your boss than to me if you can't keep my little secrets. When the chips are down it's not my interests that you are going to protect.

The second dialogue

C: Hello, I've been thinking about our last conversation: I've a few more questions I would like to ask – is that OK?

SW: Yes, that's fine with me.

C: I think I understand about when you would keep what I tell you secret, but how would I know that you had done it?

SW: I suppose you would just have to accept my word that I had not told anybody.

C: That's OK, I think I can trust you, so if you told me you wouldn't tell anybody else then I would believe you. I am right, aren't I, you wouldn't tell anybody else except in the cases we talked about? So I can trust you?

SW: I'm very pleased to hear you say that.

C: What if I had the kind of social worker that I didn't trust: could I find out if the social worker had kept my secrets?

SW: It is very difficult to check up on what a social worker does.

C: Why? Surely it shouldn't be?

SW: But you want to know how to make your social worker account to you for how that person behaves in handling your confidences.

C: Shouldn't the social worker have to tell me if my information is given to someone else?

SW: Well yes, of course, but I don't think the law makes this absolutely necessary. If the social worker told the police you wouldn't have to be told that this had happened.

C: But that is unfair, it is my information. I am the one who can give permission for the social worker to tell somebody else. Surely I ought to be able to say if I wanted to release a part of the information that I had given to a social worker?

SW: Yes, you ought.

C: If something goes wrong with an operation that a doctor has done I can complain to the Medical Council – I think it's called that. Is there anything like that for social workers?

SW: No, not yet. There has been some talk about setting one up. The idea was first suggested almost 20 years ago. It is closer to being created now than it ever has been before. . . .

C: That's not much use to me, I need something now – is there nothing else?

SW: If you were lucky you might be part of a social work project that was managed locally.

C: What do you mean and how would that help me?

SW: Some social workers are managed by local groups of clients and interest groups who decide on general policy and advise professional social workers what needs to be done and how to do it.

C: That's all very interesting and worth while, I'm sure – but how does it help me?

SW: Usually where social workers work in this way they would be expected to give a regular report to the management committee.

C: Yes, but I still don't see how this could help me.

SW: It could. Suppose your management committee, in discussion with the social workers, had strong feelings about keeping information confidential; you could agree a local policy about it. You could agree that no information would be divulged without the committee's approval or the agreement of whoever the information was about. Then you and anybody else in your part of the city would know that information was not being given to others.

C: That sounds fine, but what would happen about what we were talking about last time?

SW: What do you mean, exactly?

C: Suppose the courts wanted information?

SW: I'm afraid the social worker would still have to tell them what they wanted to know, but you would have more information about what the social worker was doing.

C: How?

SW: As well as the reports that the social worker gave to the management committee you would also be able to ask the social worker questions about what that person was doing.

C: If I didn't live in an area that had one of these committees, what could I do then?

SW: You can complain about your social worker; you could complain that he or she was giving away your secrets and breaking your confidences. All social services departments have to have a complaints procedure.

C: That would be rather a serious step to take. Besides which, it depends on the social worker having done something wrong – and also I've got to find out first that something has happened.

SW: Yes that would be very difficult to do, because, as you say, it is quite possible that you would not know what is being done with information about you.

C: So social workers have all the power; they can decide what to do with information about me and there is no way that they can be controlled. Surely there must be something that stops social workers behaving just as they please?

SW: Yes, of course there is. Many social workers work for local government and so they are responsible to the elected officers of the council. So by going to the polls you have some influence over these social workers in your city.

C: It's not very much is it? It doesn't help me with my problem in bringing social workers to account for how they use information about me.

SW: Perhaps it does. Many social workers have to justify their actions to the elected councillors. It's rather like how it was with the locally managed project that we were just discussing.

C: You might say that, but councillors have a lot to think about. They won't have the time to worry about my little concerns. Besides, you can't tell me that it is the same to have someone answer to somebody else. Don't you think it's better if the social worker can be responsible directly to somebody like me – somebody who makes use of social workers?

SW: Yes, I agree that would be best but it's not always possible.

C: There is one more thing that I don't understand.

SW: Tell me and I will try to explain if I can.

C: Is there no other way that social workers have to explain their behaviour than to elected councillors? They have so many other things to do.

SW: Yes, you are quite correct. Social workers have managers who are responsible for what the social workers do.

C: Do the managers tell social workers how to behave and what to do with information about me?

SW: It's not quite as simple as that. The social worker asks the manager for advice, and if things are really difficult they will often decide what to do together.

C: I keep thinking about the information about me. If the social worker and a manager were going to talk about me then the social worker would have to give the manager a lot of information about me – without me knowing anything about it.

SW: Yes, you are quite right!

C: But that's not fair! I thought that if I had given information to a social worker it wouldn't be discussed with anyone else.

SW: Yes, but the social worker might need to share the information with other people in the agency where the social worker works. There could be many reasons to do this: to get resources for you, to get advice or perhaps if what you had told the social worker was very serious the social worker might need a more senior person's agreement to decide how to help you.

C: This all seems very unfair. I gave some information to an individual, and now you tell me that many different people where the social worker works might be able to see the information and that I have no control over who sees the information inside the social worker's agency.

SW: It must seem like that – but remember your information is still being treated confidentially.

C: How do you mean?

SW: Well when you told the information to the social worker, you didn't just give it to the one person, you gave it to the whole organization. It's a bit like when you tell a priest you are also telling God.

C: No, it's not! God already knows. I thought I was telling one person, not a hundred.

The third dialogue

C: I was very angry at the end of our last conversation.

SW: Why was that?

C: It seemed as if I had been cheated; I expected some things and when we talked I realized that I had been wrong. I have some more questions, is that OK?

SW: Yes, go ahead.

C: I know that social workers keep files on people like me. Can I at least see what is in the file? Then I would know what my social worker thinks about me – I feel as though I would have some control if I could see my file. Do I have the right to see it?

SW: Yes, you can see it: the government has passed a law allowing you to see your file.

C: Can I see all of it?

SW: No, you can only see those parts of the file that contain information about you. There might be information about other members of your family; it would not be fair for you to see that information. Just as you might want to keep information about yourself from them, so information about them is kept from you.

C: Is that the only kind of information I can't see?

SW: More or less. Some information given by other people, such as doctors or the police, may not be available for you to see.

C: If the information they have is incorrect can I change it?

SW: Yes, if it is factual information about you, but if it is that you have one opinion and your social worker has another opinion then this can't be changed.

C: This is good. I know that a lot of information is on computer these days – can I still see what is kept about me on a computer?

SW: Yes.

C: I can't believe that you are giving me as much good news as this – after the previous conversations when I seemed to have very little influence over social workers. Using my powers to see my files I can really call the social worker to account, can't I? But I suppose it might not be as rosy as all that. If people know that the files are open I suppose they will be very careful about what they write down?

SW: Yes, I think you are correct.

C: I have been thinking about what you are saying, and it's not enough just to be able to see what is written about me after it has been put in the file.

SW: How do you mean?

C: I mean I want to be able to control what goes into the file in the first place. If I've got to go to the City Hall to see my records and then check them I won't want to do that very often, will I? I bet a lot of people would never do that because it would be too much trouble. So the social workers still win, don't they? If they say they have a system to let people see their files, well they have, but it's not giving people much is it, if it's hard for them to use the system. A lot of people around here couldn't get to the City hall, could they?

SW: I suppose you are right, it would be difficult for some people.

C: What I want is something that will give me control over what is written about me all the time. Is that a possibility then?

SW: Yes it is in some places. Again it depends on where you live.

C: Why? Tell me more about this!

SW: Some social workers are experimenting with different ways of keeping records about people. They would decide with the person what would be put in the record and might even write it jointly. This gives people as much control as possible over what information is kept about them. Of course it can't work where children are too young to understand what is written about them or where other people can't understand for whatever reason, such as substantial intellectual impairment.

C: This sounds like the kind of system that I want to use with my social worker. It seems so unfair that it is only available in some parts of the country. How do I influence my social worker to follow this kind of approach?

SW: Now you are asking very difficult questions indeed! I don't think I have an answer. But the first step must be to get information about what is happening to your case, what your social worker is doing.

C: The next step is to change it.

Comment

. . . In the dialogues, the attitudes and behaviours adopted by the social worker defined the nature and texture of the relationship between the social worker and the client. This was not a relationship where both had equal access to information, or to decisions about what happened to information, nor were there easy mechanisms for the client to hold the social worker to account. The social worker had the power to define the boundaries of the relationship between them. Part of the reason for this is that the nature of the relationship between the client and the social worker is as much a relationship between an individual (the client) and an organization (the social work agency). Partly it is also because social work is not a profession that enjoys statutory guarantees about privileged information.

In the dialogues, the nexus that unites confidentiality and accountability in their operation in practice is power. During the dialogues it is evident that the social worker usually has the power to define what information will be treated as confidential, just as the means for the client to hold the social worker accountable are defined through social work processes. Oddly, if social workers were paid by their clients, the client would have a mechanism to make the social worker accountable. . . . Nonetheless patients, without payment, are able to choose the doctor with whom they wish to register, so perhaps there is an argument to suggest that clients should have stronger rights to choose their social workers and to change them if dissatisfied. All too often, however, social workers are acting as representatives of their employing agency, and enabling the client to change to another social worker may lead to a change in presentation rather than of substance. The dialogues illustrate that there are some other mechanisms to increase the accountability of the social worker to the client, but these are not widespread. Ways to give clients power to define and defend their interests need to be developed. . . .

The dialogues present a conventional view of confidentiality which appears to be shared by both client and social worker. Confidentiality is seen to be about the social worker keeping information that the client has provided, and the difficulty of not divulging that information. . . .

In much of this literature confidentiality is presented as a problem for the practitioner trying to ensure that professional ethics and legal requirements coincide; as Gutheil (1990: 606) writes:

> What does one do if the law (statute regulation) dictates one path, and one's ethical mandates point another way: e.g., when the law compels a disclosure of sensitive information and one's ethical promptings urge silence?

We may ask where the client's interests are in defining the operation of the principles of confidentiality. There is in this literature little evidence of joint decision-making between clients and social workers about issues of confidentiality. By locating the problem as an issue for the social worker, professional power is maintained and reinforced, with implications for the nature of the relationship between social workers and clients. Using confidentiality in this way forces 'distance' between the client and the social worker, enhancing the status of the professional as being the competent person in the relationship to decide on such issues. It reinforces the power that the social worker has over the client. . . .

Coda for practice

. . . We now need to create dialogues between clients and social workers to define mutually desired and desirable relationships around key points such as confidentiality and accountability and to promote structural developments in social work practice. Here are some questions for practitioners to consider about their practice which may help both to define the boundaries of relationships with clients and to create dialogues:

1 In my work with clients how am I accountable to the person I am working with? Is there a mechanism that makes me directly accountable to that individual?
2 How do I see myself as being accountable to the client?

3   Do I keep information from the client? If so, what sort of infor-
    mation and why, and, most importantly, does the client know that
    I keep information to myself?
4   How do I treat the information that a client gives to me? What are
    the rules that I operate? How far does the client have a say in
    what happens to the information?
5   In the final analysis where does my loyalty lie: to my client or to
    my employer? If the client gave a piece of information about a
    serious matter to me in strict confidence, would I be able to keep
    and maintain that confidence?
6   What changes would I like to see in this aspect of practice?

References

Clark, C.L. with Asquith, S. (1985) *Social Work and Social Philosophy*, London:
    Routledge and Kegan Paul.
Coulshed, V. (1990) *Management in Social Work*, Basingstoke: Macmillan.
Gutheil, T.G. (1990) 'Ethical issues in confidentiality', *Psychiatric Annals*, 20 (10):
    605–11.
Timms, N. (1983) *Social Work Values: An Enquiry*, London: Routledge and Kegan Paul.

23

N. Black and E. Thompson

Obstacles to Medical Audit: British Doctors Speak

Although some doctors in the UK have audited their medical practice for many years, it is only in the last few years that a concerted effort has been made to get all doctors to participate. This initiative has been led by professional associations, such as the Royal Colleges, and encouraged by the UK Department of Health. The reforms of the National Health Service (NHS) which commenced in April 1991 included a commitment to medical audit and this has been supported by designated funding, distributed through the regional health authorities (and equivalent bodies in Scotland, Wales and Northern Ireland) and the Royal Colleges.

Much of the current enthusiasm for medical audit is based on a belief that it is an effective means of improving the quality of medical care. Published accounts of audit tend to confirm this belief (Eisenberg, 1986). However there may well be some publication bias; audits that fail to improve the quality of care are less likely to get reported. It has been suggested that concern about the effectiveness of audit acts as a deterrent to doctors' involvement in audit (Baron, 1983). Other potential obstacles to audit that have been suggested include: a reluctance to judge peers (ibid.); the danger of reducing public confidence in doctors (ibid.); a belief that doctors have been auditing their work for years (Paton, 1987); inadequate data and information systems (Paton, 1987; Gumpert and Lyons, 1990); a lack of time (ibid.); the fact that the process can be threatening, boring (Gumpert and Lyons, 1990) or require highly specialized medical knowledge (Jessop, 1989); the educational needs of senior and junior doctors differ (Packwood, 1991); and suspicions about managers' interest in audit (Tomlin, 1991).

These suggested obstacles have largely been based on the personal views of the respective authors. . . .

First published in *Social Science and Medicine*, 36(7): 849–56 (Elsevier, 1993). Abridged.

Unless the views of doctors are recognized and addressed, no amount of funding, persuasion and directives will prove successful in implementing effective medical audit. This study set out to discover and chronicle the views on audit of doctors working in general (internal) geriatric and accident and emergency medicine. Knowledge of their opinions and experiences should provide a more realistic basis from which to assess the measures most needed to fully implement audit.

Methods

Interviews were carried out between August and October 1991 in four NHS district general hospitals in south-east England. These hospitals were taking part in a large study of the cost-effectiveness of an audit of the appropriate use of thrombolytics in people admitted with chest pain. Selection of hospitals for the study was based on the doctors having both an interest in the subject and a willingness to participate. Although the four hospitals are fairly typical of district hospitals in England, their agreement to participate suggests there may have been some selection bias in favour of audit.

All consultants and junior medical staff working in general medicine were invited to take part. In addition, in each hospital, one consultant and two juniors in geriatric medicine plus one consultant in accident and emergency medicine were asked to participate. Sixty-two interviews were conducted by one of the authors (ET), about half with consultants and half with junior doctors. . . . This included all the relevant consultants (except for one who was 'too busy') and about 50 per cent of junior staff. Those junior doctors not participating were either on leave, not interested or said they did not have sufficient time. It seems probable that the non-respondents were less supportive of audit than the respondents.

The interviews were relatively unstructured and lasted between 15 minutes and 1 hour. Respondents' views were sought on the following aspects of audit: its purpose; its impact on relationships between doctors; its help in day-to-day work; its impact on quality; the extra work it generates; its educational role; its effectiveness and usefulness. Notes were taken during the interview and supplemented by additional notes made immediately afterwards. The data were analysed using the method of constant comparison (Glaser, 1964).

Results

Before discussing the various obstacles that respondents identified, it is important to recognize that many doctors expressed a good deal of enthusiasm for audit. Their concerns and criticisms should be considered in this context. Here we have focused deliberately on the worries they had, since it is these which are of most importance in developing better methods of implementation. Generally speaking, adverse comments were made in the hope that difficulties could be overcome and audit could be strengthened. The obstacles to audit that the respondents identified can be grouped into four categories: perceptions of the need for and the role of audit; practical considerations; the effects of audit; and anxieties about the use of audit. Each will be considered in turn.

Perceptions of the need for and role of audit

Most doctors accepted the need for audit and identified it with good doctoring. However, rather than seeing it as anything new, they felt that they had been carrying it out for years, starting long before the recent spate of interest from government, professional associations and managers. The only change had been formalization of their existing activity:

> We have been doing audit for a long time. Clinical meetings have been going on for as long as I can remember. It is nothing new, we are not big stupid buffoons who do not question what we do. By its very nature the medical profession is a very self critical group. Audit is a more formal version, sometimes too formal. (Consultant)

> I think it has always been going on in people's heads. There is nothing new about audit. Now it's all written down and it's made more of an issue. (House officer)

> (It's a) myth that we've never been doing it before. (Registrar)

While such widespread existence of audit should be encouraging to its proponents, most of the activities referred to were actually unsystematic, irregular, unstructured discussions of clinical subjects with no clear agenda for action of attempts to reassess the problem after improvements in practice had been attempted.

A second perception that could impede the development of audit was suspicion about the motives behind the current encouragement from government. Many respondents seemed to feel that cost containment rather than improved quality of care was the real motive. Doctors' belief that improvements in quality could only be achieved by increased expenditure simply served to increase their incredulity regarding government motives. For example, they felt consultations would need to be longer in order to ensure patient satisfaction and more time would be needed to write legible notes and to ensure that discharge summaries were dispatched promptly. Some felt that government and managers would be prepared to use audit information to reduce resources and yet would not be prepared to increase recourses if they were needed.

> I'm suspicious of the motives for audit. The package that it came in . . . it's like trying to squeeze more blood out of a stone. (Consultant)

> The latest reforms came in a packet. It's definitely a way managers can control their budget. (Consultant)

> Do you want the truth? I think it's a government intervention, a political tool to discipline doctors and make them do more work. It's another initiative imposed by the Conservative government, well Mrs Thatcher really, to discipline doctors. Its an important political weapon with which to divide the NHS. . . . You may have caught me on a bad day! (Consultant)

Doctors who held such beliefs were sceptical about the real motives of their colleagues who were undertaking audit:

> I think it attracts those who want to have less to do with patients and more to do with politics. It is for those doctors who are not so busy. It attracts them. Good doctors are always busy because they have many patients to see. This is rather rude but it's like the saying – those who can, do and those who can't, teach. (Consultant)

. . . A third potential problem was that many felt audit should be confined to administrative rather than clinical issues. This was partly because they perceived clinical aspects as being too difficult to audit and partly because variations in clinical practice were seen merely to be a reflection of differing approaches to medicine, differences which should be accepted, if not actually encouraged. In contrast there was considerable support for auditing administrative matters.

> Case review generally reveals things such as wrong GP's address, no letter to GP and so on. It's nearly always a clerical problem such as the wrong address and so on. The management of patients is good. It's usually other things such as a lost letter to the GP and then the patient ends up with the wrong drugs. (Registrar)

> I do think audit should look at the management of things, the functioning of the hospital. There's a lot of red tape and bureaucracy in the hospitals and I think that when audit was set up it was set up to audit this. Also I think with medical conditions there are always reasons for and against, always arguments . . . it's difficult to reach a consensus. If audit looks at better and easier ways of management then I think that the goal is clear and achievable. . . . (Senior house officer)

The emphasis on administrative problems rather than clinical ones led to a fourth intriguing perception of the role of audit: the question of who exactly was being audited. Since the junior staff carry out the day-to-day duties of clerking and managing patients, juniors felt that more than anything else it was their work that was being monitored – and duly resented the fact:

> I know it has to be done but . . . err you get it in the neck a bit, really. It's enough strain as it is without added hassle . . . you're the one that's on the ground, the one who admitted him. (Senior house officer)

> At audit meetings we look at topics such as GI (gastro-intestinal) bleed or case review . . . we look at the notes, whether they are dated, tidy, are they filed? It's probably important but it's very tedious. . . . Often it comes down to almost the handwriting. (Senior house officer)

Many consultants shared this view unapologetically:

> The purpose of audit is to check standards, to look at the junior doctor's management and see whether it is acceptable. To look and see whether they have overtreated, undertreated . . . to review ongoing management. (Consultant)

. . . Finally, there was a common, recurring perception that audit sought to turn medical practice from an individualized, subtle art into an unthinking, routine activity based largely on guidelines and rules. Many doctors believed that such dependency upon guidelines would have adverse effects for doctors, destroying the initiative of juniors who would no longer think through the logistics of treatment but pick up a form and tick the appropriate box. Some doctors also believed that the presence of guidelines meant that they were obliged to comply with them, even when they felt that it was not appropriate in a particular case.

> I haven't been practising long but sometimes it's best to follow your own instincts. As you get more senior you have to think of medicine as an art. I'd hate it to be constrained with form filling and following regular guidelines. (House officer)

> I feel you should do what you are happy with. You should not be foot-marching into something you do not agree with. (Consultant)

Others recognized the value of audit and therefore the need for compromise but still worried about the introduction of strict guidelines:

> If everything was rigid, then some of the fun would be taken out of medicine. We do need some framework, but would not want it to get too regimented. (Consultant)

Practical considerations

. . . Given the potentially sensitive nature of audit, it is desirable that it takes place within a cooperative, supportive environment. The need for this together with the dangers of carrying out audit in a hostile environment were clearly recognized:

> Doctors should not feel threatened. It's not a question of slagging each other off. It's criticism which should be constructive. (Consultant)

> No one would have the bottle to criticize with any degree of aggressiveness. You wouldn't. It would be professional suicide. You wouldn't want to anyway. (Consultant)

> At meetings you can get peer encouragement and bullying. It depends how supportive the group is. If you have a group who were already at each other before audit, well then audit will make it worse. (Consultant)

. . . Even if conflicts are avoided, fear of them can still inhibit criticism and thus reduce the potential effectiveness of audit. Juniors, in particular, could feel unable to challenge their seniors:

> I do think that the junior staff don't join in much. I think you feel a bit intimidated . . . you don't really like to criticize the consultants. (House officer)

While juniors' dependence on their seniors for future jobs made them reluctant to criticize consultants, some consultants, in their turn, felt inhibited due to their lack of medical knowledge in particular areas. They felt it inappropriate to audit their colleagues unless they were a specialist in the field under consideration. It was, therefore, much easier for everyone to focus on organizational issues where knowledge and experience were more equal. . . .

Moreover, even if the working environment was conducive to audit and doctors felt no inhibition about criticizing their colleagues, audit still imposed an additional burden of work – a third practical problem:

> I get a bit annoyed with central government when they say you must do audit, but they do not understand the different constraints upon doing audit. (Consultant)

> There are two problems with audit and that is time and money. This change has been added to the health service with no resources to put it into shape. That part of it has not been thought through. It's piling more responsibilities on us. The secretaries are very busy and have not got time to pull more notes. The facilities are not there. (Consultant)

Lack of time was exacerbated by other concurrent health service reforms that had led to an increase in demands on consultants' time. Activities such as resource management and collecting clinical information all imposed their own load. Thus, although the introduction of audit officers and assistants was generally appreciated, it was felt there was still insufficient time for analysing results and preparing for meetings. As a result, seeing more patients or spending more time teaching juniors were viewed by some consultants as possibly more effective uses of their time. . . .

Medical audit had also created extra work for the junior staff, who already felt over-committed. While the juniors agreed with the principle of audit they had other priorities too and felt that it was impractical for them to get too involved. If protocols were not filled in the success of audit projects could be jeopardized:

The trouble is the juniors have to do it all. When you've had 20 admissions and then some psychiatrist asks why we hadn't filled in the forms . . . it's difficult. (House officer)

Well I'd get more involved if it was taken out of our time, not if it took up extra time in our day. If half a day was devoted to audit, then that's fine. (Senior house officer)

In addition, some juniors felt that the extra work imposed on them was for someone else's benefit:

We're at the front line. We're managing patient care. On top of that, audit creates extra things for us to do. We do all this so they can write up a paper of get their name added to something. (House officer)

. . . A fourth area of practical difficulty arose from doctors' limited knowledge and understanding of audit. This was partly revealed, as has already been seen, by respondents' beliefs that they had been auditing their work for years, despite a lack of use of criteria, standards or reassessments. . . .

Lack of understanding of audit was not universal. There were many doctors who knew about the audit cycle – the need to establish criteria of good quality care, set standards, see if those standards were being achieved, implement changes and then reassess to see if the quality of care had indeed improved. Despite knowing what they should be doing, many doctors recognized that they were failing to carry out audit properly:

Really we talk about audit rather than do it. (Senior house officer)

. . . One consequence of this was that many doctors were highly critical of audit meetings.

There were two principal criticisms: dull administrative topics were selected rather than issues of clinical practice and often no decisions were made or action taken to improve the quality of care.

At [previous hospital worked at] I didn't go to any meetings. At [another previous hospital] it was even worse. So boring. We used to have to hand in our bleeps so no one could escape. It was so boring. We looked at dull topics, like discharge letters and we concluded that we weren't doing them quick enough. (Senior house officer)

The best thing about audit is the sandwiches at lunch. (Registrar)

. . . Some consultants were well aware of their juniors' lack of enthusiasm for audit meetings and were attempting to improve the situation:

I think it has to come from the top. There is no point telling the juniors to get involved if the consultant does not. I expect the registrar to be involved, in some areas I regard them as being more experienced than me. I think it is important for juniors not to look at it as some sort of ivory tower. That takes time. (Consultant)

I have a checklist so everyone feels obliged to attend. I worry about the meetings . . . that the juniors feel that they are a waste of time. I think the difficulty is in getting audience participation . . . now I'm trying to get the juniors involved in thinking up a programme and to actually lead the meetings. (Consultant)

While such strategies may increase junior participation, nothing can at present be done to change the sixth practical difficulty – junior doctors' relatively short contracts of employment means that completing the audit cycle would usually take longer than their stay at the hospital:

At grass roots level you resent having to write up all the forms and then you move on after six months and don't really see the changes or benefits that come out of it. (Registrar)

Finally, lack of participation is not a problem confined to junior staff. As has long been recognized, audit fails to touch some of those that it is meant to reach. Respondents felt that it was too easy for consultants not to participate as it was voluntary. If was felt that those that needed auditing most would not participate.

In the past anyway I think good doctors practised audit and bad ones haven't. (Consultant)

It is, however, superimposed on an already heavy workload. Those that need disciplining don't go. Good doctors have an academic and intellectual audit of their own. (Consultant)

Effects of audit

. . . Is audit effective in improving the quality of care and if so, is it the most cost-effective approach? Even the most ardent supporters of audit seemed to be uncertain as to its effectiveness:

With things like audit it is an act of faith. To practice it you have to be convinced . . . it's difficult. (Consultant)

Take the quality of the notes. You find that they [juniors] make more entries, they are more legible. Whether or not this means that there is an improvement in patient care is difficult to say. The problem with audit is that the outcomes of audits aren't necessarily reflected in the outcome for the patient. Maybe that will come later. (Consultant)

I have no evidence. It's a gut feeling. If we're completing the cycle, then it should improve care. (Senior house officer)

Not surprisingly, those with little sympathy for audit were convinced it was ineffective or could even directly harm the quality of care:

Rubbish. That's it. That is what I think. They think we are looking at how we manage ourselves. I think that nothing ever happens. (Consultant)

Pharmacy did an audit on resuscitation and as a result . . . a new policy was adopted. They told some people, but not us. On one of my wards a patient needed resuscitation and my staff went to the equipment and things were not there that are usually there. Audit did not cause that, but it was a consequence of audit. (Consultant)

The ineffectiveness of audit was, as has already been seen, frequently blamed on the failure to complete the audit cycle. Audit seemed to repeatedly reveal the same problems with the quality of care, but there was no evidence that matters were actually being corrected. Such failures were attributed to a lack of organization, poor management or the need for additional resources. . . .

Some doctors were also concerned about the cost-effectiveness of audit, given the cumbersome nature of obtaining information in the NHS, the great commitment needed and the possibility of improving practice through other, possibly better, means.

> More and more time is given up to go to meetings that weren't done before. It is assumed that this is all good news and no one is questioning whether they are beneficial and what they are replacing. (Consultant)

> I could learn that [the subject of the audit] from a paper in five minutes, instead of sitting through hours of audit meetings. Few people would argue with that. (Consultant)

> I think it is good, useful but is it the best thing to do, to spend money on? (Consultant)

> It's gone a bit mad. Everybody wants to audit everything. I think it's a good thing but if they paid us double, doubled our numbers then there would be no need to audit. (House officer)

Finally, there is the danger of doctors appearing to change their clinical practice to produce better audit results while in reality continuing to practise in the same way. In one of the hospitals, a house officer admitted that juniors had decided to modify their entries in the case notes in order to influence the audit results and maintain the appearance of reaching their targets.

Anxieties about the use of audit

While doctors' principal concerns were about the current practice of audit, many were anxious about the uses to which audit might be put in the future. Their anxieties covered the potential of audit to be used to intimidate doctors, further growth in expenditure on audit, medico-legal implications and an increasing involvement by managers and politicians. . . . Some doctors felt that audit would increase rather than decrease their vulnerability to litigation.

> The more structured and formalized it [clinical practice] becomes, the more it becomes an issue for medico-legal purposes. . . . I can see more lawyers using failure to comply exactly with agreed guidelines as negligence. (Consultant)

In the future, the legal medical implications (is my worst fear), because that is the way that some people earn a living. For example, you may follow 90 per cent of guidelines and if you do not follow 10 per cent because of clinical discretion will you be sued? (Consultant)

Finally, it has already been seen that some doctors were convinced that managers' and politicians' interest in audit was motivated by cost containment. There were even greater anxieties about the future behaviour of managers and governments:

There is a lot of suspicion between clinicians and management. Doctors will fiercely defend their actions. They do not want to be dictated to by administration. I don't think that management should interfere, tell us how to run our clinics and so on. If a doctor is not seeing enough patients then fair enough, management should tell the silly man to pull his socks up. (Consultant)

I don't think management should have access to all data. They should have access to information that they need to manage. If management had authority to move around, I mean to get information and make decisions, they wouldn't understand what clinical medicine is about. The reason I'm saying this is because I've been rather disappointed with management. They don't really understand what medicine is like. (Consultant)

However, not all consultants took the likelihood of such developments so seriously. Two respondents took a much more cynical view:

If you have been here as long as I have, then you usually find a way around things. (Consultant)

If think it's a phase in the NHS. It's a bit like TV franchises, the poll tax. It'll soon die down. It's a pain experiencing it. I think audit will change shape and form many times until it becomes disreputable. It's a shame because it distances doctors from enjoying their jobs. I don't want audit to occupy any more of my time. I think that there will be a new buzzword next year. (Consultant)

Discussion

Doctors have many criticisms of audits. This should not make proponents of audit despondent, as most critics accepted the general aims of audit and shared its objectives. Their criticisms were levelled more at the way audit was being implemented than at the principles of the approach. On the other hand, it would be equally foolhardy to be complacent and dismiss the criticisms as ill-informed comments born out of the respondents' self-interest.

Nineteen potential obstacles grouped into four categories have been identified. While some of these confirm previous anecdotal reports by writers on audit, several have received little or no attention. Before considering the practical implications of the findings, we wish to make two general observations. The first concerns the validity of the data. Should we believe what the doctors say? Much of the material can only be taken on trust. The recurrence of similar views from different doctors, often working in different hospitals, suggested that a particular opinion or experience was neither unique nor fabricated. For some issues, we were able to confirm the respondents' comments. For example, examination of the minutes of audit meetings revealed that no attempt was being made to complete the audit cycle. This was confirmed by attending the meetings. For other issues we cannot be so confident. Reports of junior doctors having dreadful, humiliating experiences at audit meetings generally seem to occur to 'other people at other hospitals'. It's possible that such accounts are the medical equivalent of urban myths, always happening to third parties elsewhere.

The second general observation is related to that of validity. Hundreds of accounts of audit by doctors have been published, ranging from general discussions of methods to descriptions of specific projects, yet all the authors speak about their subject in a strikingly different way from the doctors interviewed for this study. Why is this? Partly it may be due to selection – authors of audit articles tend to be enthusiasts and successful audits are more likely to be reported than failures. A second factor is the contrast between public rhetoric and personal experience. We found this in our interviews. On initial questioning, respondents tended to provide well-accepted definitions of what audit was and why it was important. It was only after this 'public rhetoric' had been produced that doctors started to give us their views based on personal experience. A similar contrast has been demonstrated in research into lay people's views of health and disease (Cornwell, 1984).

What then are the main lessons to be learnt from this study? The first is that factions or interest groups in organizations may subsume new initiatives for their own purposes. . . .

A second lesson that emerges is the extent of medical complacency that exists. This is best illustrated by the confidence with which doctors declare that the principal (or even only) problems affecting health services are administrative and organizational rather than clinical. . . .

A third lesson, and one that has previously been noted (Baron, 1983), is that many doctors are not convinced about the value of audit. They repeatedly question the opportunity cost of their time, audit staff and other resources, and resent being forced to undertake audit. . . .

Finally, doctors seemed to confuse a knowledge of medicine with a knowledge of audit. . . . What they didn't appreciate was that audit is largely about asking questions about how and why medicine is being practised in the way it is. It is not necessary to know the correct answer; it is necessary to have the courage to ask simple, revealing questions.

Through interviews with practising doctors, this study has produced a taxonomy of their beliefs and attitudes. It would now be
possible to quantify how rarely or widely held such views are by
means of a quantitative study. Some of the range of obstacles to audit
could be overcome by simple practical measures and others by
improving doctors' understanding and skill at conducting audits.
However, many problems would remain which will only respond to
more profound changes in the beliefs and attitudes of doctors. The
difficulty of achieving such change should not be underestimated.

Acknowledgements

We would like to thank all the doctors who participated in the
interviews, Mike Robinson and Phil Strong for their comments; and
the Department of Health for funding. This study was carried out in
collaboration with the Research Unit of the Royal College of
Physicians (London).

References

Baron, D.N. (1983) 'Can't audit? Won't audit!' *British Medical Journal*, 286: 1229–30.
Cornwell, J. (1984) *Hard-Earned Lives*, London: Tavistock.
Eisenberg, J.M. (1986) *Doctors' Decisions and the Cost of Medical Care*, Ann Arbor:
    Health Administration Press.
Glaser, B. (1964) 'The constant comparative method of qualitative analysis', *Social
    Problems*, 12: 436.
Gumpert, R. and Lyons, C. (1990) 'Setting up a district audit programme', *British
    Medical Journal*, 301: 162–5.
Jessop, J. (1989) 'Audit: all talk and no action?', *Health Service Journal*, 31 August:
    1072.
Packwood, T. (1991) 'The three faces of medical audit', *Health Service Journal*, 26
    September: 24–6.
Paton, A. (1987) 'Audit long overdue', *Health Supplement*, 3 (September).
Tomlin, Z. (1991) 'Grasping the nettle', *Health Service Journal*, 27 June: 31–2.

24

E. Scrivens

The Accreditation Experience

. . .

The King's Fund organizational audit

The King Edward's Hospital Fund for London, an independent foundation whose mission is to improve the quality of management in the NHS, has developed the nearest thing to a national accreditation system in the United Kingdom. This scheme has evolved from an interest in the experience of other countries with accreditation. In the early 1980s the Fund sent a multidisciplinary team to look at the Joint Commission on the Accreditation of Healthcare Organisations system (Maxwell et al., 1983). The JCAHO standards were tried out by two pilot hospitals but this development lay fallow for a while. Later the Fund set up a process of peer review for a small number of hospitals, and adapted the standards from the Australian system. This developed into what is now known as the King's Fund Organizational Audit Scheme. This is a scheme which, although it incorporates advice from the medical profession and colleges, is not dominated by them. The 17-member board includes representatives from general practice, the United Kingdom Central Council for Nursing, Midwifery and Health Visiting, the Royal Colleges of Physicians, Surgeons, and Obstetrics and Gynaecologists, the Professions Allied to Medicine, the Institute of Health Services Management, the National Association of Health Authorities and Trusts, the Independent Healthcare Association, and the National Association of Community Health Councils. In addition there are two consumer representatives, one from the National Consumer Council. And finally there are observers from the Royal College of Nursing, the Conference of Royal Colleges, the NHS Executive, and the Health Advisory Service.

This is the most extensive scheme in existence. Its clients are acute general hospitals and teaching hospitals, all large institutions with

First published in *Accreditation: Protecting the Professional or the Consumer* (Open University Press, 1995), pp. 50–68. Abridged.

many beds and also many independent (private hospitals) which tend to be relatively small and specializing in elective surgery. The final reports are qualitative, highlighting areas of good practice and deficiencies. Recommendations are made for improvements, but it has no graded outcome. The scheme is different from any others reviewed in the UK and abroad, in that survey managers are employed who help the organization with its preparation. Unlike all other accreditation systems, the Board does not assess the individual reports returned to participating organizations. The activities of the Board are restricted to the overall workings of the operation and the standards. The surveyors, usually three working for three days, are health service practitioners, a doctor, a nurse and a manager. Hospitals pay a fee to participate – the scheme is run on a not-for-profit basis and is self-funding.

Because of its origins, the emphasis has remained on self-improvement: on professional peers learning from each other during the surveying process. This is reflected in the fact that the King's Fund audit does not award a pass or fail or attempt any sort of accreditation award or grading, following the visits of its surveying teams but merely reports to the hospital concerned about what it has found. . . . There has been no attempt, as yet, to introduce outcome indicators. Changes are, however, being planned: the King's Fund Organisational Audit Scheme is about to adopt the accreditation label, to offer pass/fail awards and to revise its standards to emphasize patient outcomes.

Like its counterparts overseas, the King's Fund is also extending the scope of the services it covers. It is moving into other service areas, notably community hospitals and primary care services.

Hospitals contact the King's Fund Organisational Audit Unit and make an application to enter the organizational audit process. The growth in popularity of the audit means that some hospitals have to go on a waiting list until there is a slot available for them. But once accepted the hospital is then supplied with the manual of standards and a coordinator from the King's Fund is assigned to the hospital to help it through the 12 months of preparation for the final survey. The manual is then issued throughout the organization to managers who set about involving staff and ascertaining whether the standards are met. A steering group is appointed from within the body of hospital staff who supply the necessary management controls and motivation for staff. To encourage staff to understand the process and to feel involved, most hospitals hold open meetings where the steering group can talk about the process and what is involved. The King's Fund encourages participating organizations to go through a mock survey a few months prior to the survey which enables the organization to see how well it is doing. After 12 months of preparation, the surveyors (usually three: a doctor, a nurse and a manager) then visit for about three days to review the hospital against the standards. A timetable is arranged for the surveyor visits by the hospital and all necessary documentation is sent to the surveyors a week before the survey.

The surveyors normally meet with the management team early on the survey day to introduce themselves and to discuss any issues. They are then taken individually to meet the relevant staff and to visit wards and departments. In the course of the visits, they discuss the standards with the managers and their staff, and discuss aspects of interest with any members of staff they meet. Normally a night visit occurs so that the night face of the hospital can also be seen. The surveyors write down their impressions and note compliance with the standards as they go around the hospital and at the end of each morning and afternoon begin to compile their reports. On the evening of the final day of interviewing the surveyors work together to draft the outline of their report on the performance of the hospital. On the final day of the survey, the surveyors meet with the executive team and inform them of their detailed findings. Then there is usually an open, public meeting with any members of staff who wish to attend, where the surveyors report their general impressions.

The coordinator takes the draft report away and within a few months, after approval by the King's Fund board, the report, with commendations for good practice and recommendations for improvement, is sent to the hospital. It is then up to the hospital what it does with the recommendations. Most will institute processes to encourage staff to act upon them. And after three years, the hospital decides whether it wishes to repeat the process.

The Hospital Accreditation Programme

The Hospital Accreditation Programme (HAP) was the first accreditation scheme to develop in the UK and in some ways is the only true model in that unlike the King's Fund it awards an accreditation status. Its clients are community hospitals which provide non-acute care (mostly nursing, rehabilitation and minor surgery), frequently to rural communities who have restricted access to the large acute hospitals. The scheme was derived from the Canadian model and its standards were first published in 1988 (Shaw et al., 1988). It awards graded scores offering one or two years' accreditation, with the possibility of non-accreditation. The Board which has membership comprising representatives of the Royal College of General Practitioners, Anaesthetists, Surgeons, Obstetricians and Gynaecologists, and Nursing, plus the rehabilitation professions, the English National Board for Nursing, the National Association of Health Authorities and Trusts, the Institute of Health Services Management, the Community Hospitals Association, the British Geriatrics Society, the Independent

Health Care Association and the Community Health Councils, awards the final accreditation score. Surveys take one day, are pre-planned and organizations have to prepare themselves for the process. The scheme is self-funding, with participants paying for the costs of the survey. The surveyors (normally two are in attendance) are practitioners working in community hospitals or general practitioners who review the process. The standards focus only on organizational processes and make no attempt to incorporate clinical standards. However, in line with all other accreditation systems, the scheme has been updating its standards to emphasize linkages between hospital departments.

The survey process in the HAP is very similar to the King's Fund in most respects (Hayes, 1992). The community hospitals receive the manual containing the standards six months before the survey is due to be conducted. During that time, the hospital staff work on the standards to assure that they conform with them. In many cases, the hospital managers will contact colleagues in other hospitals to check ideas with them. On the appointed day, two surveyors review the hospital against the standards, meet with the staff to give their general impressions at lunch-time and at the end of the day. The surveyors then write their report and when this has been passed by the HAP board and accreditation status decided upon, the hospital is issued with a certificate and a report showing good practice and recommendations for improvement. After one or two years (depending upon the status awarded) the hospital has the opportunity to repeat the survey before accreditation lapses. This is therefore a continuing process of examination.

The experience

Interviews were conducted with the managers who had participated in either of the schemes to ascertain the impact of the accreditation process and the views of managers towards the process. The 17 managers interviewed for the HAP were managers of small community hospitals, ranging from 9 to 40 beds. The 27 managers taking part in the King's Fund scheme were chief executives of acute hospitals ranging in size from 200 to 600 beds. In addition, a detailed study of two hospitals participating in the King's Fund scheme was undertaken by members of the accreditation study research team. A comparison of the views of managers from the King's Fund and the HAP shows a remarkable similarity in the perceptions of the experience. Whether the organization is a large acute hospital or a small rural one, the work involved, the stresses and strains caused to the organization and the benefits to be derived are reported as being nearly identical.

The motivation to seek accreditation

Although participation in accreditation schemes is theoretically voluntary, for most health service staff, the perception of the voluntary nature of participation is limited. The decision to apply lies in the hands of the chief executives of independent trusts, although a small number felt that they had been forced into this by their purchasers. The managers of the community hospitals, who are part of a larger management organization, rarely had the opportunity to choose not to participate.

> The Unit General Manager talked to the manager of the scheme and we were volunteered to sign up. The same manager had only just decided to go on the programme. We felt we were a flagship and would like to join. (HAP)

> We didn't apply. The previous locality manager decided it would be a good idea and applied. It was discussed with us. She 'sold' the idea to us. (HAP)

A number of managers felt that they wanted to enter the accreditation programme to compare the performance of their hospital with others. A recurrent theme is that hospital managers of both large and small institutions feel isolated in their work and want to be able to compare their management with their peers.

> The reasons for going for it were two-fold. First there was a recognition that for the future there needed to be some sort of benchmarking and league tables. We wanted to influence that, so we needed to understand it, and therefore had to do it. It was an opportunity for the organization to take stock. It is a good way of testing out whether the hospital was working as a hospital or had clinical directorates which caused the hospital to split up. . . . There were many who felt there were some benefits to show a wider audience. It would show that our hospital was a good place. (King's Fund)

> At the time, I think that the answer was merely that we would know where we stood. And on the side of the survey where we didn't expect to do well, we figured that would give us an action plan, an agenda to instigate improvements. It's independent and relatively inexpensive. (King's Fund)

In addition, the larger hospitals saw it as means of controlling the conflicting demands placed upon them by a number of different purchasers.

> There were two main reasons. One was, we price ourselves on high standards and therefore we wanted to test the theory, if you will, against a nationally recognized scheme. And two, as a hospital that has a lot of purchasers who could all impose their own quality standards, we thought we could take the initiative . . . rather than responding to 15 different sets of criteria, we could just say, there, we've done it to an independent national standard. (King's Fund)

Preparing for accreditation

It is generally accepted that preparation for accreditation is onerous, at least the first time. It is also accepted that probably the greatest value of accreditation lies in the preparation. There was little difference in the responses, whether the hospital is small (some community hospitals are only 10 beds) or large (acute units can have as many as 600 beds).

> Really it allowed us the opportunity to self-assess, to see these are the standards, how far do we go to meet them, and where we don't what action will we take to put it right. In many ways, this caused a certain amount of grief, to tell the truth, because we were very honest. (King's Fund)

> We had to write policies for everything . . . we didn't possess any. We decorated the whole place purely for accreditation. In their questionnaires each head of department had to identify shortcomings and met to discuss what we could do. Some things we just couldn't, but we tried to see what we *could* do to meet the standards. (HAP)

Many hospitals, particularly the small ones, did not have information in the appropriate format. Most had been managing with very little information and the requirements imposed by the accreditation standards generated a lot of work. In both the King's Fund and the HAP systems the standards were cascaded through the hospitals, requiring staff in all departments to pull together the information.

> All the forms went out to the various members of staff. We had to have the information from central sources with statistics which we needed. Nevertheless the staff came up with the goods and on the day were complimented on the information we had managed to get together. There were 25 people involved; nursing staff, catering, admin. More or less everyone had something to do with the nurses. Medical staff were not involved last year but this year I will give it to one of the purchasers. (HAP)

> We involved all the nurse managers, all the clinical directors, all the department heads. It took an awful lot of my time to manage the dissemination of standards, actually physically going through them. It was very time consuming – a lot more than we were led to believe. (King's Fund)

Therefore, a major benefit from the requirement to provide information before the visit was that managers were able to review and amend existing information systems. They reported some surprises in the information they reviewed. It was apparent to them that if they had not been required to provide the information they would never have examined it. The information questions had changed between years one and two of the programme and the changes were felt to be a great improvement. The managers did point out that collecting the information took a tremendous amount of time and effort, which they often reported was very rushed.

The first time they were useful because I realized what I hadn't got. But it made a lot of work for me. I had to rush around and create things. (HAP)

Motivating staff is a major management task. Many managers found that they had to work very hard to instil enthusiasm and interest in the staff. Much depended upon their approach to the exercise. Leadership from the top of the organization turned out to be very important in demonstrating the commitment to a quality initiative.

[Our staff were] not enthusiastic at all. There was a certain amount of feeling threatened – especially to start – when the standards were first seen and identified as unachievable. (King's Fund)

Mixed: on the whole they found it an interesting challenge and rose to it. The value was more in areas where people found they weren't as good as they had thought after all. (King's Fund)

All accreditation systems are dependent upon considerable amounts of data collection. This is partly due to the demands of the standards for policies and procedures, partly due to the laborious task of checking compliance with the standards. Any organization going through accreditation for the first time expends a considerable amount of energy galvanizing staff to find the information. The most activity went into the writing of documents and policies for the surveyors to examine. A major benefit of the accreditation visit was that it required the collation of policies and statistical information which in many cases had not been collected before. Managers reported that they had used accreditation to encourage team work between the staff in the hospital. It provided a useful opportunity for different departments to come together to discuss issues within the hospital. It was also vitally important that the staff owned the accreditation process.

In particular, the doctors found it hard to accept the process. Many were very resistant to it and were not interested in getting involved. And without medical support, the exercise is of limited value. However, most managers found that by running special workshops, using noticeboards and newsletters for communication, and showing enthusiasm, staff, including the clinicians, could be won round.

We had to do lots of presentations to staff to get them to take part. We had a noticeboard. We had to organize a special meeting for the King's Fund to come up and meet the medical staff. The doctors felt they couldn't understand what it was about and wanted convincing. (King's Fund)

The standards

As the accreditation systems have attempted to cover the whole range of hospital (and health service) activity, the standards have multiplied in number, resulting in literally thousands of standards. But they do offer a definition of good practice and a starting place for assessing the quality of organizational processes for most staff who would find it difficult to decide the components of good practice.

> It is like going to an encyclopedia. You have to be bothered to look. You might not agree with all of them but they are good thought provokers. (King's Fund)

All the accreditation systems, including the King's Fund, have found it necessary to revise the standards continuously to reflect new views of health care and service design. The rapid pace of change in the health service demands a lot of an accreditation scheme to keep it up to date and relevant to those delivering the services.

The survey visit

The value of the accreditation survey visit is the linchpin of success for accreditation systems. The surveyors, in effect, make or break the accreditation process.

> The two who came were delightful. They made every member of staff feel very comfortable and not threatened. They were very positive about the whole day and that was important. I felt I could go out and tell my girls 'well done'. They had put their utmost into it and the way information was asked of them really helped them. (HAP)

> It was the Spanish Inquisition. The GP surveyor was very complimentary and made good suggestions but his manner was inquisitorial and efficient. The nurse was a bit warmer. We were told they wouldn't get in the way but they took a lot of time. The sister in casualty and the midwifery superintendent were absolutely shattered afterwards. The domestic and catering assistants weren't asked anything although they were all prepared to talk. They were very disappointed about this. I don't know what we would have done if there had been an emergency. (HAP)

> The surveyors were very fair, accommodating, personable people – and it is important that they do have the credibility themselves as individuals. (King's Fund)

All systems have found that the credibility of the surveyors is crucial to the success of accreditation. If the surveyors are not of high enough status, if they are not well qualified or if they appear to make irrelevant comments or ask the wrong questions they can bring the whole process into disrepute.

> The one who didn't go down very well was the private manager. He'd worked in the NHS for a very long time before he went to a private firm, but unfortunately, because of his private sector experience, he didn't have the credibility. (King's Fund)

> We felt that by and large the survey team were not up to the job, in the sense that they came from much smaller organizations. They didn't appreciate the political dimensions of a large hospital. (King's Fund)

We had problems with the nurse surveyor. She was a top manager but she told the managers that the nurses would benefit from a standard cardigan. It blew her credibility. (King's Fund)

The surveyors have to use their judgement to assess which areas of the hospital to concentrate their energies upon. They have limited time to review the processes of highly complex organizations. In the case of HAP, an unsatisfactory final grading was frequently contested by the participants who felt that they had not been reviewed objectively.

If you look at it [the report] you can see that we were marked quite highly . . . got mostly credits. So what criteria did they use that we should not have been accredited? We felt on the whole we'd done quite well. It's all a question of judgement, isn't it? But I think this hospital was actually much better than another I know that got two years' accreditation. (HAP)

The UK, with its less well developed commitment to accreditation, demonstrates a greater degree of scepticism about the value of surveyors. A number of hospitals have preferred to 'go it alone', obtaining the standards and limiting their involvement to self-assessment. There are different views about the benefits to be derived from this approach. It seems unlikely that the organization can inspect itself as adequately as others can. It is harder to structure the exercise and the process and requires considerable self-discipline. It is also impossible to gain the credence given by an external assessment.

The UK also shows the substantive difference in the experience of accreditation according to the size of the organization. The community hospitals reported that the survey day was a nerve-racking experience. Everyone said how tired they had felt at the end and experienced a feeling of anticlimax. Their main concerns were that the surveyors did not talk enough to the staff who had become very involved in the preparation for the day and had wanted to participate. And that sometimes the surveyors missed pieces of information which gave the impression that some things were not being done when they were. This reveals the highly personalized nature of the survey to a small hospital where accreditation was felt to be a 'family affair'. The same feelings were reported by the smaller private hospitals which had been through the process.

This contrasts significantly with the experience of the larger hospitals. The chief executives claimed that the surveyors disappear into the fabric of the hospital to emerge days later. Many staff did not even know the surveyors had been around. Although the standards applied may be identical, and the surveyors' approach the same, the reaction of the institution may be very different. Staff are 'hyped up' to the survey visit and have expectations which frequently exceed the surveyors' ability to deliver, in terms of meeting and talking with everyone.

> I think there was a great deal of build-up to the survey. We pointed out to
> them not to be disappointed if they didn't spend a lot of time in their area.
> But they were. (King's Fund)

> The general view was that it was less than we expected. At the end of the
> day it was a bit of a let-down . . . not so much in terms of the work that
> went into it, but in the survey week. (King's Fund)

> It wasn't the most pleasant of days. When they left it was like a wedding
> day without the disco. (HAP)

> There was a tremendous anticlimax. Even though we prepared people to
> see organizational audit as ongoing, the surveyors came and then they
> were gone. Some departments had done remarkable amounts of work, and
> on the day itself, there was a fleeting visit. They didn't even see the
> surveyors, some of them. (King's Fund)

For the community hospitals, where the hospital had been referred
for a future visit, or the accreditation status awarded was less than
the maximum number of years, the managers felt they might have
been unfairly judged by the surveyors.

Reports and recommendations

The final report which communicates the findings in written form is
equally contentious. The level of detail contained in the document is
an important finale to the survey visit. The HAP experience was that
a number of the managers felt that these reports were too short,
particularly in cases where the hospital had been referred. Managers
felt that the reasons for the accreditation status awarded were not
explained well enough. Many of the managers spent a considerable
amount of time trying to reason out why they had not received a two-
year accreditation. This was significant in the cases of managers who
had encouraged their staff by telling them they were 'going for gold',
for two-year status. They felt they needed information to explain to
their staff what had gone wrong. Not surprisingly, those who had
received two years' accreditation were less interested in the fine
detail of the report. But if there is a duty of education placed upon
the accreditation programme, it is vitally important that final reports
are accompanied by explanation and suggestions for improvement.

> The report sets out an action list. You have to agree what you are going to
> do and put dates on which these things will be done by. (King's Fund)

The distribution of the report around the participation organization
varies, often depending upon the result conveyed and the reactions of
the staff to the accreditation status awarded. A number of the
managers in the community hospital scheme confessed to having
waited a while after receiving the report before telling staff its content.

The King's Fund managers, although not pressured by accreditation status, behaved in a similar fashion. There was a reluctance to make departmental managers feel that they were being criticized for their performance. So reports and recommendations were divided up, with only the relevant sections being handed to individual managers.

> Very, very useful. The report has been a bible . . . everyone's had it and knows what we must look at. Always being mindful that the GP and nurse who wrote it were not infallible. It's been a very useful tool for managers to enhance the quality. Very nice to go to the Trust with the report in hand and point out what's been highlighted as not so good. (HAP)

External reviews do raise expectations among the staff which cannot always be met. Not only do staff expect to be talked to during the visit, they also expect consistency between the verbal reports and the final written report. Managing participating organizations' expectations turns out to be one of the hardest tasks.

> We did encounter one problem. . . . We had surveyors who visited a few directorates and they made their verbal report although they didn't mention it in the final written report. (King's Fund)

> Some departments were left out of the written report and were fed up with the fact that they felt ignored and we had some serious morale problems after that. (King's Fund)

The participants' perceptions of the benefits of accreditation

Whatever the size of the organization, the preparation for at least the first accreditation visit appears to take considerable time and work. The organizational standards demand policies and procedures which in many cases have to be decided and written. Much depends upon the desire of the managers to write usable policies. The greater the concern about applicability, the more necessary it is for managers to gain the interest and cooperation of staff. So in some organizations, the process of applying for accreditation becomes one of involving staff and gaining their commitment to the idea of quality and its implementation. The participation in accreditation systems therefore becomes more of a management tool and takes as many resources as managers wish to use. . . .

> It helped us focus on quality. It would have taken us a lot longer to have a 'culture of quality' in the organization. It was a good vehicle to provide us with an overview. (King's Fund)

> It recognized the need to get clinicians involved in the process. It galvanized the staff to think about quality issues. It did make them update policies and procedures. It did get people to work together. (King's Fund)

. . .

> They didn't tell us anything we didn't already know but it was good to hear
> it from the King's Fund. (King's Fund)

In the small community hospitals of the HAP scheme, accreditation
forced the managers to look at the whole of the hospital rather than
at discrete departments or functions within the hospital. A number of
the managers were new in post and they felt that working through the
accreditation process had helped them get a feel for the managerial
tasks and responsibilities they were facing. In the larger hospitals
participating in the King's Fund, the managers were more likely to
have greater experience. For them accreditation served the purpose of
creating a more coherent focus on quality for their staff. It became a
symbol of commitment to quality initiatives. . . .

Another benefit of accreditation, found in all schemes, is network-
ing and support between managers in different hospitals. Entering
the programme gave managers a reason to contact colleagues in other
hospitals. Not only did this produce a sense of collegiality among
participants, fostering new friendships and generating an excuse to
visit other sites, it also alerted managers to good practices which
were growing up in other hospitals. Interestingly, in the smaller
hospitals there was no sense of competition between the hospitals but
a growing sense of camaraderie. The competitive element was
supplied by trying to achieve the status of two-year accreditation. In
fact a number of managers were distressed that their colleagues in
other hospitals had failed to achieve the two-year status. There were
stories of visits to other hospitals to learn how to organize the day
and make the appropriate preparations, of borrowed curtains, and
advice on how to keep the surveyors happy – such as feeding them
a good lunch. The larger hospitals in the UK, facing greater
competitive pressure, did tend to look further afield than nearby
hospitals.

The difference between the impact of accreditation upon the community hospitals and the larger acute units is striking in the UK. . . .

The managers of the large acute units were less likely to 'sell'
accreditation on this basis. They emphasized the need to make it a
non-threatening exercise, encouraging staff but not allowing failure
to be seen as criticism. Care must be taken in interpreting these
differences. One interpretation is that the community managers were
protected from the need to consider competitive strategy by their
relatively lowly place in the strategic hierarchy. But the community
scheme carries with it accreditation status and therefore the risk of
failure is inherent within the accreditation process. . . .

One recurring issue raised by managers, across both the community and the King's Fund schemes, was that the surveyors made
recommendations which require expenditure and in many cases the

hospitals did not have resources to make the recommended changes. ... In a number of cases, particularly the community hospitals whose managers have limited powers and even more limited budgets, this caused the managers to question the usefulness of the exercise: 'What is the point of being told to do things you cannot do anything about?' However, a number of community hospital managers saw a main purpose of the accreditation process as putting information to unit managers about the need for improvements, and as a means of arguing for more resources. Some managers felt that the surveyors should convey this information directly to senior management in order to ensure that the information had the desired impact. Equally a number of acute unit managers saw opportunities from the recommendations of the King's Fund to argue with their purchasers for more resources. The King's Fund outcome was seen as a vindication of management difficulties, enabling greater discussions between the purchasers and providers about capital investment and service development.

The positive effects of being told you are good enough were felt to create signals not only inside but also outside the hospital. The general public could be informed of the success of their local hospital.

> We put it in the local paper. We sent copies to the Community Health Council and the purchasers; but we don't think the purchasers noticed. (King's Fund)

Purchasers, too, in theory could be told of the relative success of their providers. Such is the theory. The community hospitals, frequently under threat of closure, were able to use a successful accreditation outcome to inform the general public of the tragedy of closure. ...

The larger hospitals were less likely to adopt such a strategy, again probably because the King's Fund did not carry any convincing measure of success. Furthermore, the larger hospitals also discovered the need to have a purchaser interested in, and capable of understanding accreditation. Although in a few cases the purchasers were asking for accreditation, few were interested in the results *per se*. The provider units accused their purchasers of ignorance of the purpose and the processes of accreditation. ...

But it was also true that most providers were unwilling to share the reports emanating from accreditation with their purchasers. They feared that purchasers would seize upon recommendations and begin to use them to control the work of providers. This ambivalence can be attributed to the poor relationships most acute unit providers have with their purchasers in the internal market. The providers' greatest fear was that of interference from purchasers in their day-to-day management. Accreditation reports in many cases were too detailed to be shared with purchasers. ...

References

Hayes, Jackie (1992) 'Accreditation in community hospitals', *Health Direct*, 19: 11.

Maxwell, Robert, Hardie, Robin, Rendall, Max, Day, Margaret, Lawrence, Hilary and Walton, Neville (1983) 'Seeking quality', *The Lancet*, January (1/8): 45–8.

Shaw, C., Hurst, M. and Stone, S. (1988) *Towards Good Practices in Small Hospitals*. Birmingham: National Association of Health Authorities.

25

C. Corkish and B. Heyman

The Resettlement of People with Severe Learning Difficulties

> The world in which we live is not always safe, secure and predictable. It does not always say 'please' or 'excuse me'. Every day there is a possibility of being thrown up against a situation where we may have to risk everything, even our lives. This is the real world. (Perske, 1972: 24)

This chapter is based on a research project which is examining quality of life issues for people with severe and profound learning difficulties who are currently resettling from a long-stay institution. . . .

Cultural and domestic factors mediate the ways in which people with learning difficulties encounter risks (Perske, 1972; Edgerton, 1975; Edgerton et al., 1984; Edgerton, 1988; Heyman and Huckle 1993a, 1993b). This research, in general, portrays adults as restricted by their care environment, and family carers have been represented as trying to maintain their offspring in a childlike state (Richardson, 1989; Richardson and Ritchie, 1989). However, this view of the family carer role discounts as irrational parents' fears about the dangers which they see people with learning difficulties as facing, and overlooks cultural variations. Heyman and Huckle (1993a, 1993b) found that adults with relatively mild learning difficulties who came from better-off, two-parent families, generally had less autonomy and were more protected than those from poorer, single carer, families. Ironically, the children from more prosperous families appeared to be achieving less of their potential with respect to everyday living skills.

Cultural beliefs, material wealth, ethnic origin, parental marital status, the gender of the main carer, and of the person with learning difficulties, the health status of both, and the local environment may influence family attitudes towards risks. People with learning difficulties cannot learn how to manage risk for themselves unless they are given the opportunity to practice. Incompetence resulting from lack of practice reinforces the impression that they can never learn. Conversely, the view held by many parents that their offspring have

First published in *Risk, Health and Health Care* (Arnold, 1998), pp. 215–27. Abridged.

reached the limit of their potential, and therefore should not be exposed to additional risks, should not be dismissed *a priori*. . . .

Formal carers' perspectives on risk management

Life in any environment, inescapably, entails risk. However, paid carers who take decisions on behalf of people currently undergoing resettlement are faced with a risk-management dilemma. At one extreme, environments which maximize safety may severely limit individuals' life experiences. At the other, environments designed to enrich life experience may generate demands on a person which they cannot, currently, manage safely. Professional care staff need to develop environments that optimize the balance of autonomy and safety, and to identify ways in which service users' existing skills can be improved upon, so that the zone of acceptable risk-taking can be expanded.

In theory, more personalized care can be provided in smaller community homes. However, paid carers who wish to enhance service-user autonomy have to continually appraise and manage situations involving potential risk to individuals with severe disabilities. If, for example, a client wished to visit the local public house, the carer would need to assess the risks entailed on the basis of previous knowledge of the individual's capabilities and anticipation of possible negative outcomes. The carer would then need to attempt to plan to meet *all* anticipated contingencies. In practice, restrained by staffing and other resource limitations, formal carers may be tempted to access local facilities by taking all the residents out collectively. Although service-users may value such activities, they do little to promote personal autonomy or competence.

When adversity does strike, judgements about the actions of responsible staff may be subject to hindsight effects. Fear of punitive action by employers and professional bodies, and of litigation, can dissuade formal carers from exposing service-users to avoidable risks. Anecdotal evidence from colleagues, and press reports of staff negligence, can serve to reinforce an atmosphere of uncertainty, while formal carers have very little personal incentive to allow service-users to take risks. Not surprisingly, they often adopt a risk-minimization strategy.

Staff balance resident safety and autonomy in different ways. A few of those responsible for the different residences within the hospital studied took service-users on regular weekend trips to a large shopping centre, 11 miles away, or to a more local swimming pool and pubs. Staff who adopted this line saw access to the local community as relatively easy to obtain. One staff member wrote that the hospital was 'rather central, walking distance to local shops, on a regular bus route. Hospital has contract with a local taxi firm', and that 'Residents are accepted in local community.'

Most hospital formal carers, however, rated accessibility as a major problem which limited external activities, and highlighted the disabilities of the residents. As one staff member wrote: 'Most residents are disabled and use wheelchairs [for] most trips out, visits to shops even local are made by taxi or bus. Distance for wheelchair users too far.' This staff member also took a much more pessimistic view of community integration, stating that there was 'very little contact with local people'.

Variations in staff attitudes may have arisen because of differences in the disabilities of service-users living in particular residences, since similar clients tended to be grouped together. One ward, for example, catered for the more elderly population. However, each residential area housed at least a few individuals dissimilar from the rest, who needed extra support when engaged in potentially hazardous activities. Given the need to manage groups of residents *en masse*, the balance of personal development versus safety tended to be struck at the level of safety which was deemed appropriate for the most vulnerable members of the group. One staff member responded to the questionnaire items on risk management and community access as follows:

> Normality can only be taken so far, depending upon the type of resident living within the home. Abilities differ dramatically.

This carer had had to cope with an increased number of people who had challenging behaviours moving on to the ward as the hospital rationalized its resources. These individuals, although a minority, needed a greater level of support, taking staff away from the rest. This 'lowest common denominator effect' may intensify when residents move out into community facilities and are exposed to new internal and external hazards.

How should professional carers differentiate between acceptable risks and dangers to be avoided? The rational individualistic model of care, which many hospital and community establishments purport to employ, would utilize information from a wide variety of sources. Details of individuals' skills, physical and mental state, history and personality would all contribute to an assessment of their present abilities. Risks could then be considered in relation to environmental hazards. For the fictitious character . . . who wanted to visit a local pub, the relevant information might include his knowledge of geography, purchasing skills, drug-alcohol contraindications, ability to manage alcohol consumption, mental state, previous experience of the pub and general demeanour. Knowledge of the fictitious public house, especially its safety for the individual concerned, would figure largely in the equation. As a result of this calculation, the level of necessary support could be determined, or an alternative provided if necessary. In this way, probabilistic reasoning could be used to shift the balance from dangerousness to risk for the individual.

Unfortunately, such individualized risk appraisal cannot be achieved in current conditions. Care staff do not enjoy the luxury of making decisions solely on the basis of information about individual service-users and their environment. They have to consider issues such as professional accountability, staffing ratios, previous experiences, political pressure, the needs of other service-users and relatives' demands. However, as people who have learning difficulties resettle from institutional into community facilities, the opportunities for experiencing healthy risk should increase. Long-stay hospitals, by their design and organization, have achieved the objective of the early reformers, to provide safe segregated care, but have generated dehumanizing, overprotective living conditions.

Formal carers working in the new community-based environment have the opportunity to break away from the old institutional culture. They should be able to find the appropriate means to restore the balance between risk, and safety for each individual, provided that the institutional mentality does not merely relocate as the hospitals close. . . .

Family carer perspectives on risk

Professional and family carers differ considerably in their attitude to risks. Family carers, most commonly parents, looking after a relative at home may worry continually about their relative's personal safety, and fear for their future after the carer has died. The close relatives of people who have lived most of their lives in hospital face different issues. Direct responsibility for day-to-day care has been transferred to formal carers, who make judgements about the persons' risk-taking capabilities from a different viewpoint. Although concerned for residents' welfare, they are unlikely to have the same degree of emotional involvement as family members. They can appraise risks in a more detached way, but have to take into account the requirement to manage groups of vulnerable people, and the risks associated with professional accountability.

Some residents within the hospital were originally admitted through necessity, for example following the death of the main carer. However, the majority moved to the hospital as a result of decisions made by their next of kin. Of the 98 residents being resettled, 68 per cent were under 18 when they were admitted to hospital. Accounts given by the 51 next of kin who visited residents regularly suggest that their original decision to have a relative admitted was influenced by the concern expressed by health professionals and other family members about the safety and well-being of the person with learning difficulties. Having made the decision to admit their relative, family carers had to rely on the expertise and trustworthiness of hospital staff.

The impending closure of the hospital will dramatically affect those moving out. On average, the hospital residents included in the present study have spent 36.7 years (range 10–65 years) in the same environment. During this time, friendships between residents, and between residents and staff, have developed. Routines necessary to the smooth running of the organization have become well established. Residents may find resettlement difficult to cope with, and service-providers have given some consideration to overcoming 'transition shock' (Booth et al., 1989). The emotional consequence for their next of kin is, perhaps, given less attention. Many family members participating in the present research discussed their feelings and actions at the time their relative was admitted to hospital, and spoke of admission as a recent event despite the long time period which had since elapsed: a testimony to its significance for them. Of the 51 people visited, all but one expressed confidence in the hospital staff and in the quality of care provided.

Relatives' feelings about the impending resettlement were, however, more mixed. Eighty-one per cent (41) of those contacted expressed concern about the safety of their kin in the new environment, and about the ability of care staff to recognize potentially dangerous situations. Relatives cited well-publicized cases, in which individuals moving out of long-stay mental illness hospitals had encountered problems, as evidence of poor community-care practice.

A minority of family members opposed resettlement completely, and had formed protest groups which sought to maintain hospital-based care. However, none of those whose relatives had already been resettled expressed anxiety about the risks associated with the new environment. Those next of kin who had been visited by members of staff from the community home before their relative moved there were, also, generally less anxious than those who had not. Direct or indirect experience of the new environment appeared to rapidly assuage family carer apprehension. Relatives may have been reassured by the rapid erosion of risk-taking in the new community homes.

Discussion

Few of the service-users participating in the present study will ever be able to fully understand the issues involved in risk management.

Decisions affecting their health and safety will always be made by others. However, people who have severe and profound learning difficulties are capable, to varying degrees, of learning how to manage some hazardous situations successfully. For example, many residents excluded from hospital kitchens could, with support, learn how to negotiate this dangerous environment safely. Some risks must be accepted if residents' quality of life is to improve in the new community setting.

Formal carers need to find an appropriate balance between risk-taking and danger avoidance. Staff are, inevitably, influenced by factors other than the needs of individual service-users. They have to manage groups of residents, and must seek to protect their own professional status by avoiding disasters for which they would be held accountable. There is a risk that any adverse events that do occur will be subject to media amplification and overreaction, leading to the reinstitution of the hospital environment in a community setting.

Alternatively, with respect to services for the elderly, care systems for vulnerable people may respond to the dilemma of autonomy promotion versus hazard avoidance by oscillating between the two over the longer term. A trend towards prioritizing safety may eventually be corrected, perhaps in response to outside criticism, because life for residents has become too stultifying. When disasters occur, they are then blamed on the risk-accepting line, and the regime becomes more restrictive.

Closely regulated systems may be criticized for failing to promote as normal a life as possible for residents of institutions, while more risk-tolerant systems can be accused of recklessness if accidents occur.

Service-user risk-taking ability is, at present, assessed informally in the community. Safety rules commonly evolve in response to specific incidents. This reactive approach to accidents needs to be replaced with proactive planning based on detailed knowledge of individuals. It should be possible to predict how much autonomy each resident can be given in different zones of everyday living, and to plan accordingly. The establishment of formal risk-assessment procedures in community settings would help carers to design systematic risk-management programmes which balance costs and benefits and do not depend on responses to the vagaries of chance. Documented risk assessment would also protect professional carers from litigation by enabling them to demonstrate that they had employed reasonable care in taking risks. Professionals who feel confident that they have only accepted appropriate risks, in line with organizational policies, may not need to adopt protective strategies which will defeat the purpose of the community-care reforms, and provoke an eventual counter-reaction.

References

Booth, T., Simmons, K. and Booth, W. (1989) 'Transition shock and the relocation of people from mental handicap hospitals and hostels', *Social Policy and Administration*, 23: 211–18.

Edgerton, R.B. (1975) 'Issues relating to quality of life among mentally retarded persons', in M.J. Begab and S.A. Richardson (eds) *The Mentally Retarded and Society: A Social Science Perspective*, Baltimore, MD: University Park Press.

Edgerton, R.B. (1988) 'Aging in the community: a matter of choice', *American Journal on Mental Retardation*, 92: 331–5.

Edgerton, R.B., Bollinger, M. and Herr, B. (1984) 'The cloak of competence: after two decades', *American Journal of Mental Deficiency*, 88: 345–51.

Heyman, B. and Huckle, S. (1993a) 'Normal life in a hazardous world: how adults with moderate learning difficulties and their carers cope with risks and dangers', *Disability, Handicap and Society*, 8: 143–60.

Heyman, B. and Huckle, S. (1993b) 'Not worth the risk? Attitudes of adults with learning difficulties and their informal and formal carers to the hazards of everyday life', *Social Science and Medicine*, 12: 1557–64.

Perske, R. (1972) 'The dignity of risk and the mentally retarded', *Mental Retardation*, 10: 24–6.

Richardson, S.A. (1989) 'Letting go: a mother's view', *Disability, Handicap and Society*, 4: 81–2.

Richardson, S.A. and Ritchie, J. (1989) *Letting Go*, Milton Keynes: Open University Press.

26

D. Leat and E. Perkins

Juggling and Dealing: The Creative Work of Care Package Purchasing

The study

. . . The data reported in this chapter were collected in the course of a wider study of alternatives to residential care. The aim of this particular part of the study was to identify both the role of unit costs in costing a package of care, and other factors that influence the way in which care managers put together packages of care. The study fieldwork was undertaken in late 1994 and early 1995 in six selected authorities participating in the 'Caring for People Who Live at Home Initiative' which was set up by the government to encourage developments in day and domiciliary care, particularly in the independent sector. Authorities were selected to include urban and rural and different levels of development of the independent sector. In each authority semi-structured interviews were conducted with four care managers involved in constructing care packages for a range of client groups. Additional interviews were undertaken with other budget-holding officers, contracts officers and financial allocation panel members.

Care managers constructed and purchased care packages within broad centrally directed policies and practices concerning purchasing in the independent sector. However, there were important distinctions between policy and practice; and between policies and practices in relation to different user groups and different services. In addition, there was an important distinction between policy and practice pre- and post-autumn 1994.

First published in *Social Policy & Administration*, 32(2): 166–81 (Blackwell, 1998). Abridged.

Pre-autumn 1994

Policy in relation to purchasing in the independent sector varied in terms of both its explicitness and its approach. In one authority there had been an explicit policy statement that in-house services should always be the first port of call, and purchasing in the independent sector should only occur if in-house services were unavailable. This was the policy, but in practice 'It's not worth the paper it's written on' because resources to in-house services had not increased and services were fully booked. In other authorities managers reported a positive explicit policy encouraging purchasing in the independent sector. But, whatever the policy, managers reported strong institutional and cultural barriers to purchasing in the independent sector at the time. In one authority care managers described the notion of care packages and purchasing from private care agencies as 'like something off another planet'.

In the early months of 1993, purchase in the independent sector was hampered in some authorities by the state of the market. For some user groups and some types of service independent sector provision simply did not exist. This was most likely to be true of services for groups other than elderly people, but availability also varied within and between authorities. As one local authority purchaser explained:

> When community care came in in 1993 we were dealing mainly with in-house services because the private sector hadn't got its act together. In the rural areas there was no private sector home care to purchase so we had to get it from in-house providers. When the private sector began to flourish we were able to go to them, although we were purchasing mainly domiciliary care and residential and nursing care.

Purchasing in the independent sector in these early months after implementation of the Act was also constrained by care managers' lack of knowledge of availability of independent sector providers. Even if such providers were available, and care managers knew that they existed, purchasing might still be constrained by lack of confidence and trust. As one care manager said: 'I knew that a few existed but I didn't know them. It was very much taking leaps in the dark at that stage and that's quite a difficult thing to do with other people's care.'

In all of the authorities studied, this situation changed during 1993. More providers became available, sometimes with the active stimulation and support of the social services department. Although availability of independent sector provision increased in most authorities, certain types of service for certain user groups remained in very short supply.

Purchasing in the independent sector gathered pace as care managers gained knowledge of available providers and more confidence in their reliability. One care manager remembered: 'You started off knowing no one. But then you used a few and they were OK so you used them again. You began to develop a relationship and an understanding and you built up a little list of agencies you went to as your first port of call.' Most of the care managers interviewed reported that by the autumn of 1994 more independent sector providers had entered the market (though this was still uneven within and between authorities), and knowledge, relationships and confidence were becoming established. Purchasing from the independent sector was taking off. One care manager summed up the situation towards the end of 1994: 'You couldn't purchase in the independent sector everywhere but where you could – where they existed – you probably did it. At the least you seriously considered doing it, which was a major change in itself.'

Further development of purchasing from the independent sector was constrained not only by unavailability (for some services and user groups) but also, and increasingly, by the lack of spare capacity in new, small agencies. The effects of limited capacity in agencies were exacerbated in some authorities by care managers' desire, and/or explicit departmental policy, to purchase as much as possible of any care package from one agency in order to maintain continuity for the user by keeping the number of agencies involved as low as possible.

The effects of these constraints were somewhat offset by the resources available to develop and sustain independent sector agencies. One care manager explained: 'I'm not saying for one moment that we were profligate with care but we could, at that stage, afford to be fairly flexible, pay their price without haggling and make it worth their while in terms of, say, total hours purchased.' As a consequence some packages were expensive, above the comparative cost of residential care or even nursing home care and well above net costs. Furthermore, in some authorities emphasis on spending in the independent sector increased as the need to fulfil the conditions of the Special Transitional Grant (STG, requiring 85 per cent spending in the independent sector) became more urgent.

Briefly, by the late summer of 1994, in some authorities there were signs of a rosy dawn for the NHS and Community Care Act reforms. Purchasing in the independent sector was developing, new providers were entering the market, relationships and trust were growing – and statutory provision, though still largely dominant, was experiencing the chill wind of competition. And then came the frost of autumn 1994.

Post-autumn 1994

At different points in autumn 1994, authorities experienced varying levels of pressure on their budgets as it became clear that STG moneys had, or were going to, run out. This was dealt with in a variety of ways including raising eligibility thresholds for care;

introducing limits, or reducing existing limits, on the value of any individual care package; cutting the cost of existing care packages by x per cent; requiring that all newly arranged services be provided in-house or designating the independent sector as a 'last resort'.

These approaches had various effects on constructing and purchasing care packages. In some authorities, in-house services were, in most cases, already fully booked or were only available mid-morning. For new users in-house services were effectively available only if someone died, went into hospital or reduced their care for other reasons. In some authorities care managers reported that in-house care had not been available for months, and suggested that users should be cautioned to 'book early to avoid disappointment'.

Even if new purchasing in the independent sector were permitted, care managers still faced the difficulty of reduced maximum limits on spending on care packages. If there were any in-house care available at any time (e.g. mid-morning) they attempted to get what they could from in-house services and then top up with purchases in the independent sector, 'boxing and coxing and juggling around to cobble something together'. In order to stay within the new required limits and to reduce the cost of existing packages, care managers could reduce the quantity of care purchased or, in some authorities, they could attempt to maintain quantity but reduce cost by asking providers to reduce prices.

Unsurprisingly, purchasers reported resistance from independent sector providers to any attempt to reduce prices. But in some areas care managers reported that: 'Once they realized we were serious and we really would go elsewhere or that it was that or nothing, some of them were prepared to bargain.' Some care managers suggested that, for the first time, shopping around in the independent sector became a real possibility as previously overstretched agencies began to have spare capacity.

By the beginning of 1995, the combination of lower maximum limits for domiciliary care packages and the limited accessibility (for different reasons) of in-house and independent sector services was, some suggested, in danger of re-creating the perverse incentive to residential care. Predictions of a 'big comeback in residential care' were not uncommon. In some authorities care managers reported that residential care home owners and managers were now telephoning the authority to ask for business when previously the phone was in the other hand. Furthermore, some homes were now prepared to accept Income Support prices which they had previously rejected.

Budgets and financial limits

There were at least two levels of control over spending on care packages. One level controlled total spending on purchasing care packages (budgets) in a department, district/area or team, and the other controlled spending on each individual care package. In theory, there had to be some mechanism linking spending on individual care packages to total spending within budgets at different levels.

Controls over total district spending on purchasing Control over budgets for total spending on purchasing care packages varied between, and to some extent within, authorities. Budgets devolved to district or area level were primarily composed of STG moneys. There were plans in some authorities to engage in further devolution of budgets to teams, but in one authority budgets previously devolved to teams had been 're-centralized' to district level.

Although budgets had been devolved, what this meant in practice varied. Some respondents claimed that there had been no clear budget limits at district level. In addition, some complained that indicative team budgets were the necessary, but missing, building blocks for workable district-level budgets. So, for example, in one authority, the situation was described as follows:

> In theory, the district manager knows when the district overspends. If there is a problem at district level that may be because of a problem across all the teams, and that must be shared at district level. The team manager is responsible for not overspending and if he overspends the DM (district manager) will want to know why. But currently the team doesn't have a notional budget. From April this year (1995) we will have.

Some complained that they did not have either the information or the training, or both, to manage budgets. The importance of limits, ongoing information and training were illustrated by another respondent:

> It would only be helpful to have budgets if they were reliable. I haven't even got a calculator and I have no administrative support to check my figures. Basically we are still going on intuition and guesswork. So we meet every week, discuss what we've got and try to make decisions on the basis of some kind of allocation that is in our heads. For example, we know that we can't do more than one drugs case every week.

The lack of information for budget monitoring and management underlines the finding of other studies (Hawtin and Smith, 1994; Lewis et al., 1996). One particular problem in monitoring spending concerned ongoing commitments and end-dates of placements/ services. In this respect, care package construction and purchase resembled trading in futures, in organizations where management understanding, information systems and controls were ill-adapted to the work of those spending the money.

Controls over spending on individual care packages Control over spending on individual care packages occurred via two main mechanisms: allocation panels/teams and financial limits on individual care packages.

In most authorities allocation panels met at least weekly. In some authorities they were largely a final check on arrangements made by care managers, within clearly laid down eligibility thresholds and financial limits on the cost of any individual care package. One care manager described her allocation panel as: 'More or less a rubber stamp. As long as the person is clearly within the new tighter eligibility category and as long as you're within the new lower limit then you're pretty safe in assuming it will go through.'

In other authorities, allocation panels were more interventionist in both controlling spending and in rationing and approving individual packages. One allocation panel member described this type of approach:

> Care managers come to the allocation meetings saying they have assessed an individual's needs and this is what they are. If the client is in category C he/she would not receive a service. But in relation to A or B we would say we have a responsibility to fund some care. The issue becomes how do we therefore fund the package in the most cost-effective way. There may be other ways in which we could fund it and there may be other ways in which we could provide it without any cost to us – for example, by suggesting a voluntary organization – and that is how it would be resolved.

In some authorities, allocation panels had changed their way of working over time. As demand increased and larger numbers of care packages were being constructed, some allocation panels became overburdened and began to delegate approval of some or all care packages within agreed limits.

Creative purchasing

Purchasing policies, budgetary arrangements and financial limits formed the framework within which care managers worked. One fundamental factor in creating a care package was the availability and accessibility of supplies of care regardless of its source. As we shall discuss below, care managers attempted to 'stretch' the available fabric of care by various means.

Comparing costs

As Lewis and colleagues have noted, providers' systems are not geared to producing information about costs in the manner required by purchasers (Lewis et al., 1996). One of the issues in which we were especially interested in this study was the role of unit costs in the creation and purchase of care packages. What information was available to care managers on unit costs and how did they use this?

Availability of information on unit costs varied between authorities, with some care managers equipped with information on the unit cost of every in-house service. However, as one care manager pointed out: 'Information on the cost of in-house services isn't really very relevant in that the cost of in-house services isn't costed against your budget so in that sense it doesn't matter.' In general, however, even if in-house services were not costed against the budget, their cost was included in any limits on the total cost of an individual care package, and were included for independent living funds (ILF) calculations.

Estimates of unit costs of in-house services varied in their level of detail and 'realism'. Information on such costs might or might not include a full scale of costs detailing prices for daytime, evenings and weekends. This information was, in theory and in some cases in practice, important in both calculating the cost of a care package and juggling the contents, as well as in comparing costs with those in the independent sector. The 'realism' of in-house costs was also important for the purposes of comparison with the cost of independent sector services. But as one care manager commented:

> The costs on in-house home care are £6 per hour which I'd guess is a pretty optimistic figure. In theory it seems to me it's a case of market rigging because that's then the benchmark for the others. But in practice it doesn't matter much at the moment because in-house care simply isn't available.

Information on costs in the independent sector also varied. Whereas the cost/price of in-house services was centrally set, if at all, that of independent sector services was frequently whatever the individual agency charged. In some authorities there was no systematic official information available, but care managers reported that, 'You soon get to know how much is charged and for what. You build up your own price lists in your head if not on paper.' In one authority, which was unusual in having developed an approved provider list for home care agencies, that list also gave unit costs of services from each approved provider. This included out-of-hours costs but all costs quoted were inclusive of travel and any other 'extras'.

Care managers raised various issues in discussing the value of information on unit costs in constructing care packages. One of the most important was that of real availability, i.e. if a service is, in effect, not available then its cost is of little relevance. but other issues were raised which were more narrowly concerned with the complications involved in using and comparing information on unit costs of different services and providers. As one respondent put it: 'If you think that constructing and costing a care package is about listing the services and then putting a price beside each one, multiplying by however many units, you're wrong. It's not that simple.'

Travel costs In some cases these were included in the quoted unit cost (especially for in-house services), in other cases they were not. If they were not, they obviously had to be calculated in relation to the number, and distance, of separate journeys rather than the number of hours of care provided. Especially in rural areas this could significantly affect the cost of care. But there was a further complication explained by one care manager:

> If travel is not included then it can change as the worker changes, or if the worker's work sequence changes. It would be much easier if the price was all inclusive and stayed the same for us, but then the agency would be bearing the cost and the uncertainty and they might not be prepared to provide, or might stop if their work pattern changed. It would probably reduce what little choice there is for users in rural areas.

Scales of charges for out-of-hours work, and the definition of out-of-hours As one care manager explained:

> You can look at two sets of prices and one looks a lot more expensive than the other. But then you look closer and find that the cheaper one charges extra for evenings and weekends whereas the other doesn't. Or you find that both charge extra for evenings and weekends but the one that initially seemed more expensive charges less than the cheaper one. And then on top of that you find differences in when 'evenings' or 'weekends' begin.

Using information on unit costs involved knowing exactly what you wanted to purchase and when, as well as the exact composition of the total purchase. A further difficulty was that having established that this provider gives the best value, given the total composition of the purchase, that total composition may change, e.g. the user may require more care during the day and less at weekends, thus altering the calculation of costs and benefits of choosing this provider.

The way in which units are multiplied and the effect of this on total cost One provider may charge £y per hour for evenings and overnight care; another provider may charge £y + 1 per hour for evenings up to 10 p.m. and a total charge for the whole night which may be less than £y × 8 hours charged by the first provider. The cost of night care was affected not only, or primarily, by the cost per hour but by the unit of calculation and the 'fit' between that unit and what was needed by the user.

The minimum chargeable unit This was an issue of particular importance to many care managers in putting together and costing packages of care. As one care manager explained:

> One of the most difficult things is when you need a quick check visit, or someone to put the lunch on the table. It may take 15 minutes and you might want two or three per day, but some providers won't do it unless they can charge you for an hour, and some have a minimum two-hour

charge for the first hour. From their point of view that's probably fair enough, but from mine it gets expensive. But a few providers will do it, or they will only charge for half an hour. So you might go to a provider who has a high price per hour but if they'll do a check for half or even a quarter of that then they're obviously cheaper than another one who has a lower cost per hour but insists on a one-hour minimum. On the other hand, they may only be willing to do the quarter-hours if they're also getting the rest of the package, or some other package close by – and then you may be paying the higher rate for other things and it may work out more than if you'd just paid for the full hour at a cheaper rate.

Although in the past some care managers had been able to get 15-minute visits from in-house home care, this service was no longer generally available. In some authorities in-house services were fully booked and, in others, in-house home care now refused 'to be dumped with all the 15-minute calls' and demanded a minimum one-hour contract.

Changes in price   There were different controls in different authorities to prevent this happening, and different penalties for the provider. But it was rarely a simple case of raising prices in an obvious direct way. What purchasers might describe as raising prices, providers might explain in terms of inappropriate assessments of either user needs or time required.

The effects of grant-aid to voluntary organizations   Grant-aided voluntary organization services were usually in effect 'free' to budget-holders in that they did not represent a cost to the budget. If they could access such services this was clearly an advantage to budget-holders and, indirectly, to care managers. However, as one manager pointed out:

> As a budget-holder funding via grants is an advantage to me but it's also a disadvantage in two ways. One is that I can't plan properly. If Mrs A is receiving 10 hours of service from a grant-funded voluntary organization and she dies and Mrs B, with exactly the same needs, moves into her house it doesn't follow that I can give her 10 hours of service because Mrs A's death hasn't given me any hours or any money. The second disadvantage of grants and block contracts is that the price you pay today may be quite different from the one you have to pay tomorrow for exactly the same service. That's true in two senses. If I get someone a place at x day centre today I may pay nothing because they have a block contract for 20 places and there's one place left. Tomorrow there are none left under the contract so I have to pay the full amount. And in grant aid you're getting these places for nothing or at prices which are subsidized by the grant – but next year if grant aid is phased out I've no idea what we will be paying.

Listing these complications in using the comparing unit costs gives an over-simplified picture. In reality, the complications interact with and feed each other, requiring the care manager to juggle one set of considerations against another. Unit costs were only part of a complex equation in which prices were negotiated, total cost juggled in the context of budgets, financial limits and real accessibility, and all that balanced with quality considerations.

Dealing and juggling

In some authorities care managers were required to obtain three quotes before agreeing to purchase any services in a care package. But the procedures for checking up on this varied. For example, in one authority all three quotes were supplied to the contracts division; in another authority, the care manager was only required to record the accepted quote. But, in an important sense, the formal requirements prior to statement and acceptance of quoted prices miss the dynamic reality of purchasing care.

Creating a care package is, in many respects, very little like going to a supermarket and buying goods off the shelves up to a maximum total spend. Some care managers described constructing care packages in ways which resembled street or stock markets, rather than shops. They talked about 'wheedling' and 'persuading', 'doing deals' and 'juggling'. Prices were regarded as open to negotiation, depending not least on the quantity purchased. They were searching for ways of getting more for less – not necessarily by driving down prices from providers but by using in-house and other (e.g. grant-aided voluntary sector) resources which were not charged to the budget, even if they were included in any limit on the total cost of the services in any one individual's basket of care.

One care manager described the process: 'You go to a provider and say "Look, I need this care here, can you do it and what will you charge?" And they quote a price and if it's going to take you over the limit then you start dealing. You might take out the evenings and hope you can cover that from somewhere else or you might add in the evenings and say "If I pay your price plus £x will you do the evenings as well?"'

Another care manager described the way in which it is misleading to look at purchase of any one care package in isolation from purchase of others. 'You may want an hour's care in a village. The provider wants a minimum two-hour price because of the travelling. So you try to find another care manager who wants the other hour. You hear people shout out: "I've got an hour's care in Greenfield – what will you pay me for it?"' This is not playing shops, it is trading on the stock of care exchange.

Quality considerations

Quality considerations were a thread running through the juggling and dealing discussion above. At the time of our interviews, most care managers were working without developed formal approved-provider lists. In the beginning, finding good providers had been a matter of 'trial and error' but care managers reported that they were now starting to develop their own list of trusted providers. However, several stressed that this was very much a personal matter related to personal experience of the purchaser and the user.

Continuity was one of the most frequently mentioned considerations relating to quality of care. In several authorities the initial policy had been to restrict the number of agencies involved in delivery of any one care package to one or two. Since autumn 1994 this policy had been relaxed, and the aim was now to provide the necessary care by whatever means possible.

Care managers did not necessarily believe that continuity of care workers was always a major dimension of quality from the user's viewpoint. As one remarked:

> It depends on the user and on the task. Some people may rather like having some variety, new people to talk to, a bit of a change, whereas for others a stream of different people coming into your house may be very confusing and upsetting. But it also depends on the task. If it's very intimate then building up a relationship with one person and having continuity is important.

Restricting the number of agencies involved in delivery of a care package was only part of the problem of ensuring continuity of care. One agency may send a different care worker every day and, conversely, two agencies may send only two different care workers. In general, care managers were reluctant to use agencies which did not provide continuity and stability of care workers. However, as one care manager pointed out: 'In the end there's not a lot you can do about it. If I took the contract away then I'd have to find another agency which would be another change and the same thing could easily happen again because they're trying to juggle limited staff, cover absences and do the best they can with the staff they've got.'

Quality care for some groups was defined in terms of encouraging independence, and this was seen as an approach not readily available from in-house or external agencies. Some care managers believed that an enabling approach to caring could be encouraged by training. But in the independent sector, they suggested, the combination of low wages and high turnover among care workers, along with the need to use carers in other settings, and the small volume of enabling care purchased, gave agencies no incentive to invest in training.

Some care managers suggested that it was often necessary to trade quality against flexibility. For example, some said that the quality of care for severely disabled people was often higher if purchased from nursing homes providing a home care service. But diversified nursing homes were, they pointed out, often not very flexible because of in-home demands. Similarly, care managers suggested that, in some cases, in-house services provided higher-quality care but lacked flexibility in 'opening hours' (e.g. no care before 8 a.m.) or tasks.

Some care managers suggested that, in the final analysis, quality considerations were about having a degree of control over what was provided, when, how and by whom. Quality could not always be specified or known in advance. What mattered was being able to influence, to make complaints, adjustments and changes with confidence that these would be dealt with. But as some care managers pointed out, the influence and the sanctions available were limited because they were not purchasing enough from most agencies to really have much influence or control.

One final issue in relation to quality was frequently raised in interviews – pay and conditions of independent sector care staff. Several care managers questioned whether quality should be seen solely from the user's viewpoint: 'I'm not sure whether quality is just about the product or whether it also needs to take in the worker. Can you say this is a quality service if the care staff are working for a pittance?' Apart from any moral scruples care managers might have in purchasing care from agencies paying low hourly rates and with poor employment conditions, some saw employment conditions as directly affecting quality of care. Low pay, lack of employment benefits and security were seen as linked to high turnover and lack of training for care workers. Care managers also suggested that users found care workers' conditions unsettling: 'It's upsetting for the user because, of course, care workers talk about it and that makes the user feel that they can't expect much or they worry that the worker will leave.'

Approved provider lists, requiring certain employment conditions for care workers, were seen as one solution to this problem – but a solution with other costs. Apart from 'fixing' prices in over-simple ways and reducing flexibility, approved provider lists were seen as likely to restrict choice for purchasers and users. In addition, such lists may generate a spurious confidence in the quality of those agencies included on the list.

Conclusion

This chapter has suggested that the creative work which goes on in the 'space' between assessment of need and purchase of services has been neglected. That creative work goes on in a market in which supply, demand, availability and prices play an important part; but it also takes place in a wider social and political context in which values, trust, information/knowledge, budgets, policies and relationships influence purchasing outcomes. Care managers work creatively within the resource and process factors noted by other authors (Wistow et al., 1994).

References

Hawtin, H. and Smith, P. (1994) *Community Profiling – Auditing Social Needs*, Buckingham: Open University Press.
Lewis, J., Bernstock, P., Bovell, V. and Wookey, F. (1996) 'The purchaser/provider split in social care: is it working?', *Social Policy & Administration*, 30 (1): 1–19.
Wistow, G., Knapp, M., Hardy, B. and Allen, C. (1994) *Social Care in a Mixed Economy*, Buckingham: Open University Press.

27

M. Harris

Instruments of Government? Voluntary Sector Boards in a Changing Public Policy Environment

During the 1980s and 1990s a number of profound changes in public policy have affected charities and other voluntary agencies working in the field of social welfare in the UK. The post-Second World War dominance of governmental agencies in welfare service provision has been replaced by 'welfare pluralism' and a 'mixed economy of care' in which the commercial and voluntary sectors are expected to work alongside governmental agencies in providing mainstream services. Concepts such as 'markets', 'consumerism' and 'competition' have been increasingly applied to relationships between and within welfare agencies, and between agencies and individuals. Contracting has become a widely employed mechanism for channelling funding from the governmental to the voluntary and commercial sectors. Trends towards 'deinstitutionalization' and 'community care' in social provision have increased the pressures to find facilities in the 'independent' sector for people who formerly would have been in governmentally funded and governmentally provided residential care (Wistow et al., 1992; Deakin, 1994; Salter, 1995; Lewis and Glennerster, 1996).

These shifts in public policy have altered the nature and scale of work undertaken by voluntary and charitable agencies. Increasingly they are engaged in direct provision of services – funded in whole or in part by governmental agencies – rather than in self-help, advocacy, or community development activities. And emphasis has been placed on professionalism, 'value for money' and responding to the most severe cases of social need such as the most dependent older people and children 'at risk' (Billis, 1993; Lewis, 1993). Voluntary agencies have found themselves in a competitive environment with new or increased responsibilities for the use of 'governmental' money, the care of vulnerable people and the employment of growing numbers of staff (Billis and Harris, 1992).

First published in *Policy and Politics*, 26(2): 177–88 (The Policy Press, 1998). Abridged.

At the same time, there have been rising demands for voluntary agencies to demonstrate more 'public accountability' and to submit to closer scrutiny (Commission of the Future of the Voluntary Sector, 1996). The efficiency of voluntary agencies has been the subject of governmental reports (Woodfield, 1987; Home Office, 1990) and there have also been changes in legal and other regulations affecting charities (Middleton and Lloyd, 1996). Concern amongst governmental funders about the proper use of 'public' money has been reflected in wider coverage of voluntary sector issues in the mass media – with emphasis on cases of mismanagement and incompetence (Fenton et al., 1993).

There is growing evidence – from the United States as well as from the UK – that as voluntary agencies expand their role in response to shifts in public policy and as they come under increasing public scrutiny, they undergo important changes to their organizational structures, to their work and accountability systems and to their internal groupings (Billis, 1993; Gronbjerg, 1993; Smith and Lipsky, 1993; Lewis, 1996; Taylor, 1996). This chapter explores the ways in which the changing public policies of recent years have been experienced by one key internal grouping of voluntary agencies – their governing bodies. These comprise people who serve on a voluntary basis and they are variously referred to as 'boards', 'councils', 'trustees' and 'management committees'. The 1991 National Survey of Volunteering suggested that about 7 million adults in the UK were involved in this way in voluntary sector governance (Hedley and Rochester, 1992).

Three main data sources are used: work by the author and colleagues on the links between public policy and the performance of local voluntary agencies in the UK (Billis and Harris, 1992); an exploratory study of the way in which voluntary boards were affected by the introduction of the 'contract culture' (Harris, 1997); and findings from a study (the voluntary governing bodies study or VGB study) of how recent trends in public policy have been perceived by the boards of local voluntary agencies. Quotations from this latter study are used throughout to illustrate key points.

The next section reviews the ways in which public policy can impact on the functions which voluntary boards perform within, and on behalf of, their agencies. The chapter goes on to examine in more detail the practical implications for boards of the changed and changing public policy environment in social welfare. The data offer some important lessons for those who seek the successful implementation of public policy.

Public policy and board functions

The functions performed by the boards of charities and other voluntary agencies can be broadly classified under five headings: being the employer; formulating and monitoring adherence to agency goals; securing and safeguarding resources: being the point of final account-ability; and providing a link or buffer between the agency on the one hand and its external stakeholders and environment on the other hand (Harris, 1996). Although changing public policies have affected performance of all these, the impact has been greatest, it seems, with respect to the resource and accountability functions.

Thus, boards may now have to take the lead in funding negoti-ations with governmental agencies. As 'arm's length funding' and general purpose grants have been replaced by contracts and 'service-level agreements' with governmental funders, board members have been drawn into lengthy, specialist and complex negotiations and have had to act as 'intermediaries' between governmental agencies and their own paid staff (Centre for Voluntary Organization, 1996). Boards have also had to deal with the implications of cuts in funding – often themselves the result of public expenditure constraints. VGB study interviewees described their boards as constantly preoccupied with the uncertainty of governmental funding. They were concerned about their relationship with governmental bodies, with the resources their agencies would receive in the future, with the need to compete and 'jostle' for funding, and with attempts to diversify funding to avoid dependence on public sector agencies: 'it's always a fear; we wonder what assistance we will get'; 'the greatest nuisance of all, constantly trying to find new sources of funding'.

In this context, voluntary boards can feel the impact of changed *central* government policies towards the support and financing of *local* government:

> Any legislation [by national government] which cuts down money to local government means more work [for us].

> They [local government department] are always pulling in the reins tighter.

Some voluntary agencies have tried to diversify their funding sources in order to shield themselves in the future from the full impact of public policy changes and public expenditure constraints. But this can cause further problems for boards who have then to conform to a range of differing monitoring requirements. Many board members struggle to get to grips with the sheer complexity of their agency's funding situation: 'for us it's a question of balancing funding from XYZ charity with other funding which may have different time scales . . . jiggling and juggling'. In general, senior members of boards cooperate with paid staff in ensuring that funders' monitoring requirements are met. But in smaller voluntary agencies with few paid staff it may fall to board members themselves to provide the often detailed information required:

At the last monitoring visit, the Grants Officer wanted to know how many games of dominoes members had played in the inter-borough competition, how many outings and holidays were organized, number of telephone calls made, numbers of callers to the office, numbers of people receiving the newsletter and number of publicity leaflets distributed.

In the larger voluntary agencies, board members may need to keep in close touch with the day-to-day work of paid staff in order to ensure that governmental funders' requirements can be met. As signatories of contracts, boards have become more aware of their role as monitors of their agencies' work and as the point of final accountability for both the quality of services and the proper use of funds (Hedley and Rochester, 1991; Russell and Scott, 1997). Recent publications have also highlighted the heavy sanctions available for those boards which do not live up to expected standards of accountability (Tumin, 1992; Sargant and Kirkland, 1995).

[Frequent monitoring visits from funders] make more work for the committee in checking up that things are done.

. . . When public expenditure cuts leads to cuts in grants or to more stringent contracting conditions, for example, boards may bear the brunt initially in negotiations with the funder and then in their employer role: having to support staff through difficult meetings and adjustments or tell them that their posts are to be altered or terminated. One VGB interviewee described what happened when difficulties between the health authority and the local social services department over joint finance led to late payments and her committee had to work out how much it would cost to make some of the staff redundant:

Suddenly you are the employer. It may not be nice. . . . It's slightly daunting to realize at the end of the day I am responsible for X number of people.

. . .

Maintaining appropriate levels of expertise

Boards may struggle to maintain levels of expertise sufficient to enable them to respond appropriately to changes and complexities in public policy. This is not only a matter of being able to understand new laws and regulations, but also a matter of being able to understand the financial, accounting and monitoring implications of purchase of service contracts and 'community care' policies.

What was in the past a fairly straightforward matter [understanding the financial situation of the agency] has become very complicated. The committee is being asked to deal with very technical matters, legal and financial.

> Very few people on the committee, unless they are professionals, under-
> stand the implications of community care . . . it adds to the mystification.

They also need to acquire sophisticated negotiating skills since the
creation of a welfare 'market' demands an entrepreneurial approach
to governmental purchases (Centre for Voluntary Organization, 1996;
Russell and Scott, 1997). Boards which comprise both user representatives and people who are welfare professionals may become polarized between those whose prime concern is meeting local and specific
needs and those who are knowledgeable about the 'contract culture'
and who want to push the voluntary agency towards embracing it.

> [The contract has] . . . created much more of a them and us; those who are
> there because of professional knowledge and those who are there because
> they are users and love the service.

. . .

Maintaining services for vulnerable groups

As a result of the moves to 'a mixed economy of care', many voluntary
agencies which were formerly providing services that complemented
or supplemented governmental provision have moved into the
'mainstream' of service provision for their client group (for example,
people with mental illness or drug addicts). Often such services are
funded by short-term contracts with no guarantee of renewal. While
they were pleased to have secured the contracts, many VGB
interviewees, aware of the vulnerability of their agency's clients,
reported that their boards were increasingly concerned about finding
funding to ensure the continuity of services. In line with their role as
guardians of their agency's mission and representatives of their
agency's stakeholders (Ben Ner and van Hoomissen, 1994; Harris,
1994), boards feel an ongoing concern about the welfare of those to
whom they provide services. But this can be at odds with the market
principles underlying current public welfare policies which assume
that services will be provided by whichever agencies are most
efficient and 'competitive' at any one time: 'We began in the voluntary
sector tradition of people having sympathy with an idea . . . [but now]
you are actually operating with a very serious role.' In those agencies
where service users or carers are members of the board, the threat to
the funding of valued services can be experienced as a major and
personal anxiety.

Maintaining board autonomy

In a public policy climate in which governmental agencies tend to see
the voluntary sector as an instrument through which governmental
policies can be implemented (Billis and Harris, 1992; Commission on
the Future of the Voluntary Sector, 1996), boards find themselves

struggling to maintain their freedom to identify, advocate and meet needs in their own way in the face of demands from public sector funders:

> You have other people on your back with their own criteria for assessing whether what you do is good or bad.

> The borough is increasingly pressing to have everything down in black and white . . . we have found that increasingly intrusive.

The struggle to maintain independence once voluntary agencies become 'providers' for governmental 'purchasers' can become overwhelming and can raise questions for boards about their own role and the role of their voluntary agencies.

> [We have to] . . . come to a decision about the role of the organization: is it to be a statutory [governmental] body, a voluntary body, to do preventative work or only work in acute cases?

> For us it's about autonomy and us laying our own priorities. It's them setting the agenda, which has brought out issues like are we an independent organization or are we just a service provider?

> . . .

> [The local authority representatives on the board] became monitoring officers and it was made very clear that this was now a contractual relationship. They no longer had the time to be an adviser, a friend. . . . We feel put upon. We haven't adjusted and don't want to. We feel much more inspected, regulated, mistrusted. We just want to be left to get on with it.

Maintaining a longer-term vision

When boards become nervous about funding and project continuity, discussions at meetings about the immediate future and day-to-day organizational survival tend to crowd out consideration of other important issues, particularly strategic discussions about long-term goals and purposes.

> People currently have to react to necessary things and can't think creatively about the service provided.

> We have been consumed in the last three years with the funding situation, contracts and changing from a registered charity to a company limited by guarantee, and by the need to produce things such as a complaints procedure, users' charter, equal opportunities policy and so on.

> You always think you can just deal with an issue, then have time to stand back and consolidate. But you just get over one thing and something else looms around the corner.

By contrast, in periods when funding had been more secure and the demands from the environment less insistent, VGBs had: 'time to spend discussing quality and type of service and general operational matters'.

Recruiting new members

Some studies (for example Tumin, 1992; Marsden, 1996) have suggested that potential board members can be frightened off by a public
policy environment which places emphasis on voluntary sector
accountability. However, our own empirical evidence is closer to that
of Russell and Scott's findings (1997) on the impacts of contracts on
volunteers. It seems that rather than concern about responsibilities
and accountabilities, a more usual source of problems over recruitment and retention of board members is the increasing *complexity* of
board responsibilities as voluntary agencies move into larger-scale
and mainstream welfare provision: 'People are asked to deal with
issues that are difficult to understand and outside their expertise;
they need to have some sense of purpose and see some result.' Again
like Russell and Scott, we also found that this complexity has led
some agencies to narrow the range of people they consider suitable for
board membership; increasingly they look for people with specialist
skills, especially 'business' skills (Marsden, 1996) – for whom there is
much competition: 'They [people with specialist experience] are either
already committed or aren't interested.' Involving service users in
voluntary sector governance is particularly challenging (Hardina,
1993; Brophy, 1994; Harris, 1994). Special efforts have to be made
to recruit user members and non-professionals and then help them to
come to grips with the complexity of the work and responsibilities:

> There is a difficulty in getting users to become committee members. A lot of
> them are not committee people and wouldn't normally think of going on a
> committee . . . they represent the non-professional part of the committee
> who find it difficult to understand what the discussions on finances are
> about.

> [Parental involvement] is problematic and is something we are trying to
> deal with . . . their feeling of them and us, our feeling of not being able to
> use professional jargon.

. . .

Demands on personal time

Funding concerns and rising external demands have the effect of
increasing calls on the volunteer time of individual board members,
particularly the more senior ones. Growth in the numbers of paid
staff does not necessarily alleviate this problem. Although the latter
may take over some of the more onerous accountability-related tasks
as voluntary agencies grow, this can be counterbalanced by the
increasing amounts of time needed for board members to attend
meetings to develop strategies; to negotiate contracts; to comprehend
complex funding arrangements; to liaise with other agencies; to

manage staff; to prepare funding applications; and to lobby funders: 'Committee membership takes up more time than it used to . . . preparation for committee meetings, liaison with other organizations, funders . . .'.

Some VGB interviewees painted a picture of committee members under constant pressure to deal with new challenges and adapt to the changing environment: 'I was happier when there was more time, less pressure, and the committee could take time to see issues in a more leisurely fashion'.

The need for board members to give more of their voluntary time can be a special problem because of the personal circumstances of many of those who volunteer for board service:

most people work full time and aren't available.

People work longer hours and that squeezes the time and energy you have left at the end of the day.

[members of the VGB who are carers] have enough to do looking after their relatives without additional worries.

Anxiety and insecurity

Public policies which result in insecure funding and onerous account-ability demands can induce insecurities and high levels of anxiety amongst board members. Some of the VGB interviewees suggested that they and other board members just tried not to think about their responsibilities as they would be overwhelmed if they did: 'we would be scared out of our lives if we really thought about it'. But for many individuals, anxiety and insecurity is a constant part of their board membership. One VGB Chair, who sometimes took annual leave from his paid job in order to fulfil his board commitments, talked of the increasing demands made on him as his agency took on more work and more staff: 'A few years ago I'd never have woken up at night worrying about something [to do with the board].' Another VGB interviewee recounted a sense of being overwhelmed with responsi-bilities. He talked about being 'increasingly nervous' about the many responsibilities faced by his board and said that in the last few years he had had 'a sense of increasing responsibility' about matters such as Health and Safety regulations; charity law; responsibility for vulnerable clients; and the need for insurance. He felt that an increasingly litigious, less trusting, punitive climate had developed as public policy had changed: 'The sense of responsibility has become significantly greater . . . we may suddenly be in deep trouble.'

Senior members of boards are especially affected by stress and anxiety. . . .

Demoralization

When members of boards feel that their agencies are being unfairly treated as a consequence of public policies such as expenditure constraints and demands for tighter accountability, feelings of resentment build up and combine with anger about what is demanded of volunteer board members:

> We feel we are being let down [by the health authority] though we are providing a service for their patients.

> [We feel we behave] in a most faithful manner but our effort is not matched because of bureaucratic ideas within the Council.

The cumulative effect may be individual demoralization:

> Some people are asking why we have to do this [conform to monitoring requirements] when we are an independent organization. . . . Why are we giving our time for nothing if we're not being allowed to make decisions?

> They don't seem to accept that people are volunteers and give a lot of time to the organization . . . at the end of the day people are still volunteers . . . it isn't everybody's idea of fun volunteering.

The next step can be defection from the board as people find that their membership is not pleasurable, but, on the contrary, anxiety- and stress-provoking: 'Most of the time it isn't fun . . . if people are considering giving time voluntarily, they want to enjoy what they do'; 'Running voluntary organizations is not fun any more.' . . .

References

Ben Ner, A. and van Hoomissen, T. (1994) 'The governance of nonprofit organizations: law and public policy', *Nonprofit Management and Leadership*, 4 (4): 393–414.

Billis, D. (1993) *Sliding into Change: The Future of the Voluntary Sector in the Mixed Organization of Welfare*, Working Paper 14, London: Centre for Voluntary Organization, London School of Economics.

Billis, D. and Harris, M. (1992) 'Taking the strain of change: UK local voluntary agencies enter the post-Thatcher period', *Nonprofit and Voluntary Sector Quarterly*, 21 (3): 211–26.

Brophy, J. (1994) 'Parent management committees and pre-school playgroups: the partnership model and future management policy', *Journal of Social Policy*, 23 (2): 161–94.

Centre for Voluntary Organization (1996) *Contracting Trust: The Case History of the Negotiation of a Service Level Agreement*, London: London School of Economics.

Commission on the Future of the Voluntary Sector (1996) *Meeting the Challenge of Change: Voluntary Action into the 21st Century*, London: NCVO Publications.

Deakin, N. (1994) *The Politics of Welfare: Continuities and Change*, Hemel Hempstead: Harvester Wheatsheaf.

Fenton, N., Golding, P. and Radley, A. (1993) *Charities, Media and Public Opinion*, Loughborough: Department of Social Science, University of Loughborough.

Gronbjerg, K. (1993) *Understanding Nonprofit Funding*, San Francisco: Jossey Bass.

Hardina, D. (1993) 'The impact of funding sources and board representation on consumer control of service delivery in organizations serving low-income communities', *Nonprofit Management and Leadership*, 4 (1): 69–84.

Harris, M. (1994) 'The power of boards in service providing agencies: three models', *Administration in Social Work*, 18 (2): 1–15.

Harris, M. (1996) 'Do we need governing bodies?', in D. Billis and M. Harris (eds) *Voluntary Agencies: Challenges of Organisation and Management*, London: Macmillan.

Harris, M. (1997) 'Voluntary management committees: the impact of contracting in the UK', in P. and J. Kendall (eds) *The Contract Culture in Public Services*, Aldershot: Arena.

Hedley, R. and Rochester, C. (1991) *Contracts at the Crossroads*, Rugby: Crossroads Care.

Hedley, R. and Rochester, C. (1992) *Understanding Management Committees: A Look at Volunteer Management Committees*, Berkhamstead: Volunteer Centre UK.

Home Office (1990) *Efficiency Scrutiny of Government Funding of the Voluntary Sector: Profiting from Partnership*, London: HMSO.

Lewis, J. (1993) 'Developing the mixed economy of care: emerging issues for voluntary organizations', *Journal of Social Policy*, 22 (2): 173–92.

Lewis, J. (1996) 'What does contracting do to voluntary agencies?', in D. Billis and M. Harris (eds) *Voluntary Agencies: Challenges of Organisation and Management*, London: Macmillan.

Lewis, J. and Glennerster, H. (1996) *Implementing the New Community Care*, Buckingham: Open University Press.

Marsden, Z. (1996) *A Beneficial Experience: A Study of Business People on Voluntary Management Committees*, Working paper 17, London: Centre for Voluntary Organization, London School of Economics.

Middleton, F. and Lloyd, S. (1996) *The Charities Acts Handbook*, Bristol: Jordans.

Russell, L. and Scott, D. (1997) *Very Active Citizens? The Impact of Contracts on Volunteers*, Manchester: Department of Social Policy and Social Work, University of Manchester.

Salter, B. (1995) 'The private sector and the NHS: redefining the welfare state', *Policy & Politics*, 23 (1): 17–30.

Sargant, N. and Kirkland, K. (1995) *Building on Trust: Results of a Survey of Charity Trustees*, London: Trustee Services Unit of the National Council for Voluntary Organizations.

Smith, S. and Lipsky, M. (1993) *Nonprofits for Hire: The Welfare State in the Age of Contracting*, Cambridge, MA: Harvard University Press.

Taylor, M. (1996) 'Between public and private accountability in voluntary organizations', *Policy & Politics*, 24 (1): 57–72.

Tumin, W. (1992) *On Trust: Increasing the Effectiveness of Charity Trustees and Management Committees*, London: National Council for Voluntary Organizations/ Charity Commission.

Wistow, G., Knapp, M., Hardy, B. and Allen, C. (1992) 'From providing to enabling: local authorities and the mixed economy of social care', *Public Administration*, 70 (1): 25–45.

Woodfield, P. (1987) *Efficiency Scrutiny of the Supervision of Charities*, London: HMSO.

PART V

CONSTRUCTING: PROFESSIONAL IDENTITIES

A theme running through this book has been the uncertainty, insecurity and challenge that characterize the experience of today's professional. Traditional hierarchies are crumbling, old notions of professional identity are under assault and professional support structures are no longer what they were. The loss of familiar certainties has coincided with the blurring of role distinctions and demands for multiprofessional collaboration. Pressures to be more efficient coexist with new social policies which challenge notions of professional accountability and regulation. Demands for flexibility and innovation in ways of working are now widespread. All of these challenges to professional identity have forced professionals to examine who and what they are and to question what they could be in the future. This part of the book explores dimensions of their quest to create new identities.

In the opening chapter, Della Fish and Colin Coles argue that professionals are currently tormented by two incompatible views of professionalism – views which are underpinned by contrasting values and ideologies. They draw upon Schön's distinctions between the technical rational and professional artistry view of professionalism. *Technical rationality* views professional practice in terms of clear-cut, expert knowledge, rules, behaviours and routines. The *professional artistry* view, on the other hand, recognizes the complexities of practice and acknowledges that any knowledge is contingent, dynamic and problematic. Practice, they suggest, involves risk and improvisation – where 'learning to do' is achieved only by engaging in and reflecting upon doing.

Gray Southon and Jeffrey Braithwaite similarly distinguish between types of professionals as they critique the current 'reforms' propelling professionals towards more technical procedures. They argue that the introduction of performance measures and standardized treatment protocols actually undermines what is central to professional practice: its high levels of complexity and uncertainty. Taking up cudgels on behalf of professionals, they urge those behind the current reforms – managers, trusts and the government – to do more to value the central role played by professionals.

The next two readings emphasize the continuously evolving nature of professions. Mike Saks offers an intriguing account of how professions emerge out of broader socio-political and historical contexts. Applying neo-Weberian ideas of social closure, he views professionals as privileged groups who have managed to monopolize social and economic opportunities in order to maximize their status and rewards. He traces the way in which different professional groups have been more or less successful in their push to professionalize through their training, organizations and legislation. The dominant position of the medical profession is contrasted with that of the subordinate semi-professions who continue to engage in 'turf-battles'. In his fascinating historical narrative, Stephen Rashid pursues the twists and turns of the debate about whether or not social workers should similarly embrace professionalization. He shows how, from its beginnings in the voluntary sector, social work in the UK emerged within a strong statutory framework that itself placed limits on professional autonomy. Since then, evolving currents of thought and changing political and economic realities have pushed social work in different directions. At times social workers have been exhorted to professionalize and extend their knowledge base. At other times, a combination of political and managerial forces has resulted in pressures to de-professionalize.

The next two chapters focus on the wider structural implications of changing professional practice. The authors call for professional bodies urgently to review their standards and provide guidelines that are more relevant to future developments.

Sue Dowling and her colleagues describe the not unusual situation where a nurse takes on the work previously the province of a doctor. Compiling a composite case study, they document the confusions of accountability that can occur. Is the nurse accountable in her own right or is the doctor accountable for delegated work? Where is the line to be drawn between responsibilities as a professional and as an employee? How would the issue be seen in the case of a legal claim in relation to negligence or battery or a complaint against the trust by a patient? The importance of doctors and nurses being equal partners in planning new divisions of labour and the necessity of legal advice and managerial support are stressed. Keeping the patient properly informed is vital. There are challenges here for the bodies that register professionals to work together in new ways to recognize and facilitate such new forms of work.

Luis Archer turns attention to the ethical, social and legal implications of new medical discovery and knowledge. As he points out, the use of genetic information to anticipate future disease in individuals creates new ethical dilemmas for professionals. Do you tell someone they will die of cancer aged 48? Do you pass on that information to an enquiring employer? Should the person's daughter be advised to abort her baby to avoid propagation of the gene? New codes of practice, which guide and protect professionals and service users alike, cannot, Archer persuasively argues, be postponed: they are needed now.

The final chapter offers a vision for professional practice in the future. Celia Davies addresses the provenance of professionalism, exploring how today's notions of professionalism are tied to a long tradition of masculine ideas which stress the mastery of knowledge, control, detachment, competition and autonomy. She applies these concepts to the issue of caring, comparing the traditional 'professional work' of men with the 'supportive activities' of women. She notes how women have enabled men to function in their arm's-length way, clearing up after fleeting medical encounters. However, the structures which helped reinforce these traditional notions of professionalism are now breaking down. In their place, Davies argues for a 'new professional' – one who is committed to reflective, participatory, empowering, collaborative practice.

A combination of new structures and evolving ideologies has resulted in many changes to professional practice where old professional models are being dislodged. Whilst professionals are subject to many pressures that are not within their control, they also have an opportunity to shape their own future, to decide who and what they want to be. Has the time come to embrace a new professionalism?

28

D. Fish and C. Coles

Seeing Anew: Understanding Professional Practice as Artistry

. . . We believe that the health care professions of the late 1990s and those who work in them are tormented by two incompatible views of professionalism. Clear manifestations of both these views are visible – for those who look – in currently emerging approaches to professional development across health care. Understanding these is, we believe, the first step to seeing professional practice anew and to recognizing the responsibilities that this new view brings with it.

On the one hand reflective practice is being hailed as the way forward in professions like nursing, where many professionals now treat it as a shibboleth, believing that it is a new term for thinking about one's practice which they have 'always done'. Yet, coincidentally, continuous quality improvement (CQI), and total quality management (TQM) have also become hot issues in health care as a whole (Berwick, 1996; Taylor, 1996) and there are demands that bureaucrats should impose system-wide procedures, such as protocols and guidelines, which will require professionals to follow rules and enable them apparently to stop thinking for themselves (see Fish, 1998).

Beneath such conflicting initiatives, then, we suggest there lurk two different views of what a professional is and how a professional should behave, and these in turn are influenced by two very different sets of values. Following the work of Schön (1983, 1987), we see these as the technical rational view of professionalism (which cashes out into a competency-based approach to practice which accepts the bureaucratic system-wide constraints of professionals) and the professional artistry view of professionalism (which, as we shall see, leads to a more serious form of reflective practice than is currently commonly found in heath care).

First published in D. Fish and C. Coles (eds) *Developing Professional Judgement in Health Care: Learning through the Critical Appreciation of Practice* (Butterworth Heinemann, 1998), pp. 30–43. Abridged.

It seems to us that the technical rational view is held broadly by the public (which includes the press and politicians but who are also the pool from which health care's clients and patients emerge). But, we would argue, professionals recognize that this view does not fit with their experience and that the professional artistry view represents ways of thinking about professional practice which those who know it from the inside recognize as more nearly what practice is actually like. Schön first drew attention to these views, they were first published in this form by Fish (1991) and have been explored further by us, in Coles (1996, 1997) and in Fish (1995, 1996).

Two views: their overall notions of professional practice

The technical rational (TR) view of professionalism catches health care practice up into the late twentieth-century behaviour of labelling everything in mechanistic terms. It views professional practice as a basic matter of delivering a service to clients through a predetermined set of clear-cut routines and behaviours. The metaphor of 'delivery' has become so common that it appears as an unquestioned part of discussion in both health care and education. Yet some would point to the insidiousness with which the term — drawn from commercial and market-driven activities like getting the newspapers, milk and bread to customers' doorsteps — has gained acceptance for describing the activity of working with patients/clients. Its acceptance shows just how far members of the public and we as professionals have been seduced by the idea that technology and business are a paradigm of all useful human activity. And its most pernicious influence is its penetration of our subconscious with the idea that the 'deliverer' (the professional) is someone who must not tamper with the goods (the package) he or she is delivering, but is simply an agent for conveying safely something created by one body to another. The term 'delivery' then is thus both a major means to, and a key signal of, the success of the downgrading of professionalism, via a TR view of it. Indeed, for education Carr and Hartnett (1996) demonstrate how deep these issues go by tracing in detail the deintellectualization of policy in relation to that profession. Some strong parallels between what has happened in education and in health care can be deduced from their work.

The TR approach to health care, of prescribing and proscribing all the practitioner's activities, is flagged as being able to cut down considerably the risks incurred when professionals make more of their own decisions. Here the ever-present threat from accountability has been allowed to push the practitioner into such a defensive frame of mind that he or she is constantly in a 'no-win position', where both to act and not to act are equally likely to invite litigation, and where it is only possible to defend activities which come within the pre-specified rules. And it assumes that practice is a relatively simple interaction in which the practitioner gives and patients and clients receive, and which can be perfected.

By contrast, those who espouse a professional artistry (PA) view of professionalism believe that the TR view is a deficit view of professionals and denies the real character of both professionalism and practice. They argue that far from being simple and predictable, professional practice involves a more complex and less certain 'real world' in which, daily, the professional is involved in making many complex decisions, relying on a mixture of professional judgement, intuition and common sense, and that these activities are not able to be set down in absolute routines, or be made visible in simple terms, and certainly are not able to be measured, and which because of this are extremely difficult to teach and to research.

Their view of the activities of a professional

The TR view, then, characterizes professional activities as essentially able to be pre-specified and susceptible to being broken down into their component parts. Such parts are all regarded as 'skills' and are thus viewed as being able to be mastered. The TR view further regards being a professional as being essentially efficient in 'the' skills, and submissive in harnessing them to carry out other people's decisions. Such skills, it is assumed, can be listed beforehand, and are now commonly referred to as competencies, or, sometimes, 'performance outcomes'. The identification of these skills, which are superficially reassuring in their ability to be seen and measured, makes professional accountability superficially easy. Thus, competencies or 'outcomes' have for some time now dominated many courses of preparation for professional practice and are currently proposed as the basis for university courses and for staff development in the professions. In this way the technical rational view of professionalism and the competency-based approach to practice is rapidly gaining ground as the only view.

The PA view, by major contrast, sees behaving professionally as being concerned with both means and ends. Here, professional activity is more akin to artistry, where only the *principles* can be pre-determined and practitioners may in practice and for good reason need to choose to go beyond them, just as, say, good artists often go beyond or break artistic conventions in order to achieve an important effect. Thus, in this view, practitioners are broadly autonomous, making their own decisions about their actions and the moral bases of those actions (for which, of course, they are accountable). In the PA view, the *activities* of the professional cannot be pre-specified, just as a painter cannot tell you what the picture he or she is creating will be like until it is finished.

Thus, too, the characteristics of 'good practice' are regarded as context specific because, again like the artist, the professional has to harness on the spot professional judgement as to what to do since every situation is to some extent unique. Further, the PA view recognizes that there are many components of professional activity (just as there are many things involved in artistic activity) and not all of them are able to be distinguished one from another, and some of them are tacit. There will, of course, in any piece of professional practice be of necessity routine and unreflecting parts of daily professional life, but loss of sight of fundamental principles on which one has come to believe that one's practice should be founded is (to adapt Golby, 1993: 5) at once a loss of professionalism. In this model, then, the professional is not less accountable, but is in fact accountable for more – for skills of course, but also for much more important moral and ethical matters that underpin their decision-making and judgement. Here, to be professional is to be morally answerable for all of one's conduct, and for one's conduct as a whole, not just for parts of it.

But this brings with it the problem of how to render visible the invisible, and how to view the whole not just the parts. How can one 'see' the moral basis of one's judgement? Such a problem is acute when the invisible is – as we shall argue professional judgement indeed is – the very centre and the distinguishing mark of one's professionalism.

Our contention is that it can be made visible by articulating one's practice in full, that is, articulating not merely the surface fact, the observable 'doing' of professional practice, but the invisible depths below it. We also believe that if professional practice is akin to art, it is entirely appropriate in capturing and investigating professional activities to draw upon artistic means of investigation and of expression, because art is concerned with conveying the subtleties and ineffable aspects of life, and does so without first needing to attempt to atomize it (see Fish, 1998). The attempt to think about practice is sometimes characterized as 'reflective practice', but it is not often seen as rigorous, and in our experience until now it has rarely involved the serious level of enquiry and deep consideration of the artistry of the professional that we are arguing for.

Their views about professional expertise

Thus, the TR view believes in the centrality of rules, schedules, prescriptions, whereas the PA view believes that, as in the work of the artist, so in the work of a professional, practice starts where the rules fade (because the rules rarely fit real practice). Thus, the PA view relies on frameworks and rules of thumb, rather than rules. The TR view emphasizes diagnosis, analysis, and efficient systems. It believes in detailed job specifications, protocols and guidelines, that is, in being able to analyse a professional role down to the last detail. The PA view, by contrast, believes instead in interpretation of details, acknowledges the inevitable subjectivity of setting them down, and comes to an understanding of professional activities by means of appreciation (as in the critical appreciation of art and music). It wishes to encourage not narrow efficiency but creativity and the right to be wrong. The TR model assumes that knowledge is permanent, able to be totally mastered, and is thus worth attempting to master. The PA view is that knowledge is temporary, dynamic and problematic, and that it is more useful to know processes than to know facts.

Their views of professional practice

The professional artistry approach sees professional practice as complex. Just as a painting, a poem or a piece of music demands a response to its entirety which would not be satisfied only by analysing it technically into its component parts, so professional practice needs to be understood holistically. This inevitably raises deep questions about what is involved in professional expertise seen as artistry. The following might well be raised:

- How is practice (which is artistic in nature) learnt and how can it be improved?
- How far is self-knowledge significant?
- In the exercise of artistry, how can we come to understand better the thought and action involved?
- How can we investigate artistry in ways that aid our understanding of it?

By comparison, those who subscribe to the TR view would argue that professional practice need not be that complex, has for too long been surrounded by mystique and has now advanced to the point where goals can be set by society for professionals whose role is purely instrumental. For example they might point to the very language of health care today, including 'clinical guidelines; clinical outcomes; health outcome individualisation; health technology assessment [which] all form part of NHS (National Health Service) strategies for improving the effectiveness of the service it provides'

(Culshaw, 1995: 323). They would argue that this shows that the professional's role can indeed by analysed technically and rationally in terms of activities and skills (though in the end this can lead to an obsessive intention to tie things down further and further in the inevitably vain attempt to try to cater for all eventualities).

Their views about how to improve practice

The TR view of professional development sees it as a simple matter of providing skills training. Practice, in TR terms, is easily learnt. But the PA view sees the TR approach as unable to meet the real situation of practice which is messy, unpredictable, unexpected. The PA view recognizes the importance in practitioners of the artistic ability to improvise (an ability often *diminished* by training and routine). Also, because practice is rapidly changing, it requires the practitioner autonomously to be able to refine and update his or her expertise 'on the hoof', which is what reflective practice is about (and what professional development should be about) and which those who subscribe to this view would argue is more cost effective than endlessly changing the system. Here, to improve practice is to treat it more holistically, to work to understand its complexities, and to look carefully at one's actions and theories as one works and, subsequently, to challenge them with ideas from other perspectives, and to seek to improve and refine practice and its underlying theory. Here, the professional is working towards increased competence (but not towards acquired competencies, see Fish, 1996). Those committed to the TR view, however, would argue that this is all too woolly (because it admits of less certainty). Further, it does not please politicians (who represent professional views to the public in simplistic terms because they do not fully understand the complexities of professional practice and do not share the values and perspectives of professionals). Politicians undervalue the professional artistry view of practice and the reflective practitioner approach that it brings with it because its fruits may show up less clearly in the short term since it emphasizes aspects that are not simple, visible behaviours. But in fact it offers in the long term scope for deeper-rooted improvements, which are owned by the professional.

Their views about theory

But it is, perhaps, in its views about theory that the TR model is most highly specific and – for us – the most suspect. It sees theory as 'Formal Theory' produced by researchers who stand apart from the practitioners. This formal theory is to be learnt and then applied to practice. It regards practice as an arena in which to demonstrate previously worked-out theory. By contrast, the PA view is that theory is implicit in (underlies) all action, that (as for the artist) both action and theory are developed *in practice*. This means that refining practice involves unearthing the theories on which that practice is founded and that formal theory aids the development of practice by challenging and extending the practitioner's understandings. This view (that with the help of reflection theory emerges *from* practice) enables the professional to examine and develop personal theory as it arises from that practice. Such personal theory is implicit in all action but needs to be unearthed from beneath it in order to be acknowledged, understood and used to inform decisions about later action. It is also able to be refined by recourse to further practice and to the wider view of theory offered by other theorists and researchers.

The TR view, then, emphasizes the 'known', and is in tune with present trends in that it celebrates certainty and hard evidence. By contrast the PA view recognizes the value of uncertainty, humility and critical scepticism and is willing to accept the notion of mystery within human activity. It regards the activity of the professional as not entirely able to be analysed down to the last atom, even if the routinized craft skills on which artistry is based are able to be specified. It regards professional practitioners as eternal seekers rather than 'knowers'. It sees the activities of the professional as mainly open capacities which by definition are not able to be mastered. (The test of an open capacity is that the learner can take steps which he or she has not been taught to take, which in some measure would surprise the teacher and perhaps the learner.)

The professional artistry view, then, sees professional practice as an art in which risks are inevitable if there is to be any creativity, where learning to do is achieved only by engaging in doing and reflecting upon the doing, and where improvisation, enquiry into action and resulting insight by those involved in it generate a major knowledge base.

This idea goes back to Greek thought where the term 'praxis' (which approximates to the kind of professional practices we are describing) is, as Aristotle argued, action in which the end product is not an object but is the realization of morally worthwhile good (see, for example, Carr, 1995). Thus, in health care for instance, the good that practitioners seek is health and perhaps education (and the health care educator is certainly concerned with both 'goods'). Such good cannot be *made* outside the practice and then delivered to it, but can only be done within it. That is, the ends cannot be absolutely designed in advance of engaging in the practice. Although they might be *formulated* in theory, they are not fixed, but are mutable and develop as the practice develops. And they are only intelligible in terms of the traditions of good (health and education) which are being practised. Professional judgement is at the centre of this.

These ideas have profound significance for *preparation* for practice in health care at all levels from undergraduate (pre-registration) training, in learning to carry out day-to-day work in practical situations, through to lifelong professional development itself.

The notion that the details of practice cannot be pre-determined fiercely challenges the orthodox assumption that health care practitioners need to be well prepared for practice by being trained in routines and given knowledge to apply *in situ*. In fact, ironically, such routines, which are designed to provide a good basis for practice, can be very dangerous for patients and undesirable for practitioners. Routines can obscure the realities of real practice for and with the individual patients. Those who see their practice only through the veil of such routines, will only *perceive* it as routine – even when it is not so. Learning routines and applicatory knowledge is also undesirable for practitioners because the 'auto pilot' nature of routine and the application of knowledge obliterates the detail from which practitioners could learn by thinking about their practice both during it and afterwards. The need for practitioners in health care to appear as experts who are 'unshakeable', then, is not best provided for by preparing *for* practice, by being equipped with pre-determined routines. It is better met by being prepared *to* practice, by being alerted to the messy and complex nature of practice, by treating the knowledge one has as adaptable, and by being made conscious of principles upon which one's practice is based and of the need to use these to 'make meaning' in the particular situation. It is about being prepared to meet and work with the unexpected.

It is for this reason that it is not possible in health care and education to train student practitioners in all they need to operate their practice. And it never will be. It is not that we currently lack the right knowledge and technology to train practitioners in 'the right procedures', and that we shall 'crack' this in time. The entire idea is a chimera. It may be true in terms of scientific and technical knowledge that when we have more factual knowledge we shall be able to put it into practice and thus improve our end product. But that is not true of practice (or praxis), as all practitioners really know at heart. Here, the improvement of practice itself is an improvement of *understanding* and comes as part of the doing and the reflection upon it. Improvement of practice is entirely in the hands of the practitioner.

Their views about quality

Each model also gives rise to a particular view of quality. The TR model speaks in the language of quality assurance and control. It

Table 28.1 *Two views of professional practice*

The technical rational (TR) view	The professional artistry (PA) view
Follows rules, laws, routines and prescriptions	Starts where rules fade, sees patterns, frameworks
Uses diagnosis, analysis	Uses interpretation/appreciation
Wants efficient systems	Wants creativity and room to be wrong
Sees knowledge as graspable, permanent	Knowledge is temporary, dynamic, problematic
Theory is applied to practice	Theory emerges from practice
Visible performance is central	There is more to it than surface features
Setting out and testing for basic competency is vital	There is more to it than the sum of the parts
Technical expertise is all	Professional judgement counts
Sees professional activities as masterable	Sees mystery at the heart of professional activities
Emphasizes the known	Embraces uncertainty
Standards must be fixed. Standards are measurable and must be controlled	That which is most easily fixed and measurable is also often trivial – professionals should be trusted
Emphasizes assessment, IPR, inspection, accreditation	Emphasizes investigation, reflection, deliberation
Change must be managed from outside	Professionals can develop from inside
Quality is really about the quantity of that which is easily measurable	Quality comes from deepening insight into one's values, priorities, actions
Technical accountability	Professionals' answerability
This is training	This is education
It takes the instrumental view	It sees education as intrinsically worthwhile

Source: This table was first published in this form in Fish (1995: 43).

places emphasis upon visible performance. It seeks to test and measure these, believing that technical performance is all-important. Thus the model is behaviourist, emphasizes fixed standards, controls professional practice via inspection and individual performance review, and believes that change can be imposed from outside the profession and that quality is measurable. It is characterized by 'a centralist surveillance of standards' (Carr and Hartnett, 1996: 176). Ironically though, it holds the professional practitioner accountable only for his or her *technical* expertise. This is because it unconsciously but inevitably denies the existence of professional judgement and a moral dimension to professional practice (or perhaps believes that it is only a matter of time before it is expressed in simplified procedures as clinical reasoning already is). It also has the effect of demotivating the professional by reducing the challenge that autonomy offers, and turning practice into a factory-like monotony and the practitioner into a delivery agent.

By contrast, the PA view sees that there is more to professional practice than its surface and visible features, more to the whole than the sum of the parts, more to competence than an accumulation of competencies. It believes in the unavoidable significance of professional judgements in professional practice, holds that the most easily measurable is often also the most trivial, and that issues involving moral complexities are never resolved by resort to empiricism.

Most importantly, the PA view wishes to harness investigation, reflection and deliberation (and, we would add, appreciation) in order to enable professionals to develop their own insights from inside their own practice. It holds that this is a better means of staff development than change imposed from without. In short, it believes that quality comes from deepening insight into one's own values, priorities, actions. Under this model it is possible (and necessary) to talk about wide professional answerability rather than narrow technical accountability. This makes professionals responsible for the moral dimensions of professional action, and for reflecting upon, investigating and refining their own practice. It enables practitioners to own their practice and to enjoy improving it.

Table 28.1 offers a summary of the points in our argument. . . .

References

Berwick, D.M. (1996) 'A primer on leading the improvement of systems', *British Medical Journal*, 312: 619–22.

Carr, W. (1995) *For Education: Towards Critical Educational Enquiry*, Buckingham: Open University Press.

Carr, W. and Hartnett, A. (1996) *Education and the Struggle for Democracy: the Politics of Educational Ideas*, Buckingham: Open University Press.

Coles, C. (1996) 'Approaching professional development', *Journal of Continuing Education in the Health Professions*, 16: 152–8.

Coles, C. (1997) 'Training and the process of professional development', in *The Cambridge Handbook of Psychology, Health and Medicine*, ed. A. Baum, C. McMannis and S. Newman et al., Cambridge: Cambridge University Press. pp. 325–8.

Culshaw, H. (1995) 'Evidence-based practice for sale?' *British Journal of Occupational Therapy*, 58: 233.

Fish, D. (1991) 'But can you prove it? Quality assurance and the reflective practitioner', *Assessment and Evaluation in Higher Education*, 16: 22–36.

Fish, D. (1995) *Quality Mentoring for Student Teachers: a Principled Approach to Practice*, London: David Fulton.

Fish, D. (1996) 'Competence: spelling out the problem', *Journal of Teacher Development*, 5: 58.

Fish, D. *Appreciating Practice in the Caring Professions: Re-focusing Professional Development and Practitioner Research*, London: Butterworth-Heinemann.

Golby, M. (ed.) (1993) Editorial comments, *Reflective Professional Practice: A Reader* (Course 124 Papers for M.Ed. students at Exeter University), Fair Way Publications.

Schön, D. (1983) *The Reflective Practitioner*, New York: Basic Books.

Schön, D. (1987) *Educating the Reflective Practitioner*, San Francisco: Jossey-Bass.

Taylor, D. (1996) 'Quality and professionalism in health care: a review of current initiatives in the NHS', *British Medical Journal*, 312: 626–9.

29

G. Southon and J. Braithwaite

The End of Professionalism?

. . . This chapter takes a look at the nature of professionalism in terms of the task that it addresses, and identifies a basic conflict between professionalism and the principal reforms which are being undertaken around the world.

The task orientation of professionalism

The dominant sociological analysis of professionalism focuses on the privilege, power and social behaviours of distinct professional classes (Wolinsky, 1993; Mechanic, 1991). Factors such as guaranteed autonomy and dominance over other groups are prominent themes, and primary attention is paid to the historical development of professions and the behaviours of professional organizations. The focus of this chapter is primarily on the functional aspect of professionals: why professionals are needed and what roles they play. Freidson states that 'the sole generic resource of professions is, like all labour, their capacity to perform particular kinds of work' (Freidson, 1993). Seen from this perspective, professionalism becomes a set of task-oriented behaviours with associated social behaviours. Such task-related behaviours include a high level of expertise, autonomy or the freedom to control the management of each task, commitment to the task, identification with peers, a system of ethics and a means of maintaining standards (Raelin, 1986).

High levels of professionalism involve professional organizations which enable professionals to support each other in enhancing their standards, and perhaps protecting their collective reputation by ensuring the standards of their colleagues. This interaction of professionals results in social behaviours which have become the subject of much sociological analysis. However, these social behaviours are a by-product rather than the essence of professionalism.

First published in *Social Science and Medicine*, 46(1): 23–8 (Elsevier, 1998). Abridged.

A task-oriented analysis is important. If professionalism is essentially a set of social behaviours, it may be judged according to current social standards. However, if professionalism is a requirement for achieving a particular task, then it must be judged according to its ability to achieve that task. If that achievement is found wanting, then professionalism may need to be better supported and enhanced, rather than being rejected. On the other hand, if the task does not require professionalism, then professionalism and its trappings should be discarded. It is therefore necessary to be clear about the role of professionalism and the types of task that require it.

Task characteristics and implications

While many definitions of professionalism have been offered in the literature, the difficulty of addressing the essential character has been noted by Pennington (1990). He felt that the closest came from the Court of Ontario in the judgment of P. Wright in 1951:

> A profession is a self-disciplined group of individuals who hold themselves out to the public as possessing a special skill derived from training or education, and who are prepared to exercise that skill primarily in the interests of others.

The United Kingdom Monopolies Commission Report on the Professions (1970) extended this somewhat:

> The service calls for a high degree of detachment and integrity on the part of the practitioner in exercising his personal judgement on behalf of his client.

Even these definitions say more about how the task is addressed than about the task itself. We suggest that the tasks that are performed by professionals can be described by two main characteristics: high levels of both uncertainty and complexity. It can be seen how the combination of these characteristics leads naturally to the key features of professionals as discussed above.

Uncertainty

When the diversity of a task means that each case cannot be predicted, then the task itself is uncertain, and each case needs to be individually assessed. Thus, people with the skills required to assess each task must engage with the task, and be given the freedom or autonomy to act according to the demands presented. They also need to take ultimate responsibility for the task. Guiding them, however, must be general principles or ethical codes, especially if there are significant implications beyond the bounds of each case.

Complexity

When a task is very complex, it needs to be supported by well developed knowledge, skills and accepted practices. Such requirements cannot be established by each practitioner, but must be developed over time by groups of practitioners, with training carried out often through close tutelage. Continuing association with colleagues may be required to promote standards and to maintain currency. Thus, professional organizations are required as a basis for this support. Very high levels of complexity require specialization to deal with the sophisticated procedures and technology involved, with professional subgroups being required for each subspecialty.

These factors are quite generic and can be seen to characterize the recognized professions. Whether one is an engineer, lawyer, accountant, academic or a doctor, one is continually being faced with new situations which require individual assessment, and often the application of a sophisticated set of skills. When uncertainty becomes very low, even if the task is quite complex, then the task can become standardized, and can be seen as a technical rather than a professional task. This is typical of the production environment. Alternatively, a reduction in complexity, with high uncertainty, requires motivation and perhaps intelligence, though little training and support knowledge is required. The requirements of each situation can be established largely independently. Such a situation is typical in entrepreneurial and personal service areas.

Addressing tasks that feature high levels of uncertainty and complexity requires professionalism. However, to say that these features of professionals are required does not mean that they necessarily exist adequately. Lack of such features may result in inadequate professional standards. For instance, many professional organizations have been unable to maintain effective continuing education and peer review programmes that ensure the performance of all of their members.

These task characteristics also have a major impact on the nature of the organizations in which professionals work. Uncertainty and concomitant autonomy limit the scope for managerial control, since it is the professional, rather than the manager, who has much of the ultimate responsibility. Individual organizations have limited influence over their practices, as practices are defined more by the profession than the organization. These factors introduce many fundamental dilemmas concerning the management of professionals in organizations (Raelin, 1986; Mintzberg, 1979). A common solution is to see management not as controlling professional practice, but as supporting it (Quinn et al., 1996). It is notable, however, that while the special dilemmas of the management of professionals have been recognized, very little attention has been paid to it by management writers.

The task in health service provision

In medicine high levels of both uncertainty and complexity have traditionally been recognized. The range of illnesses is broad, complicated and multifaceted, resulting in practices which are unpredictable and context-dependent (Cox, 1995). There is an enormous body of knowledge that supports health services, and many sophisticated skills are required. There are many specializations, and ethical principles and peer interactions have a very important role to play. Thus, in health and principal characteristics of professionalism are firmly grounded in the character of the task.

The nature of medical practice does vary, though, and the balance between uncertainty and complexity can change considerably. For instance, a general practitioner deals with a high level of uncertainty, but tends to reduce complexity by referring difficult cases to specialists. The specialist, on the other hand, deals with complex cases and techniques, but has uncertainty considerably reduced through the referral and diagnostic processes. This difference in the nature of the task has a major impact on the style of practice and the cognitive skills that are involved. . . .

It is noted that this concept of professionalism is rooted essentially in the ability of the professional to perform specific tasks of high uncertainty and complexity rather than the status, power or remuneration involved. It means, for instance, that the movement of a doctor into management with greater power and remuneration involves a reduction rather than an enhancement of professionalism. Similarly, the establishment of clinical directorates, while giving that group greater say over their activities, will degrade professionalism if it constricts the ability of each member to address each case on its own merits.

Impetus for health reforms

There have been numerous concerns about professionalism which have been voiced in the literature (e.g. Kassirer, 1993; Newble et al., 1994). At various times critics have argued that professionals pay insufficient attention to the costs of practice. There is obvious inconsistency in medical practice, and this has led investigators to explore variation and the reasons for it. Allegations about health professionals' performance include a slow uptake of new knowledge and practice, a high error rate (Leape, 1994), interprofessional rivalries, a preoccupation with professional rights and remuneration, a lack of willingness to be accountable and, generally, a neglect of patient interests. In general, professionals have paid inadequate attention to the maintenance of their standards (Maynard, 1993) in either peer review or continuing education (Newble et al., 1994). In addition, there is a strong literature which bemoans information asymmetry between practitioners and patients and condemns supplier-induced demand. Each of these concerns has some degree of legitimacy and has been explored extensively elsewhere. In contrast, considerably less attention is paid to the skill, commitment and altruism that characterizes the behaviour of many clinicians. . . .

The reform agenda and professionalism

This situation has confronted health service policy makers and management with the need to control costs while ensuring services. The early strategies with an emphasis on cost control threatened to compromise quality, and so reformers began to implement a range of techniques, incentives and restructuring intended to ensure that health services were much more efficient, effective and accountable than they had been. These measures included establishing performance measures; classifying activities; standardizing practices via mechanisms such as clinical pathways, guidelines and protocols: formalizing accountabilities often through markets and formal purchasing contracts; providing financial incentives; and consumer empowerment (Hunter, 1993; Schieber and Poullier, 1990).

What then, is the nature of these reforms, and what is their impact on professionalism? . . . Each one of them depends on some form of assumption about the level of simplicity or predictability of the task in enabling control to be brought within the ambit of an authority, or to be able to control or classify the process in some way.

In the broader context, these changes have been brought about in an environment of widespread attacks on professionalism with little appreciation of the role that professionalism plays. Often professional organizations have been sidelined, with only muted responses on behalf of the professions themselves (Kassirer, 1993). . . . In general, these reform frameworks are based on analysis that made little significant reference to the nature of professionalism (Altman and von Otter, 1992; Harrison and Pollitt, 1994; Degeling, 1993, 1994). . . .

Certainly, there are ways in which some medical practices can be made more uniform, more predictable and less idiosyncratic. There is more and more information becoming available about the best ways to practise, and many procedures are becoming easier and more mechanical. However, there are also ways in which health services are becoming more sophisticated and more responsive to individual need. In arguing that the assumptions of the reform mechanisms are consistent with the realities of health services, one needs to consider that there are over 10,000 disease categories, and each case may have varying levels of severity, comorbidity and complication, with other significant factors such as age, gender, social circumstance and mental attitude. From the individual perspective, each one of us as a patient wants to be assessed for what we are, with our own sets of needs and values, and not merely be processed according to pre-defined categories. The provision of this service has generated vast volumes of literature and requires hundreds of different specialty professions. It results in a very complex and subtle clinical decision-making process (Wennberg, 1994; Cox, 1995) which has to date largely defied rational analysis or duplication.

A fundamental conflict

It seems difficult, then, to square the simplifications inherent in the health reform mechanisms with the realities of health services. . . . Reformers argue that they can, with sound doses of accountability, provide assurances that appropriate practices are being undertaken, that there is a low average cost per case and there are suitable levels of equity. From a patient's point of view, however, individuals want a unique, confidential service with the full scope of medicine's capabilities applied in their particular case. Policy makers want to manage and judge health services by their impact on the overall health of the community, but want to avoid the political ramifications of rationing. Finally, Freidson (1990) has noted the intrinsic conflict between professionalism and the two main organizational constructs of the reforms — markets and bureaucracies. . . .

Requirements for progress

The development of an effective health service needs, first, a proper understanding of the nature of the task, and then the character and requirements of the people that are required to undertake that task. This requires recognizing the complexity and uncertainty involved in health service, and the nature of the professionalism required (Lazaro and Azcona, 1996). That may require significant changes from the current situation in terms of numbers and specialization of professions. Moreover, it will require an enhanced sophistication of professionalism and professionals able to address the fundamental dilemmas facing health services in a way that will regain the confidence of the community and policy makers (Wennberg, 1995). It will involve issues of resources constraint, professional accountability (Emanuel and Emanuel, 1996) and the assurance of skills and ethics (Brennan, 1991). It will require approaches to health services which recognize the important factors that influence professional performance (Southon, 1994) and structures designed to engage the strengths of professionalism (Southon, 1996). These will, of course, need to be addressed in conjunction with the community, but in a framework that recognizes the centrality of professionalism, not one that implicitly rejects it.

Conclusion

The problems increasingly arising from many health reforms and the detrimental impact on professionals suggest the need to take a closer look at their relationship. A task-focused analysis of the role and nature of professionalism reveals the essential features of uncertainty and complexity. This is found to be in conflict with the simplifications inherent in many health reform techniques. However, such simplifications are found to be invalid, thus generating redundant tensions which explain many of the problems involved. If health reforms are to promote effective service delivery, they need to recognize the nature of the task and the central role of professionalism.

References

Altman, R.B. and von Otter, C. (1992) _Planned Markets and Public Competition: Strategic Reform in Northern European Health Systems_, Open University Press: Buckingham.

Brennan, T. (1991) _Just Doctoring: Medical Ethics in the Liberal State_, University of California Press, Berkeley.

Cox, K. (1995) 'Clinical practice is not applied scientific method', _Australian/New Zealand Journal of Surgery_, 65: 553.

Degeling, P.J. (1993) 'Policy as the accomplishment of an implementation structure: hospital restructuring in Australia', in _New Agendas in the Study of the Policy Process_, ed. M. Hill, Harvester Wheatsheaf: London.

Degeling, P.J. (1994) 'Unrecognised structural implications of casemix management', _Health Services Management Research_, 7: 9.

Emanuel, E.J. and Emanuel, L.L. (1996) 'What is accountability in health care?', _Annals of Internal Medicine_, 124: 229.

Freidson, E. (1990) 'The centrality of professionalism to health care', _Jurimetrics Journal_, 30 (4): 431.

Freidson, E. (1993) 'How dominant are the professions?', in _The Changing Medical Profession: An International Perspective_, ed. F.W. Hafferty and J.B. McKinlay, Oxford University Press: New York.

Harrison, S. and Pollitt, C. (1994) _Controlling Health Professionals: The Future Work and Organization in the National Health Service_, Open University Press: Buckingham.

Hunter, D.J. (1993) 'Desperately seeking solutions: rationing dilemmas in health care', _Australian Health Review_, 16 (2): 130.

Kassirer, J.P. (1993) 'Medicine at centre stage', _New England Journal of Medicine_, 328 (17): 1268.

Lazaro, P. and Azcona, B. (1996) 'Clinical practice, ethics and economics: the physician at the crossroads', _Health Policy_, 37: 185.

Leape, L.L. (1994) 'Error in medicine', _Journal of the American Medical Association_, 272 (23): 1851.

Maynard, A. (1993) 'The plane truth about doctors', *Health Service Journal*, 103 (5366): 19.

Mechanic, D. (1991) 'Sources of countervailing power in medicine', *Journal of Health Politics, Policy and Law*, 16: 485.

Mintzberg, H. (1979) *The Structuring of Organizations*, Prentice Hall, Englewood Cliffs, NJ.

Newble, D., Jolly, B. and Wakeford, R. (1994) 'Background', in *Certification and Recertification of Doctors: Issues in the Assessment of Clinical Competence*, ed. D. Newble, B. Jolly and R. Wakeford, Cambridge University Press, Cambridge.

Quinn, J.B., Anderson, P. and Finkelstein, S. (1996) 'Managing professional intellect: making the most of the best', *Harvard Business Review*, 74 (2): 71.

Raelin, J.A. (1986) *The Clash of Cultures: Managers and Professionals*, Harvard Business School Press: Boston, MA.

Schieber, G.J. and Poullier, J.P. (1990) 'Overview of international comparisons of health care expenditures', in *Health Care Systems in Transition: The Search for Efficiency*, Vol. 7, OECD Social Policy Studies, Paris. p. 9.

Southon, G. (1994) 'Professional autonomy and accountability', *World Hospitals*, 30: 4.

Southon, G. (1996) 'Health service structures, management and professional practice: beyond clinical management', *Australian Health Review*, 19: 2.

United Kingdom Monopolies Commission (1970) 'Report on the professions', in government and the professions, *Medical Journal of Australia*, 153: 242.

Wennberg, J.E. (1994) 'Health care reform and professionalism', *Inquiry*, 31: 296.

Wolinsky, F.D. (1993) 'The professional dominance, deprofessionalization, proletarianization and corporatization perspectives: an overview and synthesis', in *The Changing Medical Profession: An International Perspective*, ed. F.W. Hafferty and J.B. McKinlay, Oxford University Press: New York.

30

M. Saks

Professionalism and Health Care

The classic case of the medical profession

A discussion of the classic example of the medical profession, which can be seen to be an archetypal profession along with that of the legal profession in Britain, illuminates the application of the neo-Weberian concept of social closure in the health arena. In the 300 years immediately prior to the mid-nineteenth century in this country there was no national system of legally underwritten exclusionary closure in existence – despite such pockets of legal privilege as that provided by the sixteenth-century charter allowing the Royal College of Physicians to oversee medical practice within seven miles of the City of London. The field in fact was a relatively open one in which a broad span of therapies from herbalism and bonesetting to bleeding and purging were available from all kinds of practitioners in com-petition with each other in the market-place (Porter, 1989). In this situation, the predecessors of the contemporary medical profession – including apothecaries, surgeons and physicians in the process of forging their identities – were in a distinct minority, disunited and without consistent educational standards, even by the first half of the nineteenth century (Porter, 1987).

The 1858 Medical Registration Act paved the way for the social closure that has been the defining characteristic of the medical pro-fession in the modern context. This Act, which was passed only after much debate inside and outside Parliament, provided for the legally underwritten self-regulation of the newly unified, restrictive medical profession that formally excluded the medically unqualified from its ranks (Waddington, 1984). Critical to its self-regulatory powers was the centralized control the profession gained through the General Medical Council over education and training, the register of qualified practitioners and its own internal disciplinary affairs. Associated with this elevated occupational standing came many long-run rewards for insiders, not least being expanding income, status and

First published in S. Taylor and D. Field (eds) *Sociological Perspectives on Health, Illness and Health Care* (Blackwell Science, 1998), pp. 174–91. Abridged.

power. As such, it is not surprising that Parry and Parry (1976) have seen the rise of the British medical profession as a classic case of upward collective occupational mobility linked to the neo-Weberian concept of social closure – especially following the reinforcement of the 1858 Act by further legislation, including the 1886 Medical Act, which more starkly clarified its elevated position.

Even this legislation, however, did not formally outlaw the diminishing number of its unorthodox competitors who in Britain – as distinct from many other European countries – remained free to operate under the common law, although they could not claim to be registered medical practitioners (Saks, 1992). In this sense, the profession achieved more of a *de facto* than a *de jure* monopoly, which was pivoted on the Medical Registration Act that underwrote the exclusive rights of doctors over state medical employment. This meant that, with the subsequent establishment of the 1911 National Health Insurance Act and the 1946 National Health Service Act, the medical profession not only gained legally based self-regulation and a claim to state-enshrined legitimacy, but also managed to monopolize the market in the rapidly growing public sector. Its position of pre-eminence was further confirmed by legislation in the first half of the twentieth century that restricted the conditions – spanning from cancer and cataracts to diabetes and epilepsy – that non-medically qualified practitioners could claim to treat in the private sector (Larkin, 1995). . . .

Whatever the explanation of the exclusionary closure achieved by the medical profession, the profession had gone from strength to strength by the twentieth century on the basis of its increasingly biomedical frame of reference. This developed with the move away from 'bedside medicine' linked to the patronage system in the eighteenth century, in which rich clients had substantial control over their diagnosis and treatment. The shift was first towards 'hospital medicine' and later 'laboratory medicine' as the twentieth century unfolded – where the subordination of the patient to the doctor through the focus on the classification of disease was increased by the use of laboratory diagnosis and medical intervention without significant reference to the individual (Jewson, 1976). This emphasis on the 'scientific' paradigm of biomedicine, in which the body is conceived as a complex of cells separable into parts that could be repaired through the application of drug and surgical regimes, provided the basis of the esoteric medical knowledge on which the profession came to be founded and on which the health care division of labour expanded in contemporary Britain.

The establishment of other orthodox health professions

This development encompassed many occupational groups commonly regarded as professional – including the growing number of health administrators and managers as well as other orthodox health care practitioners. Of the latter, the groups which have exhibited the highest degree of legally enshrined closure within the marketplace are dentists, opticians and pharmacists. The 1878 Dentists Act gave the General Medical Council the power to examine and register dentists, with the formation of a Dental Board and subsequently a General Dental Council through legislation in the 1920s and 1950s respectively, closing the profession to outsiders (Nettleton, 1992). As such, dentists followed a similar trajectory to ophthalmic opticians who, with early origins in the Royal Charter granted to the Worshipful Company of Spectacle Makers in 1629, established the General Optical Council in 1958 which gave them independent professional standing (Larkin, 1983). Pharmacy shared significant roots in the past too, going back to the preparation and sale of medicines by chemists and druggists. From this practice sprang the Pharmacy Acts of the 1850s and 1860s which, among other things, gave the Pharmaceutical Society of Great Britain the statutory right to register pharmaceutical chemists and to prevent the unqualified from dispensing medicines (Levitt et al., 1995).

For all this legislation effecting social closure, however, dentists, opticians and pharmacists have nonetheless remained in the shade of medical domination as professional groups because their independence from direct medical supervision has been won at the price of being contained within their own boundaries. In this light, it is not surprising that Turner (1995) has viewed these professions as being based on 'occupational limitation' to a specific part of the body or a particular therapeutic method. He also identifies a further more common form of medical domination as that of 'subordination' in which the activities of health care occupations are formally delegated by the medical profession, with restricted scope for autonomy – as in the case of allied health professional work like medical laboratory sciences and midwifery. This is particularly well illustrated by the professions supplementary to medicine which accept patients only through referral from, and under the control of, medical practitioners in the state sector (Levitt et al., 1995). Such subjugated occupational groups were established by legislation in 1960 founding the Council for Professions Supplementary to Medicine with its seven initial boards for chiropodists, dieticians, medical laboratory technicians, occupational therapists, remedial gymnasts, radiographers and physiotherapists (Larkin, 1983).

Similar patterns of legally based subordination, mixed with the benefits of occupational closure in the marketplace, have also been apparent in the case of nurses, who constitute the largest professional group in the health care division of labour in Britain. To be sure, the professionalizing strategy of nurses certainly improved their collective position, as epitomized by the passing of the 1919 Nursing

Registration Act which created the General Nursing Council as the key regulating body for the newly forged profession. However, although this legislation has since been embellished by, amongst other things, the establishment of the United Kingdom Central Council for Nursing, Midwifery and Health Visiting which took over the registration and disciplinary function of the profession in 1983, the case of nursing reveals that size alone is no guarantee of pre-eminent professional standing, insofar as nurses remain subordinated within the division of labour by virtue of the legal monopoly that the medical profession continues to hold over diagnosis and treatment (Porter, 1992).

In this light, it is understandable that nursing and other professions allied to medicine are still frequently referred to as 'semi-professions'. Indeed, from a neo-Weberian perspective, such occupations as nursing have been viewed as examples of 'dual closure'. This is because, having failed to secure full professional closure, they are seen to combine the exclusionary device of credentialism with the usurpationary tactics of organized labour against employers and the state (Parkin, 1979), as accentuated by the significant rates of union membership among nurses (Bagguley, 1992). In this sense, it should be emphasized that the desire to professionalize can and often does involve the subordination of other less powerful occupations in the health care division of labour. This can be illustrated by the way in which nurses have historically delegated 'dirty work' to auxiliaries as part of the professionalizing project, as they continue to do today through the newly constructed role of care assistants (Witz, 1994). There are parallels here too in the manner in which groups like chiropodists and radiographers have protected their territory – in this instance against foot aides and darkroom technicians respectively – to maintain their position in the professional pecking order (Saks, 1987).

Given that the medical profession has traditionally been dominant within the increasingly pluralistic health care division of labour in Britain, a key question is how this can be explained. Functionalist commentators like Etzioni (1969) suggest that this is because the professions allied to medicine intrinsically need less expertise and training than the medical profession in a hierarchically organized division of labour. Neo-Weberian accounts, however, tend to emphasize the conflictual and fluid nature of the relationship between health professions, as opposed to the stronger connections of medicine to the ruling class that typically figure in more mechanistic Marxist interpretations (see, for example, Navarro, 1986). For neo-Weberians, this relationship is largely the outcome of interest-based 'turf battles' involving the maintenance and/or advancement of occupational position in terms of power, status and income, which may or may not have a gender dimension in a patriarchal society (Saks, 1995). The resolution of such struggles is usually seen as being mediated by the state, which in the case of health care has for long been pivoted on a medical–Ministry alliance that has helped to ensure the ascendance of the medical profession in the division of labour (Larkin, 1995). Much the same might be said of the outcome of the conflicts of medical orthodoxy with not only limited and subordinated practitioners, but also the excluded realm of alternative medicine against which it too has largely maintained its supremacy to date – notwithstanding recent moves to professionalize this area.

The emerging health care professions: alternative therapists

From participating in a thriving and relatively open field, the numbers and influence of non-medical practitioners of what became defined as alternative health care in the wake of the 1858 Medical Registration Act had declined markedly by the end of the nineteenth century. This was mainly as a result of the newly disenfranchised position of alternative practitioners and the growing legitimacy of medical orthodoxy (Saks, 1992). The increasing marginality of practitioners of therapies such as homoeopathy and herbalism, which were typically excluded from the undergraduate medical curriculum and stigmatized in orthodox medical circles (Saks, 1996), continued into the first half of the twentieth century. Although alternative therapists could still legally practise, they lacked support from the state, as highlighted by their exclusion from the fast developing public health service. This is further exemplified by the rejection of such cases as that made by the osteopaths to gain a foothold in orthodox medicine in the inter-war period, which reinforced the monopolistic position in the marketplace of medicine and allied professions (Larkin, 1992).

From the 1960s onwards, though, alternative therapies in Britain became more popular, as indicated by rising trends in consumer demand, the number of non-medically qualified alternative therapists and political support for unconventional medicine – including from parliamentary lobbies and, indeed, government itself. This followed the increasing failure of biomedical orthodoxy fully to live up to its promise in terms of efficacy and safety and the growing search by consumers for a more holistic approach to health care, involving the fusion of mind and body. When added to fears about the impact of European harmonization on the continuing common law right of unorthodox therapists to practice (Saks, 1994), the novel recent move by a growing band of unorthodox practitioners to professionalize alternative medicine becomes more understandable. There is certainly a recognizable strategic advantage to its exponents in establishing these hitherto marginalized therapies on sounder organizational and educational principles at present, even if this may not always be sought by individual practitioners (Sharma, 1995). The impact that non-medically qualified practitioners have made in this field, moreover, underlines the potentially fluid nature of the health care division of labour.

The present new-found desire for professional standing is well illustrated by the creation of the Council for Acupuncture in 1980, which brought together the British Acupuncture Association and Register, the Chung San Acupuncture Society, the International Register of Oriental Medicine, the Register of Traditional Chinese Medicine and the Traditional Acupuncture Society. The subsequent foundation of the British Acupuncture Accreditation Board served to establish among lay acupuncturists more unified standards of education, ethics, discipline and practice (Saks, 1995). Other groups of alternative therapists have also striven to increase their coherence as part of the professionalizing process, including the Society of Homoeopaths. This body has established a register and code of ethics and is seeking state recognition, not least on the basis of its accreditation of a number of homoeopathic colleges with more substantial educational programmes. Not all groups of alternative practitioners, though, are at a similar stage – as highlighted by reflexology which has thousands of practitioners, but a very diverse range of training schools with short periods of preparation for practice and little agreement on standards (Cant and Sharma, 1995).

The efforts of more strongly organized alternative therapies to gain legally underwritten professional credentials, as distinct from the more superficial trappings of professionalism, were unsuccessful up to the late 1980s. This was mainly because the government was seeking an all-embracing approach to the professionalization of such therapies, at a time when the overarching bodies that had been formed – such as the Institute for Complementary Medicine – were unable to represent the field as a whole (Sharma, 1995). The situation changed thereafter, as the government increasingly took the view that judgements should be made about individual therapies on their merits to determine their place in the health sector. This is highlighted by the case of osteopathy, which sufficiently overcame its internal divisions and put its educational infrastructure well enough in order for the Osteopaths Act to be passed in the early 1990s, following a private member's bill – marking a watershed in the development of alternative medicine (Standen, 1993).

The significance of this Act from the viewpoint of the professionalization of alternative medicine in neo-Weberian terms is that it places osteopathy under the control of the new General Osteopathic Council and establishes protection of title, a register, and self-regulation, including a prescribed set of ethical and educational standards. In so doing, it parallels legislation previously enacted to underwrite the position of other allied orthodox health care professions, although it provides no entry in its own right to state-based practice. The importance of this more limited form of social closure, however, is amplified by the fact that it was followed in 1994 by the Chiropractic Act, which established a similar basis for registration by chiropractors centred on the formation of a new General Chiropractic Council (Cant and Sharma, 1995). This suggests that the floodgates to the further professionalization of other alternative therapies could be opening. . . .

References

Bagguley, P. (1992) 'Angels in red? Patterns of union membership amongst UK professional nurses', in *Themes and Perspectives in Nursing*, ed. K. Soothill, C. Henry and K. Kendrick, Chapman and Hall: London.

Cant, S. and Sharma, U. (1995) *Professionalisation in Complementary Medicine*, Report on a research project funded by the Economic and Social Research Council.

Etzioni, A. (ed.) (1969) *The Semi-professions and their Organization*, Free Press: New York.

Jewson, N. (1976) 'The disappearance of the sick man from medical cosmology 1770 – 1870', *Sociology*, 10: 225–44.

Larkin, G. (1983) *Occupational Monopoly and Modern Medicine*, Tavistock: London.

Larkin, G. (1992) 'Orthodox and osteopathic medicine in the inter-war years', in *Alternative Medicine in Britain*, ed. M. Saks, Clarendon Press: Oxford.

Larkin, G. (1995) 'State control and the health professions in the United Kingdom', in *Health Professions and the State In Europe*, ed. T. Johnson, G. Larkin and M. Saks, Routledge: London.

Levitt, R., Wall, P. and Appleby, J. (1995) *The Reorganized National Health Service*, 5th edn, Chapman and Hall: London.

Navarro, V. (1986) *Crisis, Health and Medicine: A Social Critique*, Tavistock: London.

Nettleton, S. (1992) *Power, Pain and Dentistry*, Open University Press: Buckingham.

Parkin, F. (1979) *Marxism and Class Theory: A Bourgeois Critique*, Tavistock: London.

Parry, J. and Parry, N. (1976) *The Rise of the Medical Profession*, Croom Helm: London.

Porter, R. (1987) *Disease, Medicine and Society in England 1550–1860*, Macmillan: London.

Porter, R. (1989) *Health for Sale: Quackery in England 1660–1850*, Manchester University Press: Manchester.

Porter, S. (1992) 'The poverty of professionalization: a critical analysis of strategies for the occupational advancement of nursing', *Journal of Advanced Nursing*, 17: 720–6.

Saks, M. (1987) 'The politics of health care', in *Politics and Policy-making in Britain*, ed. L. Robins, Longman: London.

Saks, M. (1992) 'Introduction', in *Alternative Medicine in Britain*, ed. M. Saks, Clarendon Press: Oxford.

Saks, M. (1994) 'The alternatives to medicine', in *Challenging Medicine*, ed. J. Gabe, D. Kelleher and G. Williams, Routledge: London.

Saks, M. (1995) *Professions and the Public Interest: Medical Power, Altruism and Alternative Medicine*, Routledge: London.

Saks, M. (1996) 'From quackery to complementary medicine: the shifting boundaries between orthodox and unorthodox medical knowledge', in *Complementary and*

Alternative Medicines: Knowledge in Practice, ed. S. Cant and U. Sharma. Free Association Books: London.

Sharma, U. (1995) *Complementary Medicine Today: Practitioners and Patients*, revised edn. Routledge: London.

Standen, C.S. (1993) 'The implications of the Osteopaths Act', *Complementary Therapies in Medicine*, 1: 208–10.

Turner, B. (1995) *Medical Power and Social Knowledge*, 2nd edn, Sage: London.

Waddington, I. (1984) *The Medical Profession and the Industrial Revolution*, Gill and Macmillan: London.

Witz, A. (1994) 'The challenge of nursing', in *Challenging Medicine*, ed. J. Gabe, D. Kelleher and G. Williams, Routledge: London.

31

S. Rashid

Social Work and Professionalization: a Legacy of Ambivalence

To what extent should social work be regarded as 'professional' activity? Should social workers support or resist pressures to professionalize? How central, indeed, is professionalization to social work and its future as a distinct sphere of activity?

A look back at social work as it has evolved in Britain over the past hundred or so years reveals a complex picture characterized by a persistent ambivalence towards the whole issue of professionalization. From its beginnings in the voluntary sector, social work in Britain has taken shape within a strong statutory framework that has, itself, placed limits on professional autonomy. In the twentieth century, new currents of thought and changing political and economic realities have pushed social work in different directions, at times propelling it towards professionalization, while at others, challenging such aspirations.

In this chapter we explore this complex experience, taking as our starting point the definition of professional status supplied by Abbott and Meerabeau:

> Key elements in any claim to professional status seem to be autonomy or control over work, a clearly defined monopoly over an area of work and a knowledge base. (1998b: 9)

To what extent can social work in Britain be said to exert such autonomy, to enjoy such a monopoly and to draw upon such a knowledge base? And what premium has the social work community, or sections within it, placed on such goals and criteria at different points in time over the past century? In the discussion that follows, we shall find social workers in Britain seeking to professionalize, to de-professionalize and to re-professionalize, exploring a question that remains unresolved to this day.

The formative phase of British social work: voluntary and statutory roots

The voluntary legacy

Social work in Britain derived much vitality from voluntary organizations during the nineteenth and early twentieth centuries. Foremost amongst them was the Charity Organization Society (COS), now the Family Welfare Association. Founded in Victorian England, the COS had no doubts about the purpose of its work. This was to organize charity (i.e. financial help, or help in the form of the provision of material goods) in such a way as to foster a sense of independence and moral worth in the recipients. It was important to prevent them from becoming dependent on charity or otherwise morally undermined by the help offered. The connection with contemporary ideas of self-help is clear and the COS sought, like many other bodies, to help those who were prepared to help themselves. These were the people who were deserving of help, whereas others were not. The categorization into 'deserving' or 'undeserving' was imposed on the applicants, who were poor, by the Society's officials, who represented the better off and who claimed an expertise in distinguishing between the 'deserving' and 'undeserving'.

The emphasis was on helping the individual person or family. This theme recurs in social work and reflects the importance of the individual in West European social thought. Indeed it is not fanciful to characterize the Society's outlook in terms used by the Fabian Socialist, Beatrice Webb, in 1909, when she stated that the concern of the COS was to pull people out of the swamp, whereas her concern was to drain the swamp (Timms, 1983). This statement encapsulates tensions within social work which reappear periodically and which today mark a boundary between social work (especially in its statutory form) and community work/community development. The contribution of the COS to social work was its insistence on the need for systematic organization, for enquiries into the applicant's past and for records of help given.

Implicit in Beatrice Webb's remark is the focus on rescuing individuals from the swamp. This theme of rescue was common amongst voluntary organizations of the time, none more so than in the work of child care pioneers like Barnardo. Indeed Harding (1996) has argued that in child care services the 'rescue motif' has been dominant and continues to exert a strong influence. Similarly, from the 1870s the work of the Police Court missionaries, forerunners of contemporary probation officers, began with attempts to rescue drunken offenders from their dependence on alcohol and thereby from a life of crime. Interestingly the Probation of Offenders Act 1907 incorporated this voluntary activity into a statutory service, the Probation Service, whose remit widened far beyond drunken offenders. It retained the notion of rescuing impressionable youngsters and misguided or weak-willed adults from a life of crime by kindly interest and firm guidance from the probation officer. This example illustrates the way in which voluntary agencies in social work have often initiated action in a particular area and subsequent responsibility for it has been assumed by the statutory services.

A further example of the voluntary tradition is the appointment of hospital almoners in the late nineteenth century. As their name suggests, their initial concerns were with 'alms', assisting impecunious patients from voluntary funds, but the role extended during the twentieth century, as understanding increased about the impact of hospitalization and isolation from family and friends. Hospital almoners became known as medical social workers in the post-war period but until 1974 they continued to be appointed by the hospitals and therefore carried no statutory responsibilities. In 1974 they were incorporated into the local authority social services departments and had the same statutory powers and responsibilities as other social workers in those departments.

The statutory legacy

Contemporary British social work differs from that in many other countries in being predominantly a statutory activity. This is often regarded as a post-war phenomenon and is attributed to the creation of the welfare state in the late 1940s. However, the statutory tradition goes back a long way and two examples will suffice. The relieving officer who operated the Poor Law carried out functions performed by social workers today (assessing need and arranging for residential care when this is appropriate). Today's approved social worker (ASW) is responsible under the 1983 Mental Health Act for assessing the need for compulsory admission to psychiatric hospital. The ASW's predecessors were the mental welfare officer, who operated the 1959 Mental Health Act, the duly authorized officer, who operated the 1890 Lunacy Act until its repeal in 1960, and the Poor Law overseer, who was authorized to remove a lunatic to the asylum (Gostin, 1986).

This emphasis on the statutory tradition raises the question of whether social work exists to help people or to control them on behalf of society and/or the state. The debate on 'care and control' is an old one and remains current, for instance in child protection, in mental health and in work with offenders. It may be argued that frequently there is no conflict between the two, that in order to care for a severely disturbed or distressed person one needs to control him/her, or that the controlling may be part of the caring. The question still remains, however, and tensions will continue between care and control, between the individual and society. One must conclude that a statutory tradition will emphasize the role of social work as an agent of the state. Furthermore it is hard to see how major claims for professional status can be made for statutory social work, since there is little control over it and the role is prescribed by statute and/or regulation. Certainly the relieving officers and duly authorized officers would not have regarded their tasks as professional, but rather as administrative and procedural in nature.

Social work in Britain in the late nineteenth and early twentieth centuries had two major concerns: administering financial or other material relief to those in poverty, whether through statutory or voluntary bodies; and rescuing vulnerable and redeemable individuals from crime, destitution and vice. This strongly moral language would have been familiar to social workers of the period, since it reflected dominant contemporary ideas. The first has a weak claim to professional status, since it was concerned with administrative and procedural matters, the second was more akin to missionary activity and hence vocational rather than professional in nature.

Pressures in favour of professionalization

The arrival of psychiatric social work

A marked shift away from the emphasis on material need came into social work in the late 1920s with the advent of psychoanalytical ideas. Although originating in Central Europe they came to Britain from American social work and were associated with psychiatry. Drawing on Freudian ideas, psychiatric social work focused on the inner world of the patient. The social worker developed a therapeutic relationship with the patient, which helped the latter to unearth, understand and thereby resolve conflicts from the past and ease relationships in the present. The first training course for psychiatric social workers (PSWs) in Britain opened at the London School of Economics in 1929. Other courses began at the universities of Birmingham, Leeds and Manchester (with those at the last two continuing into the 1980s). Interest in psychoanalytical ideas was strengthened by the arrival in London of psychoanalysts, including Freud, in the late 1930s, as refugees from Nazi persecution. The work of Anna Freud and Melanie Klein with children influenced workers in therapeutic child care in the post-war years and continues to do so.

The numbers of psychiatric social workers were always small and they operated in specialist settings, chiefly child guidance clinics and psychiatric hospitals, but also in the Probation Service. Their influence was considerable, because of the specialized nature of their training and because they adopted a clinical model more closely than any other group of social workers. Their close links with psychiatry added to their prestige. Furthermore the interest in matters psychotherapeutic during and after the Second World War, expressed in the extension of group therapy and the development of therapeutic communities, helped raise their profile. In many ways this group of social workers had a strong claim to professional status, in that they had considerable autonomy over their work and a strong knowledge base in the psychoanalytical tradition. Whilst unable to claim a monopoly over an area of work, since they shared it with psychiatrists, they had demarcated that area clearly. Their professional body, the Association of Psychiatric Social Workers, modelled itself on medical bodies, and membership was restricted to qualified PSWs.

The emergence of the welfare state

The creation of the welfare state in the late 1940s had its roots in the social upheavals of the Second World War. This was particularly true for child care services. The experience of evacuating children from cities threatened with bombing brought a heightened awareness of slum conditions. The death of a child, Dennis O'Neill, at the hands of his foster father prompted an official inquiry in 1946 which led to the Children Act 1948. This created children's departments in every local authority, which then accepted responsibility for children in residential and foster care and also for vulnerable children living with their parents. The National Assistance Act 1948 set up local authority welfare departments, which accepted responsibility for older people and for people with disabilities.

The statutory stream of social work thus became very much part of the welfare state. It differed from the Poor Law, which it replaced, in that the legislation was formulated to allow very considerable discretion to those who operated it. Social workers were therefore able to exercise their judgement about when or whether to receive a child into care or seek the compulsory removal of an aged person. Bean (1980) has described this welfare legislation as 'therapeutic legislation', predicated on the assumption that the officials operating it would act in the interests of their clients. It hands over control to the 'experts', who are trusted by society not to misuse it. It is essentially paternalistic, leaving clients with little power to challenge the 'experts'. Bean's major concern is with mental health law but his point applied equally to child care and probation law. Under this reading, social workers become professionals by default, because society decides that they possess areas of expertise and decision-making beyond the remit of the layperson. Psychiatric social work was one example of such expertise; another was its close relation, social casework.

The new 'expertise': social casework

Social casework was not the strictly clinical model developed by the psychiatric social workers, but it made use of some of their insights.

Strongly influenced by the work of Felix Biestek, Florence Hollis and Helen Perlman and other American researchers, it focused on the casework relationship between caseworker and client, located the client's problems within his/her personality and sought to help the client by working through his/her feelings which often lay behind the presenting problem. In so doing the caseworker expected that the client's coping mechanisms would be released and strengthened.

During the 20 years between 1948 and 1968 social casework was a strong influence in British social work and its claim to expertise in the area of feelings and emotions, and their impact on family functioning, helped to advance social work's claims to professional status. Elements of social casework remain in current social work practice, for instance the emphasis on emotions and feelings, especially in working with clients of all ages who have experienced significant losses.

However, lack of attention paid to external factors, such as poverty and discrimination, left social casework wide open to criticism. To read Biestek's 1961 text, *The Casework Relationship*, today is to realize that many of the 'Seven Principles' he expounded are more relevant to counselling than to social work. This is not surprising, given the focus of casework on the client's inner world; this is the domain of counselling and psychotherapy, whose claim to professional status is less contentious. Social work has, as its name implies, much stronger links with the client's social, external world.

Pressures to de-professionalize and re-professionalize: the radical sixties and beyond

Radical social work: anti-professionalism

The upsurge of radical thought during the late 1960s brought into social work insights from sociological theories which emphasized the impact of structural inequalities on individuals and communities. The class-based nature of social work, whereby most clients were working class and poor, was stressed, together with a renewed awareness that the function of much statutory social work was social control. The prevailing orthodoxy of casework was derided in the radical social work magazine *Case Con*, which made the point forcefully that casework was a confidence trick which cheated clients by pretending to meet their needs while actually worsening their situation. Strategies were proposed, such as raising consciousness amongst clients, forming alliances with client groups through trade unions, enabling clients to set up claimants' unions to deal with Social Security officials and credit unions to obtain cheaper food.

The renewed awareness of social injustice and a determination to attempt to change it was widespread both inside and outside social work. In many ways this was an attempt 'to drain the swamp', in Beatrice Webb's terms, which rejected any notion of elitist expertise and of professionalism. Solidarity with clients against the repressive state and a breaking of barriers between social workers and clients was the aim of radical social work.

In the early 1980s the anti-racist movement gave new impetus to radical social work. It was led by black workers, who drew on their direct experiences of racism within society at large and in social work in particular. This second wave of radicalism pointed to structural, historical and ideological factors, which oppressed black people, both workers and clients. It built upon the earlier efforts of radical social work, which it criticized for focusing on class and ignoring race and gender. Issues in child care, such as transracial adoption and the over-representation of black children in the care system, provided the focus for much of the debate.

This debate was public, highlighted by some well-publicized adoption cases, where issues of same-race versus transracial placement were prominent. It came to a head in 1993, with public attacks in the media on the alleged domination of social work training by anti-racist zealots (Phillips, 1993; Pinker, 1993). Anti-racist social work was charged with being 'politically correct', oppressive and intellectually shallow. As a result of this furore, CCETSW modified its original statements in the Diploma in Social Work requirements on racism being endemic in British society (CCETSW, 1989) to a more general statement about 'discrimination, racism, disadvantage, inequality and injustice' (CCETSW, 1995). This entire episode illustrates how social work, especially in its dominant statutory form, is open to wider political pressure and attack. The inability of the training and validating body, or of the professional association, to resist this attack successfully, indicates the weakness of social work's claim to professional status.

The emergence of a feminist perspective in social work and the recognition that clients face a range of oppressions has led to attempts by social workers to develop anti-oppressive and anti-discriminatory ways of working (Thompson, 1997; Dominelli, 1998). The development of service user groups and organizations in the past decade, and the principle of working in partnership with clients, which is enshrined in the 1989 Children Act, indicate some of the changes which are still in progress. These suggest a new form of professionalism unlike the paternalistic 'expert' described earlier.

The Seebohm reorganization: new attempts to professionalize

This mood of radicalism coincided with the unification of different branches of local authority social work into social services departments in 1971, following the recommendations of the Seebohm Report in 1968. This brought together social workers in child care, those who worked with older people and with people with physical disabilities and mental welfare officers, who were responsible for people with mental illnesses and with learning disabilities. In Scotland probation officers also joined the new social work departments (note the different title), but in England and Wales they retained a separate identity within the Probation Service. As we have already seen, hospital-based social workers did not join the social services departments until 1974.

This unification was accompanied by the unification of the separate social work bodies, which formed the British Association of Social Workers (BASW) in 1971, and the creation of a new single training body, the Central Council for Education and Training in Social Work (CCETSW), in the same year. Hopes for increased recognition of social work's claims to professional status were high amongst those official representatives of social work, despite the radicalism described above. However, disputes over the criteria for joining BASW revealed wide disagreements about professionalism, which ranged from demands for open membership to demands that only qualified social workers should be admitted. Once again, social work was revealing its deep-rooted ambivalence towards the issue of professional status.

Tightening controls and managerialism

The emergence of larger, more bureaucratic and more powerful social services departments coincided with increased responsibilities as demands for child protection increased in the wake of the child abuse inquiries through the 1970s and 1980s. The growth of trade union membership and of industrial action in this period can be seen as evidence of the strains on workers and managers alike. Pressures were felt to both re-professionalize (where social workers moved into positions as managers) and to de-professionalize (where social workers experienced their role in terms of being workers).

Public concern over the highly publicized deaths of children like Maria Caldwell, Jasmine Beckford and Kimberley Carlisle, and the sexual abuse allegations in Cleveland and Orkney, was expressed in the inquiry reports that followed. This led to a tightening of child protection procedures by the Department of Health, as exemplified in the 'Orange Book', published in 1990. This may be seen as an attempt to limit the discretion of social workers and to exert greater managerial control over them. At the same time the notion that public sector managers had much to learn from the private sector became pronounced in the 1990s. Hugman (1998) has argued that the impact of managerialism, associated with New Right economic thinking, like 'value for money', and 'economy, efficiency and effectiveness' has been to weaken social concerns and strengthen the process of de-professionalization. This organizational impetus comes from government policy and is not restricted to social work; it applies to social welfare and public service more widely.

The General Social Care Council

Moves towards creating a body for social work akin to the General Medical Council or the UKCC have been slow and hesitant. This reflects doubts within social work over the desirability of such a body, which could be seen as elitist and concerned with the self-interest of its members. At the time of the Seebohm reorganization there were hopes for a social work council, but as the arguments over membership criteria for BASW showed, there was also deep ambivalence. In 1990 an influential report by Professor Roy Parker set out the case for a General Social Services Council, which would not be elitist but would be open to a wide range of staff in the personal social services. This provided the basis for protracted negotiations within the social services and government approval has been won for a General Social Care Council to be established in 2001. The shifts in terminology and the length of time between the Parker Report and the proposed date for establishing the Council indicate the lack of agreement and the slow building of consensus (Brand, 1998) within social work and the lack of political will outside it.

What will the Council do? This is not yet clear, but it seems likely that there will be a strong emphasis on service-user representation and on setting standards in order to reassure the public about the quality of service that can be expected. It is worth recalling that Parker's report was called *Safeguarding Standards* and this continues to be a prominent theme. Will it work? Many social workers will be dubious about assurances to the public when services depend on tight budgetary control, rather than on perceived needs or social workers' discretion. Doubtless time will tell.

References

Abbott, P. and Meerabeau, L. (eds) (1998a) *The Sociology of the Caring Professions*, 2nd edn, London: UCL.

Abbott, P. and Meerabeau, L. (1998b) 'Professionals, professionalization and the caring professions', in Abbot and Meerabeau (1998).

Adams, R., Dominelli, L. and Payne, M. (eds) (1998) *Social Work: Themes, Issues and Critical Debates*, Basingstoke: Macmillan.

Bean, P. (1980) *Compulsory Admissions to Mental Hospital*, Chichester: John Wiley.

Biestek, F.P. (1961) *The Casework Relationship*, London: Allen and Unwin.

Brand, D. (1998) 'Regulation and the prospects for professions', *Managing Community Care*, 6 December (supplementary issue):

CCETSW (1989) *Rules and Requirements for the Diploma in Social Work*, London: CCETSW.

CCETSW (1995) *Assuring Quality in the Diploma in Social Work – 1: Rules and Requirements for the Dip. SW*, London: CCETSW.

Dominelli, L. (1998) 'Anti-oppressive practice in context', in Adams et al. (1998).

Gostin, L. (1986) *Mental Health Services – Law and Practice*, London: Shaw and Sons.

Harding, L.F. (1997) *Perspectives in Child Care Policy*, 2nd edn, Harlow: Longman.

Hugman, R. (1998) 'Social work and de-professionalization', in Adams et al. (1998).

Parker, R. (1990) *Safeguarding Standards*, London: NISW/Rowntree Trust.

Phillips, M. (1993) 'An oppressive urge to end oppression', *Observer*, 1 August.

Pinker, R. (1993) 'A lethal kind of looniness', *Times Higher Educational Supplement*, 10 September.

Thompson, N. (1997) *Anti-Discriminatory Practice*, 2nd edn, Basingstoke: Macmillan.

Timms, N. (1983) *Social Work Values: An Enquiry*, London: Routledge and Kegan Paul.

32

S. Dowling, R. Martin, P. Skidmore, L. Doyal, A. Cameron and S. Lloyd

Nurses Taking on Junior Doctors' Work: a Confusion of Accountability

. . . A quiet revolution is occurring in the division of labour between the professions of medicine and nursing[1,2] created partly by requirements to reduce junior hospital doctors' work [3,4] and to compensate for their shortage in some specialities.[5] Nurses in particular are taking on clinical work that has traditionally been done by doctors. Our research into the resulting new roles in hospitals has made us aware of the confusion surrounding the management of accountability for the scope of these new roles and the standards that apply to them.[2,6] Certain clinicians – experienced nurses and consultants – may be at risk of complaints or disciplinary or legal action as a result of the innovatory nature of their work and the lack of clear guidance on accountability if things go wrong. We explore here some of the regulations that currently apply to doctors and nurses and illustrate, by means of a case report, some of the sources of confusion. . . .

Case report

Although the following story of a consultant-led development to reduce junior doctors' hours of work is fictional, every detail has been recorded in one or more of the eight posts studied in our recent research[2,6] and consultancy work.

Trust X created a new consultant surgeon's post without an associated preregistration house officer post. The consultants suggested that a nurse should be employed to do much of the routine work normally done by house officers. The postholder would be part of the consultant firm, clinically and managerially accountable to the consultant, and through him to the clinical director. The Trust approved the plan, ignoring their senior nurses' advice that nurses should be

First published in *BMJ*, 312 (11 May): 121–14 (BMJ Publishing Group, 1996). Abridged.

equal partners in the planning and management of the post. They conceded there should be regular meetings for supervision with a senior nurse and the consultant.

An experienced nurse, Ms Gilbert, was appointed to work with the senior consultant, Mr James. He arranged for her to 'shadow' a house officer for three weeks and learn specific skills from anaesthetists. For some weeks Ms Gilbert felt unsure about clerking routine admissions and refused to do them on her own. The house officers complained: she should 'learn on the job' as doctors did.

Ms Gilbert was uneasy about her title 'Surgical Practice Manager', which gave no hint of her identity as a nurse. She stopped using it and left off her name badge. Although she wore a sister's uniform and introduced herself to patients as a nurse with special training to do parts of junior doctors' work, they sometimes called her 'Doctor'. She did not join in ward nursing activities but behaved like the doctors, attending ward rounds, going to theatre, etc.

At the end of six months the tasks listed in Ms Gilbert's job description did not match her expanded role. For instance, she became skilled at a new technical procedure and, at Mr James's request (but unknown to the clinical director), took this over from the registrar. A senior nurse's comments that this was 'a step too far' were dismissed by Mr James, as professional rivalry; he would 'carry the can' if anything went wrong.

After some months Ms Gilbert felt isolated and unsupported. If it hadn't been for the challenge of new work she might have left. The promised regular meetings with the consultant and senior nurse had not taken place.

Ms Gilbert thought that if she required legal advice or representation she would be covered by her union's indemnity insurance. Neither she nor Mr James had given their respective insurance agencies details of this post.

Accountability for scope and standards of professional practice

The GMC and UKCC are required by statute to regulate the nature and standards of practice of doctors and nurses respectively. The GMC's guidance, *Good Medical Practice*[7] allows doctors to delegate medical care to nurses if they are sure the nurse is competent to undertake the work. The doctor remains responsible for managing the patient's care (para. 28).

In our case it is unclear whether Ms Gilbert's work would be considered 'delegated', given its inclusion in a job description for a qualified nurse. The consultant might, however, argue that he was delegating in some sense as the post operated within the framework of a surgical firm, substituting for juniors' work. For reasons of his professional regulations alone, therefore, he might ensure Ms Gilbert's accountability to him for her competence.

The UKCC's *Scope of Professional Practice*[8] describes principles to guide nurses' professional practice when taking on new roles, as in Ms Gilbert's job. These principles arise from the UKCC's *Code of Professional Conduct*[9] and associated advice[10] on accountability. The following are relevant here:

- Regardless of employment circumstances, registered nurses are subject to UKCC regulations and accountable, personally, to the council (para. 5).[8]
- In taking on new work registered nurses must acknowledge any limits in their competence and decline duties unless able to perform them in a safe and skilled manner (para. 4).[9]
- Nursing managers must ensure local policies are based on UKCC principles and that nurses are assisted to fulfil suitable adjustments to their practice (para. 25).[8]

Nurses may interpret these regulations as a major change in their relationship with doctors, removing their dependence on them for assessing nurses' competence to do work previously done by doctors.[11]

At the start of the job Ms Gilbert followed UKCC principles and refused to clerk patients on her own because she did not feel competent. If Mr James disagreed with her he should be sensitive to UKCC regulations concerning the locus of responsibility for competence when extending nurses' roles. Ms Gilbert, in turn, should appreciate that the UKCC's emphasis on nurses' personal responsibility does not exclude her being accountable also to Mr James for her competence.

Such dual accountability could be difficult to manage if there was disagreement. Finding an operational way to cope with the difficulties would, however, be in the spirit of both councils' emphasis on promoting good relationships and constructive working with other professions in health care.[7,9,10] Unfortunately neither council in its advice on multiprofessional teamwork deals specifically with respect for other professions' binding codes of conduct or the difficulties that may arise if they differ from their own.

The consultants' reluctance jointly to plan and manage this post with nurses made it difficult for the nurse leaders of the trust to fulfil their professional responsibility to ensure Ms Gilbert had the necessary professional support (para. 25).[8] In such a situation the spirit of UKCC advice[8,9,10] suggests these nurses should do everything possible to keep open their one avenue for professional support to Ms Gilbert through joint nurse–consultant supervision.

Legal accountability for civil wrongs to patients

The two main areas of civil law relevant to the changing roles of doctors and nurses are negligence and battery.[12,13,14] Generally civil legal action is directed against the NHS employer (trust or health authority) rather than the individual nurse of doctor, and it is the Trust which bears financial responsibility for paying any damages.[15] The Trust is entitled to try to recover damages from individuals at fault, but this has never occurred in practice. Nevertheless, a finding of negligence or battery against any professional is harmful personally and professionally.

Negligence and the nurse

To give rise to a negligence action Ms Gilbert must make an error which results in the patient suffering injury. In such a situation Ms Gilbert owes a duty of care to the patient – that is, she has a duty to use reasonable care and skill in the treatment. The more difficult question is to what standard of care will Ms Gilbert be held for the purposes of determining whether that duty has been breached. It cannot be assumed that because Ms Gilbert was trained as a nurse and calls herself a nurse she would be held in law to the standard of the competent nurse according to accepted standards of that profession.

In determining Ms Gilbert's standard of care, a court will look at a range of criteria including the nature of the task, the way she 'holds herself out' to patients (dress, name badge, language, socialization), and the way she is perceived by patients. If the task is traditionally performed by a doctor, and if the patient expects it to be performed by a doctor, then unless Ms Gilbert has explained her status to the patient she could, for the purposes of legal negligence, be held to the standard of the doctor in the performance of that task. This standard will pertain to all aspects of the task, including any circumstances which might arise incidental to the treatment and for which she had not been trained.

Ms Gilbert has been specifically trained in certain tasks previously performed by house officers and will probably in practice meet the standard of the doctor in the performance of those tasks. She is required to learn other jobs as house officers do, 'on the job', without the rigorous process of teaching and supervised practice and assessment to which nurses are accustomed. Inexperience will not excuse Ms Gilbert from liability. A beginner is always held to the standard of a competent performer of the task.[16,17] With respect to these tasks she will be held to that standard regardless of the innovative nature of the post.

When a patient is touched without consent a battery has been committed.[18] When Ms Gilbert has carefully explained her identity to the patient the patient can fully consent, knowing that the treatment will be performed by a nurse. Consent to touching by a specific person or profession will not act as consent to touching by any other. Without careful explanation from Ms Gilbert, a patient's consent may be invalid if, as had sometimes happened, the patient assumed from the nature of the task and the way she 'held herself out' that she was a doctor. Unlike the situation in cases of negligence, a patient need not show harm to be entitled to bring legal action; also unlike in negligence,[19] an action in battery raises the possibility of an award of aggravated damages if the patient has suffered excessive distress or if the defendant has behaved in a particularly high handed manner.[20]

Who else could be liable?

The consultant   The consultant owes a duty of care to his patients to see that Ms Gilbert does not perform any task for which she is not trained and competent. The consultant could then be found liable in negligence for allowing her to act beyond the scope of her competence or responsibility. . . . The consultant is ultimately responsible for determining Ms Gilbert's competence and ensuring that she does not exceed it.

The Trust   The Trust can become legally responsible for the negligence of the nurse or the consultant in either of two ways: through the concept of vicarious liability, or as a result of the hospital's non-delegable duty to its patients.[21]

Vicarious liability applies in relation to employees of the Trust but not to self-employed or agency staff. The Trust will be liable for any negligence or battery committed by an employee so long as the employee was acting within the course of employment. The definition of 'course of employment' is the subject of some legal debate but allows the employer to place limits on the range of tasks within the domain of employment.[22] If, as suggested by the senior nurse, Ms Gilbert's performance of a procedure previously done by the registrar was considered well beyond her expected and authorized responsibilities, she might be taken to have acted outside her course of employment,[23] which would relieve the Trust of legal liability for her practice of this procedure.

The Trust also has a personal and non-delegable duty to see that each patient is competently treated. Should a patient suffer from Ms Gilbert's practice it can be argued that the Trust was negligent in assigning her to tasks for which she had not been properly trained and which were normally done by someone more qualified.

Accountability of employers and employees to each other

The Trust as employer

The courts emphasize that the modern employment relationship is one built on 'mutual trust and confidence':[24] while employees must be prepared to adapt to new practices, an employer should provide the means for this, including the necessary training and professional and management support. Here, where Ms Gilbert was unsatisfied with aspects of the training provided, and the organization of regular meetings for clinical supervision had broken down, it might be claimed that the Trust had not provided the necessary support and was in breach of contract. If Ms Gilbert resigned as a result she could have grounds for a claim of unfair dismissal because of this breach.

The consultant and nurse as employees

Even when employees (here, the consultant) have not infringed their professional code and their action has not resulted in any commencement of legal proceedings, they may still be in breach of their employer's disciplinary rules and therefore in breach of contract. The behaviour of the consultant in relation to Ms Gilbert's work would be subject to the Trust's policies, protocols, and other rules of behaviour. By agreeing that Ms Gilbert should take over the new technical procedure from his registrar before there was agreement by the Trust, and in the absence of agreed protocols, the consultant might be in breach of trust policies and thus liable to disciplinary action.

Ms Gilbert refused to clerk routine admissions because she felt she lacked the necessary skills and knowledge. This was correct in terms of her professional UKCC regulations. However, her job specification required her to work on a surgical firm on a similar basis to a house officer. By refusing to carry out the work Ms Gilbert might be considered to be in breach of contract and liable to be disciplined.

Suppose Ms Gilbert was dismissed as a result of her stand on this issue and subsequently brought a case of unfair dismissal to an industrial tribunal. In determining fairness one of the issues for the tribunal would be to consider the adequacy of Ms Gilbert's training and supervision. This could highlight differences between the medical and nursing approaches to these, and clinicians' difficulties when developing roles between two professions with such different educational cultures.[25,26]

Conclusions and recommendations

Ms Gilbert's role might be characterized as that of a watered down doctor,[2] one of several emerging at the nursing-medical interface to meet problems in the organization of doctors' hospital work. Despite criticisms that such medically dominated posts are inappropriate for experienced nurses,[27] they appear to be increasing. Other types of expanded nursing roles exist, many located more clearly within nursing and operating within nursing management structures. We suggest that the principles raised in this chapter are relevant to all such nursing expansions, although details may differ.

Ways of reducing the risks

Doctors and nurses have to allow their roles to evolve to meet the rapid changes in health service delivery, technology, and patient needs.[28] Such innovations, however, occur in an era of escalating medical litigation,[29,30] subtle changes in the power relationship between patients and carers,[31] and policies which reinforce patients' rights to complain if adequate services are not provided.[32] It may be some comfort that there is no evidence that nurses in these new roles are more likely to make mistakes than doctors doing the same work. The introduction of crown indemnity for doctors[15] means that if a consultant or nurse in such a development were found legally negligent they would be unlikely to be financially liable for damages. Nevertheless, the stress of an official complaint can be enormous, whatever its outcome.

The dual demands of innovation and safe practice require educational and management strategies designed to make innovation as safe as possible for clinicians and employers. When addressing any ambiguities and apparent contradictions between the three areas of regulation discussed in this chapter, we must not forget that the *raison d'être*, common to them all, is the protection of patients. Our analyses suggest certain recommendations to minimize risk which complement other more general advice for managing such developments.[33,34,35]

Nurses and doctors should be equal partners in planning and managing the new roles

Because these posts bring together aspects of two very different professions both professions should be involved in the planning and management of such developments. Doctors and nurses developing such new roles should be aware that there may be different demands on each profession for accountability for the scope and standard of their practice. They require support to negotiate appropriate operational arrangements which accommodate the relevant professional regulations; clarify the nature and limits of the post; and provide means of training, supervision, and competence assessment which are mutually agreed.

Patients should be informed

There should be an agreed way of explaining the new role to patients, indicating the profession the postholder comes from and relevant training and experience for this job. The nurse's dress and job title require careful consideration to be consistent with these explanations.

Approval by employer and insurers

These posts are innovative and the work required may change within a postholder's appointment. Important changes should be communicated to and agreed by (a) all key staff concerned with the post, (b) the chief executive of the Trust (or delegate) through clearly defined procedures, and (c) the insurers of the employer and those of the consultants and nurses directly concerned. Job descriptions should be updated as necessary.

Staff need access to legal advice

However carefully these posts are planned and supported, the nurses and doctors involved are potentially vulnerable to the challenge that their practice contravenes professional regulations or aspects of the law. These staff should be advised to join an organization which can provide independent professional and legal advice and indemnity.

Need for central action

Such strategies at trust level are only a partial solution for safe innovation in clinical roles. Urgent action is also needed by the GMC, the UKCC and the NHS Executive, working together, to clarify relevant regulations, influence legal processes, and educate the public about changing professional roles.

References

1. Read, S. and Graves, K. (1994) 'Reduction of junior doctors' hours in Trent region: the nursing contribution', *Report to Trent Task Force*, Sheffield: Sheffield Centre for Health and Related Research.
2. Dowling, S., Barrett, S. and West, R. (1995) 'With nurse practitioners, who needs house officers?', *BMJ*, 311: 309–13.
3. NHS Management Executive (1991) *Junior Doctors: the New Deal*, London: NHS Management Executive.
4. Working Group on Specialist Medical Training (1993) *Hospital Doctors: Training for the Future, The Report of the Working Group on Specialist Medical Training*, London: Department of Health.
5. Medical Workforce Standing Advisory Committee (1995) *Planning the Medical Workforce. 2nd Report*, London: Department of Health.

6. Doyal, L., Cameron, A., Dowling, S. and Lloyd, S. (in press) *An Evaluation of Four New Nursing Posts in Acute Hospital Base Care*, Bristol: Policy Press.
7. General Medical Council (1995) 'Duties of a doctor', *Guidance from the General Medical Council*, London: GMC.
8. United Kingdom Central Council for Nursing, Midwifery and Health Visiting (1992) *The Scope of Professional Practice*, London: UKCC.
9. United Kingdom Central Council for Nursing, Midwifery and Health Visiting (1992) *Code of Professional Conduct*, London: GMC.
10. United Kingdom Central Council for Nursing, Midwifery and Health Visiting (1989) *Exercising Accountability: A UKCC Advisory Document*, London: UKCC.
11. Dimond, B. (1994) 'Legal aspects of role expansion', in G. Hunt and P. Wainwright (eds) *Expanding the Role of the Nurse: the Scope of Professional Practice*, Oxford: Blackwell Science.
12. Dimond, B. (1995) *Legal Aspects of Nursing*, 2nd edn. London: Prentice-Hall.
13. Korgaonkar, G. and Tribe, D. (1995) *Law for Nurses*, London: Cavendish.
14. Mason, J.K. and McCall Smith, R.A. (1994) *Law and Medical Ethics*, 4th edn, London: Butterworths.
15. Department of Health and Social Security (1989) *Claims of Medical Negligence Against NHS Hospital and Community Doctors and Dentists*, London: DHSS. (HC(FP)(89)22).
16. Nettleship *v.* Weston [1971] 2 QB 691.
17. Wilsher *v.* Essex Health Authority [1986] 2 A11 ER 801.
18. Re F [1990] 2 AC 1.
19. Kralj *v.* McGrath [1986] 1 ALL ER 54.
20. Appleton *v.* Garrett [1996] PIQR 1.
21. Cassidy *v.* Minister of Health [1951] 2 KB 343.
22. Twine *v.* Bean's Express [1946] 62 TLR 458.
23. Beard *v.* London General Omnibus [1990] 2 QB 530.
24. Woods *v.* WM Car Services [1982] ICR 693.
25. Davies, C. (1995) *Gender and the Professional Predicament in Nursing*, Buckingham: Open University Press.
26. Walby, S. and Greenwell, J. (1994) *Medicine and Nursing: Professions in a Changing Health Service*, London: Sage.
27. Salvage J. (1995) 'What's happening to nursing?', *BMJ*, 311: 274–5.
28. Harrison, A. and Prentice, S. (1996) *Acute Futures*, London: King's Fund.
29. Hoyte, P. (1994) 'Medical negligence litigation, claims handling and risk management', *Medical Law International*, 1: 261–75.
30. Dyer, C. (1996) 'Medical litigation faces British revolution', *BMJ*, 312: 330.
31. Health Service Commissioner (1995) *Third Report for Session 1994–5, Annual Report for 1994–95*, London: HMSO.
32. Department of Health (1995) *The Patient's Charter*, London: Department of Health.
33. NHS Management Executive (1993) *Risk Management in the NHS*, London: Department of Health.
34. Read, S. (1995) *Catching the Tide: New Voyages in Nursing?*, Sheffield: Sheffield Centre for Health and Related Research.
35. Royal College of Physicians of London and the Royal College of Nursing (1996) 'Skill sharing: joint statement', *J. Roy Coll Physicians Lond*, 30: 57.

33

L. Archer

Looking for New Codes in the Field of Predictive Medicine

The twenty-first century will succeed in writing the complete sequence of the human genome. The resulting knowledge will dramatically enlarge current possibilities for the prediction of hereditary diseases and other genetic traits. A series of ethical, social and legal problems will then arise, which will demand the establishment of new codes of practice.

Technical aspects

General methods for detection of genetic traits

. . . Predictive medicine aims at preventing the expression of diseases in persons carrying a morbid genetic trait. Its impact on public health is, therefore, very positive. However, there are areas of misuse which can lead to ethical concerns.

The genetic myth

The human genome analysis programme tends to create, in the public, the myth of the unlimited capacity of genetics in the prediction of future life and health.

In Greek and Roman mythology the Parcae were the inexorable three sisters who were spinning the thread of human life: Clotho (the spinner), Lachesis (the disposer of lots) and Atropos (unalterable fate). . . . They seemed to have a general power over events and were always present, spinning the thread of life.

The three Parcae are reincarnated, nowadays, in the genetic machinery of enzymes which spin the double-helical thread of DNA. The present myth announces that this magic thread encodes all our tendencies and wishes, all our future reactions and decisions, all

First published in U. Trohler, S. Reiter-Theil, E. Herych and H-K. Wellmar (eds) *Ethics Codes in Medicine* (Ashgate, 1998), pp. 273–83. Abridged.

our human destiny and individuality. It strives to make us believe that, if we succeed in deciphering our genome, we can read our future in it, as in a magic glass.

This mythic approach is a dangerous error. Even when the human genome becomes completely deciphered, human life and health remain not fully reducible to genes. Environmental factors, education, human experiences and habits have a decisive impact on gene expression. In addition, psychological motivations, cultural values and historical background also play a role in human health. Even the Greco-Roman myth of the Parcae left some room for human freedom and personal responsibility.

Public education should demythologize the powers of genetics and establish its real limits in the prediction of future diseases and life. The sometimes unproven link between genetic predisposition and disease should be explained.

Informed consent

In several cases, the prediction of a disease may have deleterious consequences on the tested subject and may conflict with his/her autonomy. Especially in the cases where no prevention or therapy are available, a positive result of a predictive test may cause severe psychological consequences or even suicide, in addition to the possibility of social stigmatization. It is questionable in which cases such predictive tests should be allowed. When allowed, special care should be taken that extensive information is given to the person involved, on the nature, possible results and consequences of the test. Only then can free consent be given. In addition, such a person should be assisted by competent counselling, before, during and after the test. In any case, the wish not to know should be respected.

In the case of children or other persons incompetent to give informed consent, a common practice allowed their parents or guardians to substitute the needed consent. This practice is, however, being questioned and the limits of parental rights are emphasized. Parents are only entitled to take decisions which are expected to be in favour of their children. They are not entitled to order predictive tests just because they wish to know the genetic make-up of their children. Only if the disease may be declared before adulthood or demands early preventive measures are parents allowed to request predictive tests.

Confidentiality in relation to family members

When a positive result of a predictive test is obtained, this information may be important for other members of the family in order for them to undergo similar tests and preventive or therapeutic measures. In these cases, the tested person should be strongly urged to allow the communication of the result to those who clinically need this information. If he/she refuses to do that, the doctor is in a difficult dilemma. The doctor either breaks the right to confidentiality or the principle of beneficence towards people in danger who need his/ her assistance. The classic answer of medical ethics gives the priority to absolute confidentiality. However, this solution may be questioned and the problem deserves urgent discussion in the perspective of new codes for the next century. . . .

Confidentiality in relation to employers

Far more stringent criteria have to be followed when the disclosure of genetic information is intended for non-medical reasons. Such is the case when employers request that information.

The problem of the access of employers to predictive genetic data of their potential or actual employees has to be discussed in relation to the appropriate balance between the rights and interests of the employers, the employees and society.

Employers are certainly interested in genetic data which may ascertain the foreseeable future state of health of the applicants for a job. The reasons for this are several. They are interested in reducing production costs and increasing cost-effectiveness of investments. For this purpose, they have to avoid inefficiency or absenteeism of the worker, loss of training investment by premature incapacitation of the worker and increased payment of health, invalidity or death insurance contributions.

These interests of the employers are legitimate. In the framework of a market economy which accepts the free enterprise system, the employers are entitled to safeguard productivity and to look for the best return on their investments. Nevertheless, these legitimate rights must be weighed against the equally legitimate rights of the employees and of society.

The employees have the right not to know, and to oppose, predictive tests. Even regarding tests already performed, they have the right to privacy and to not being unjustly discriminated against. Most importantly, every individual has the right to work, which is a fundamental element of many modern constitutions and international agreements (de Sola, 1995). Work serves the need for personal fulfilment and integration in society, in addition to being, for the vast majority of the population, the main source of income and sustenance. To deny employment for reasons not of incapacity but of prediction of a future disease or predisposition would represent severe stigmatization. This would be even more unjust than the denial to handicapped persons of special protection for the enjoyment of their right to work, which is prescribed by most laws.

The right to work should not be denied because of the prediction of a disease. Otherwise, a class of persons would be created who, although currently fit for work, were barred from employment. This discrimination is unjust for the individual and burdensome for society. These persons would have to be maintained from public funds and estimations have shown that they would cost more to society than they would to the employer.

For all these reasons, current regulations and doctrine in Europe agree that the rights of the employee, in such cases, should take precedence over the rights of the employer and that the latter is only entitled to enquire about the present, not the future, health of a job applicant. The same position was taken by the draft Bioethics Convention proposed by the Council of Europe, which in its articles 17 and 18 states that predictive tests can be performed and the results communicated only for health purposes.

A special case deals with certain working environments which can cause mutations that cause a genetic disease. This effect can act on all kinds of persons, or be specific to those individuals who have a genetic predisposition.

In the first case, work and safety rules should eliminate or minimize the risks, and genetic monitoring of the workers is advisable to confirm safety at work. In the second case it is important to identify the workers possessing a genetic predisposition, so as to limit their access to posts involving greater risk. This limitation of their right to work is justified by their right to health. But even in such cases, testing should be performed on a voluntary basis, under conditions of fully informed consent. If a worker refuses to undergo the test, his or her contract remains in force.

It is important in the latter cases that the disease is considered as occupational, since in fact its agent is environmental. Genetic monitoring and screening should not be allowed to slip into detection of hereditary diseases in general and lead to discrimination. Even more important is to avoid selection of resistant workers with the purpose of saving the expenses connected with improvement in working conditions. It would be extremely unjust to permit low levels of safety at the expense of the exclusion of a class of the working population.

The rights of society to health should also be considered. There are certain jobs in which the unexpected deterioration of workers' health could affect the safety of the public or of fellow employees. A typical example is that of an airline pilot. In these cases, predictive tests (for instance, detecting a gene predisposing an individual to heart disease) may help to prevent serious accidents and are ethically justified. However, there is the danger of over-generalizing this principle and using these predictive tests with unjustified frequency. For instance, there are no ethical reasons to justify the exclusion of a person with the gene for Huntington's chorea from being a pilot, as long as he or she is healthy (Berg, 1993). In a future code, regulations and provisions should be established to create independent bodies in charge of restricting the requirement of predictive tests for safety reasons and to defend the rights of potential or real employees no less than the right of society to safety. . . .

Confidentiality in relation to insurers

The problem of access to genetic data on the part of insurance companies is no less difficult than that of employers. In the case of life, health or other personal insurance, there is a conflict of interests between the insurer and the applicant. On the one hand, the insurer is interested in getting as much information as possible on the genetic predisposition and predictive diseases of the applicant, in order to estimate the true extent of his contractual liability and to match premiums to the health risks of the applicant. This interest is justified by the principle of free enterprise, which allows the insurer to conduct business as he/she sees fit. On the other hand, the applicant is interested in obtaining insurance without having to know or to reveal too many of his/her most intimate weaknesses. This interest is justified by the principle of privacy and by the rights not to know, of non-disclosure and of non-discrimination.

In favour of the insurer's position of free enterprise are the social interests of the community, as shown by the fact that, if many predictive tests become easily available and are routinely performed, the cost of insurance premiums for individuals showing negative results could become considerably lower and this would increase the public's general access to insurance. Also in favour of the insurer's position is the fact that insurance contracts come under the category of contracts guided by good faith. The applicant should inform the insurer of all circumstances known to him/her which might have a bearing on the assessment of the risk. This is why, in current insurance practice, insurers gather relevant information from applicants through health questionnaires (family history, etc.) and medical examinations, without opposition from most applicants. The question has only become acute with the prospect that the medical examinations will include genetic and predictive tests, which are considered humanity's most intimate bastion.

The reluctance of the applicant to be tested or to reveal information of a genetic nature is justified by the right not to know, by freedom to decide what personal information should be disclosed, to whom and when, and by the right not to be discriminated against.

Respect for the wish not to know, especially in the delicate area of predictive genetics, which has profound psychological-emotional impact on affected persons, is generally accepted and, therefore, the right not to undergo predictive tests should prevail against the interests of the insurer.

In respect of predictive tests already performed on the applicant, it has sometimes been assumed that results of these should necessarily be disclosed to the insurer. This, however, may mean that two persons with the same genetic deficiency are treated differently, just because one underwent a predictive test and the other did not. As a matter of fact, it is known that many people who have wished to undergo a predictive test have not asked for it just to avoid insurance complications.

However, the obligation to disclose the results of previous genetic tests is, in itself, questionable. Such obligation comes from the duty of contract loyalty and the requirements of good faith: both parties in the contract should share the same information. But this obligation may conflict with the individual's self-determination as regards the confidential information he/she chooses to pass on:

> Recent European legal thinking advocates that the way out of this apparently unsolvable problem is to recognize that the interest of the insured should take precedence. . . . The solution advocated by this current of opinion is based on an appeal to certain constitutional values of the social and democratic rule of law, where human dignity and the free development of personality are viewed as being clearly superior to other subordinate legal interests and values. (Yanes, 1995: 166)

The same author proposes that legislation is passed to protect the applicant's right not to disclose genetic information, without having the insurance contract rejected or affected by premium surcharges.

One recent solution adopted in several European countries has been the establishment of a temporary moratorium, during which governments and insurance companies should discuss the future use of genetic information. In the US, several insurance companies recently lost interest in requesting predictive tests, probably because these were not cost-effective. The situation may change with future biotechnological progress so continuing dialogue is necessary.

The individual right to refuse the use of the results of predictive tests for non-medical purposes may come into conflict, in the next century, with the economic mechanisms of our liberal societies. Society will then have to seriously decide on the role of solidarity in its collective organization (Comité Consultatif, 1995). Legislation should not be postponed until predictive testing becomes a widespread practice for insurance. Long before that, the threat that genetic information may be misused should lead to an early declaration on the inadmissibility of any obligation on the part of the insurance applicant to disclose such information.

Privacy and confidentiality rights may be threatened by the overwhelming progress in genetic data informatization. Data Protection

Acts regulate this matter, but their efficacy should be continuously evaluated. People should be informed that they have the right to demand that their blood samples are destroyed immediately after test results are obtained. Otherwise the samples might be used later for different purposes. In view of the fast development of data processing, a new code may be needed for stat protection.

Eugenics

In its new forms, eugenics may also be a danger in predictive medicine, and deserves to be discussed. In terms of the new technologies, eugenics may be redefined as any action which aims at lowering the risk of a genetic disease by reducing the frequency of carriers of the corresponding gene in the population (Papiernik, 1992). In this sense, under eugenic actions would fall the abortion of a heterozygous but healthy foetus able to give rise to a person who, although completely healthy, would be the carrier of a genetic disease. There are, in fact, requests for abortion in such cases of predictive diseases for future generations. It would also be considered close to eugenics to recommend abortion of foetuses affected by genes of late-onset diseases, able to give rise to persons who would live a normal life for 40 or more years. The same can be said about embryos of foetuses carrying genes that predispose or allow susceptibility to the development of certain diseases. In the north of England, selection of *in vitro* embryos has been performed destroying, upon pre-implantation diagnosis, the embryos showing the presence of predisposition genes for a late-onset disease carried by the mother. These are clearly eugenic practices.

These practices are inscribed in a general tendency and pressure towards the utopian right to a completely healthy genome. 'Many women or couples feel that genetic health almost becomes a condition that a child must fulfill' should it not meet the normative expectations of parents and society – norms that no one can rationally justify – it is his or her "bad luck" (Hacker, 1993: 305). This tendency towards the right of a fully healthy genome is scientifically utopian because there is evidence that every human person carries several defective genes in a heterozygotic state (Müller, 1950; Vogel, 1979). In addition, the so-called 'bad' genes confer, in several cases, protection against other diseases. Humanity shows a nice balance between risk factors and protective factors.

The most serious eugenic danger of predictive testing resides in the possibility that it might start being used, in the future, to eliminate healthy embryos or foetuses whose characteristics do not fit the personal wishes of the parents. This would violate fundamental rights, in addition to opposing the biodiversity of our species. This is why the Council of Europe passed a Recommendation in 1990 proposing that prenatal diagnosis and screening are approved only for medical reasons (Council of Europe, 1990).

Towards a new code

Predictive medicine is a relatively new field, especially developed by recent progress in molecular biology and human genetics. Its ethical evaluation has been codified in a variety of norms, some of which are the following: *Report* by the US President's Commission for the Study of Ethical Problems in Medicine and Biomedical and Behavioral Research (1983); *Resolution from the European Parliament A2–327/ 88* on the ethical and legal problems of genetic engineering (1988); *Report on Genetic Screening: Ethical Issues*, Nuffield Council of Bioethics (1993); *Outline of a Declaration on the Human Genome and its Protection in Relation to Human Dignity and Human Rights*, UNESCO International Bioethics Committee, 1995; *Draft European Convention on Bioethics*, Council of Europe, 1995.

All these and other documents are the final result of a great number of reports prepared by specialists, as well as of intensive discussion. Some points of these documents overlap, others are complementary. It would be desirable to boil them down to a limited number of sharp statements, which could constitute a new code of the future.

References

Berg, K. (1993) 'People who are healthy should be treated as healthy persons whatever their future disease risks are', *Revue Internationale de Droit Économique*, 1: 131.

Comité Consultatif National pour les Sciences de la Vie et de la Santé (1995) *Génétique et Médicine de la prédiction à la prévention. Avis. Rapports. (No 46)*, Paris.

Recommendation no R(90) 13, adopted by the Council of Ministers of the Council of Europe on 21 June.

De Sola, C. (1995) 'Privacy and genetic data. Cases of conflict (11)', *Law and the Human Genome Review*, 2: 147–56.

Haker, H. (1993) 'Human genome analysis and eugenics', in *Ethics of Human Genome Analysis: European Perspectives*, ed. Hille Haker, Richard Hearn and Klaus Steigleder, Attempto Verlag: Tübingen.

Müller, H.J. (1950) 'Our load of mutation', *American Journal of Human Genetics*, 2: 111–76.

Papiernik, É. (1992) 'Vers un nouvel eugénisme?' and *Vers un anti-destin?: patrimoine génétique et droits de l'humanité*, sous la direction de François Gros et Gérard Huber, ed. Odile Jacob: Paris.

Voge, F. (1979) 'Our load of mutation: reappraisal of an old problem', *Proceedings of the Royal Society of London*, B 205: 77–90.

Yanes, P. (1995) 'Personal insurance and genetic information', *Law and the Human Genome Review*, 2: 166.

34

C. Davies

Care and the Transformation of Professionalism

The concept of professionalism and its relationship to the paid work of nursing care has interested me throughout my career. Initially, however, the idea of 'care' was far from my agenda. I came to the notion of professions, as many mid-1960s sociology students did, through a study of bureaucracy. Viewed through the lens of bureaucracy, professionals were a problem. They were confident, even arrogant people. They were mainly men. They demanded autonomy on the basis of valued knowledge and expertise. Their demands were often met. All this collided with the imperatively co-ordinated system of authority that was the bureaucratic organization. The neat bureaucratic pyramid, where each office was clearly delineated in relation to others, where a system of pre-specified rules organized their relations one to another, where the work of all was seem as legitimately co-ordinated by reference to these rules, had no place for the autonomous professional. The subject of much of our study at the time was professional/bureaucratic conflict (see e.g. Davies, 1983). Organization charts with diagonal and dotted lines were drawn up proposing means of integrating professionals into bureaucracies.

We did not see at the time that theorizing is always positioned. On the one hand, our thinking about bureaucracy and hence professionalism was mediated by an American eagerness for empiricism and a highly selective and limited reading of Max Weber whose ideal-type bureaucracy provided the starting point for analysis. On the other hand, we were influenced by the management theorists. For this reason the underlying issue was resolutely about control and rarely about identity or social relations. All this of course changed. Scepticism about professions was fuelled by the radical circumstances of the 1960s. Eliot Freidson (1994) has pointed this out in his collection

First published in T. Knijn and S. Sevenhuijsen (eds) *Care, Citizenship and Social Cohesion* (Utrecht, Netherlands School of Social and Economic Policy Research, 1998), pp. 43–53. Abridged.

of essays with the title *Professionalism Reborn*. His original critique of professional dominance in medicine (Freidson, 1970a, 1970b) was an inspiration for many. The work of writers such as Ivan Illich (1975, 1977) reached an even wider audience. In the field of health more perhaps than in other areas, self-help groups, research and campaigning by service users offered an unprecedented challenge to the models of health and illness and the assumptions about care delivery offered by the professionals. Left-leaning sociologists drew satisfaction from the way in which the feminist organizations and other grass-roots activists both called on and contributed to the emerging critique of professions. User 'empowerment' became the most overworked word in the medical sociology lexicon. No small degree of confusion emerged, however, when right-wing governments, notably those of Mrs Thatcher in Britain in the 1980s, adopted the challenge to professions, argued that they had been profligate in resource use and that they needed to be subject to managerial and market discipline.

My main argument here, however, is that notwithstanding all the attacks on the professions, particularly the critique of the biomedical model of health and the calls for greater user participation and power, key elements of an old professional ideal remained intact. Sociologists concentrated on re-specifying what had been taken as attributes of professions as claims, and then on challenging whether the professions lived up to the claims they were making – to knowledge, altruism and so on. We did not enquire more deeply into the provenance of the idea of professionalism itself – what it says about ideal forms of identities and social relations, what underpinned it, and whether the underpinnings might be becoming less secure. Recent writers who have gone along this road include Richard Hugman (1991), whose work on power in the caring professions has not been given the attention it deserves and Margaret Stacey (1992) whose study of the regulatory body in medicine in the UK calls for a new professionalism and accuses doctors of operating according to outdated nineteenth-century ideals.

In this chapter I want to address the provenance of professionalism, to explore that notion of professionalism as a nineteenth-century ideal – an ideal in which gender, but also class and ethnicity are strongly implicated – and present you with some thinking about professionalism and care focusing on the case of nursing. To sketch the argument at the outset:

- Gender is a key to transforming thinking about professions.
- The ways in which we choose to handle gender as an analytic concept are crucial and
- The concept of care is central to this transformation.

Gender, professionalism and nursing care

In this section of the chapter I shall sketch an argument that is set out more fully in my book, *Gender and the Professional Predicament in Nursing* (Davies, 1995b). The background to the book was a long-standing frustration with trying to bring interests in nursing and in the sociology of professions, together. Early on, it seemed the only interpretation on offer was that nursing had 'failed' in its pro-fessionalizing project; later, this field of sociology seemed to ignore nursing, though I was very much aware that nurses were being taught (often using some old, pre-radical material in the sociology of professions) that theirs was a profession and that they should aspire to professionalism in their daily conduct. I had a vague sense, as I made a transition into the field of women's studies in the late 1980s, that gender ought to be the key that would unlock the relation between these phenomena. UK nurses at that time, however, were largely sceptical of anything that smacked of feminism and, as I found, were uneasy that someone they knew as a friend of nursing had moved into this questionable camp. I wanted to try to take the argument forward but to write in a way that nurses as newcomers to feminist debates could understand. I can summarize the route my thinking had taken by the end of the book under four headings:

- gender as an analytical concept;
- gender as embedded in both bureaucracy and profession;
- 'care' as the absent presence;
- contexts as changing.

Gender as an analytical concept

At the time I began to write, it was all too easy to sink into the mire of essentialism. If we were arguing that women had different qualities, what did we do if this did not hold up empirically, which often it did not? If women *did* have different qualities, then what did we do politically? Perhaps the sexual divisions of labour we railed against made sense after all. It seemed contradictory to celebrate womanliness yet critique it too – and so on and so on.

Yet the components of a different approach were in place. Three seemed particularly important. First, there had to be a decisive shift from regarding gender as an attribute of a person to seeing it as a cultural resource – something that could be used at different levels – in the construction of identity, in the shaping of interpersonal relations, in the logic of organizations, in the deep structure of insti-tutions. Ideas about masculinity and femininity were often embedded at many levels, saturating our lives with gender assumptions. Yet embodied women and men could and sometimes did resist, in their

Table 34.1   *Cultural codes of gender*

	Masculine	Feminine
Development of self	Separation	Relation
	Boundedness	Connectedness
	Responsibility	Responsibility to others
	Self-esteem	Selflessness
	Self-love	Self-sacrifice
Cognitive orientation	Abstract, rule-governed thinking	Concrete, contextual thinking
	Mastery/control	Understanding/use
	Emphasis on expertise	Emphasis on experience
	Skills/knowledge as portable acquisitions	Skills/knowledge as confirmed in use
Relational style	Decisive	Reflective
	Interrogative	Accommodative
	Hierarchy-orientated	Group-orientated
	Loyal to superordinates	Loyal to principles
	Agentic/instrumental	Facilitative/expressive

own lives, in their relations with each other and in the organization in which they worked. I see this separation of men and women from masculinity and femininity, together with the multiple layers/levels point, as having enormous potential especially for those who wish to do empirical work. I am still not satisfied, however, that we have got the levels at which gender can be deployed right. Second, we had to resist the equation of gender issues as things to do with women, and see gender always as a relation – and a relation in binary form – a relation that represented women as other, that took the form of A and not-A, rather than A and B. Third, we had to see it not as a noun but as a verb, 'gendering' as an active process, reproduced but sometimes resisted, supported in some contexts, challenged in others. We can perhaps sum all this up: gender is a resource, gender is a relation, gender is a verb.

But also we have to give it content. My solution was to speak of cultural codes of gender, a shared and recognizable resource drawn on often unwittingly to construct daily life and structure relations at all levels. Drawing on a wide range of feminist theorists, I drew up what appears here as Table 34.1. I referred to the cultural concepts of masculinity and femininity as offering coherent answers to the question of how to be and how to act in the world – answers that flowed from a starting point that regarded the world as populated by bounded individuals in competition with each other, and as full of people in or potentially in some connection with others (and positively welcoming and not fearing and rejecting that connection). The popular, controversial yet inspiring work that has been done celebrating what were proposed as women's ways of thinking, women's speech, women's styles of leadership and so on, was of help to me here as I struggled to try to give content to the second column, to ensure that what I was producing had the logical structure of A and B, not A and not-A.

Gender as embedded in both bureaucracy and profession

The breakthrough in seeing how this analysis could apply at the level of organizational design came when I read Roslyn Bologh's biography of Weber (Bologh, 1990). She emphasized how Weber's vision of rational-legal authority, followed through in the creation of the bureaucratic machine, was a reaction against a social order that involved the arbitrary action of a traditional ruler, intruding on the lives of subjects. This vision made a strong separation between the public sphere and the private sphere. It rendered the relations between competing individuals in the public sphere predictable, removing decisions based on the whim and mood of those in power. By creating an orderly system of positions and setting rules about their relations each to the other, by resolving conflict by resort to someone in a position further up the hierarchy, a world of what she referred to as 'hostile strangers' became bearable. Bureaucracy was a solution to the problem of masculinity – it addressed the problem of A – the problem of the bounded individual, the lone hero striving to achieve through his own skills and experience. At the top of the bureaucratic hierarchy was the distant cool articulate man, with a firm idea of the ultimate goal, keeping his own counsel, winning arguments by force of logic. Below him (since not all could be heroes) were the loyal subordinates, not necessarily strongly personally committed, but playing by the rules, expressing deference to superiors, keeping their noses clean and looking for promotion. There could be soullessness, impersonality and inflexibility, yet there was integrity and a morality in this kind of disciplined order.

It was only a short step from here – though a hard one for someone schooled in the idea that bureaucracy and professionalism are antithetical – to extend the notion of gendering as underlying bureaucracy to regard it as underlying profession. Bureaucracy and professionalism were forged in the same historical era. Professionalism if anything can be seen as a stronger celebration of a lone hero model of masculinity – and it allows more to be lone heroes. The professional (and I think here especially of the classic model of the hospital consultant) engages in a long struggle to reach the top and once there is one among equals. No doctor readily criticizes another; there is a careful protocol where referral of work across specialities is needed or a second opinion is required. Those below the classic professional, the hospital consultant, are all in training grades, on temporary contracts, moving between posts, dependent on their

seniors for making experience available and for a good reference.
Until the last decade or so, others too could be relied on to offer
deference and support – the nurses, those legislatively designated
'professions supplementary to medicine' and the administrators,
described not as managers but as 'diplomats' (Harrison, 1988) – in
their desire to provide the resources the doctors said they needed.

Drawing from the notion of a masculine gender code, I have proposed six characteristics of the gendered professional ideal:

- mastery of knowledge;
- unilateral decision process (patient as dependent/colleagues as
  deferential);
- autonomy and self-management;
- individual accountability;
- detachment;
- interchangeability of practitioners.

Where do nurses fit in relation to this? I suggest that they are
adjuncts to professions. They are the unacknowledged co-ordinators,
the supporters, the moppers up of tears and fears (including those of
the hero professional). My mistake had been to regard nurses as
engaging in separate striving against resistance about encroachment.
There is some truth in that but they also help produce the traditional
professional identity that can only be sustained by the work that they
do. As Carole Pateman (1988) had observed as she reanalysed the
social contract theorizing in political sciences, it was not just that
women were excluded from areas which men kept to themselves
(which of course they have been) – it was that they were included –
their contributions were needed to make possible the concepts of
the public world and of self and identity which underpinned and
expressed them.

Care as the absent presence

It is now possible to bring caring into the picture. Caring is firmly
expunged from the masculine gendered ideals of bureaucracy and
profession. The ideal professional is not 'uncaring', but is detached,
treating each patient or client with a correct professional concern, but
not being visibly moved, not getting bound up in their crises or their
pain. There is a parallel here with the impersonality of the bureaucrat. The bureaucrat always adheres to the rules of the organization,
processes the work in a calm and distant manner, is entirely reliable,
shows no favouritism, is interchangeable with any other in the role. I
do not think we have grasped fully the basis of these two identities

in a masculinist split between an orderly public world devoid of emotional content and a separate private world where emotions and enthusiasms, spontaneity, doubts and vulnerabilities, can be safely expressed. I do not think we have taken full cognizance of the immense distance this sets up between the identity of the distant and controlled and all-knowing and mysterious professional, the often agitated person he or she 'serves', and the others in contact with the patient or client. I am not sure we have addressed the seductiveness of the old professional ideal to all these people.

When, for example, nurses have searched for frameworks to express the different kind of care they offer, they struggle with concepts of intimacy, love and the equation of nursing with womanliness. It may be that the way the concept of emotional labour has been developed from its origins in the world of commerce (Hochschild, 1983) is not the best route for this. We need to focus more on the public/private split as creating this unnameable anxiety about the work that nurses do alongside the paragon of detachedness and decisiveness which we have all been taught to aspire to in the world in public.

A key part of my argument, as already noted, has been to point out that this old professional ideal, with its vision of an orderly, rational world in public, is a fiction. Rosemary Pringle (1989) carried out the pioneering work here in her analysis of the necessary position of secretaries in bureaucracies. Far from being a relic of some other organizational form, in providing emotional support and forms of co-ordination that are never fully conceptualized, it is secretaries who make the impossible, inhuman ideal of rational bureaucratic organization work. Nurses, I argue, are in a structurally similar place (Davies, 1995b). They function as adjuncts to the medical profession in its operation of the gendered professional ideal. In an overall process of healing, they integrate caring with curing. In doing so, they help to reproduce the traditional professional identity for the doctor because that identity can be sustained only if his or her encounter with the patient is a fleeting encounter. When we are talking about professional care (and I see this as distinct from care-work and from caregiving: Davies, 1995a), there is a division of labour in health work that calls centrally on gender to create the profession of medicine through the inclusion of nursing work as a necessary adjunct.

Could one envisage anything different? I have suggested that the old, gendered ideal could be countered point by point, thinking about a way of being that was not masculine gendered. The trick has to be transcendence – understand the link of the professional ideal with masculinity, resist the binary form of A and not-A, find a set of terms that are degendering, that will valorize the not-A and turn it into B. What this might mean is indicated in the following list. Much

remains to be done to tease out these ideas further, to work with
ideas of old and new professionalism as shaped by gender in the ways
I have suggested.

- reflectively using expertise and experience;
- creating an active community in which a solution can be negotiated;
- recognizing interdependence with others;
- collectively accountable for practice;
- engaged and committed stance towards client;
- accepts use of self as part of the therapeutic encounter.

Contexts as changing

What are the prospects for change in the direction of new professionalism? At the end of my book I analysed the context of Britain's
NHS as it was in operation in the mid-1990s. I argued that the 1980s
emphasis on managerialism and the introduction of market competition had strong continuities with the bureaucracy and professionalism that on the surface it sought to challenge. I maintained
that what we were seeing was a clash of masculinities, with new
managerialism bringing what in some ways was a more overt, brash,
aggressive and confrontational style. The new manager, I suggested,
'turns out to have many of the same characteristics as the old'.

> Like the other two, he remains distant and controlled. He take a critical
> stance towards the arguments and established practices of others, asking
> constantly for outcome data, cost information and performance measures.
> He follows his own conviction, is tough-minded in that he must take hard
> decisions about 'what market to be in', without being swayed by appeals to
> sympathy or particular cases. Above all, he is a strong and active decision-
> maker so will not dodge controversy and confrontation, be it with staff or
> the public. At his fingertips he has not the rulebook of the bureaucrat or
> the expert clinical knowledge of the doctor, but the performance infor-
> mation about the cost of the overall service, and about the performance of
> competitors. (Davies, 1995b: 168–9)

I suggested that the very overtness of this celebration of masculinity
might provide the conditions for a backlash, that already there was a
new 'gender talk' critical of the 'men in suits' and the cash register
mentality, that there was potential for alliances against it from old-
style administrators, some trade unionists and perhaps clinicians
whose ideals of public service were being challenged. I pointed to the
growing numbers of women in middle management positions uneasy
about what they could see clearly as a macho management style –
feeling strong enough to start to question a culture that boasted
about long hours of work and ask if there was not another way. I

pointed also to academic analysis raising questions about core values and concerns, doubting that a model of the consumer was right for the health field – edging very tentatively towards some reference to the need for care.

Further steps?

Since this time, I have moved in two directions. The first is to begin to think more systematically about levers for change (Davies, 1996). We can perhaps think of these at two levels. The first set are context specific. Attention here must lie with policy developments and forms of government action in particular national settings. There are moves in the UK for example, to alter the regulatory framework in which professions operate, to make changes in the organization of work and work practices within and between professional groups and to alter the educational experience that professionals receive. The second set of changes likely to dislodge old professionalism operate at a deeper level of social structure. Not only gender but class, age and ethnicity are in the process of change. Doctors are no longer drawn from so narrow a social class band; the profession has been significantly feminized at the junior levels, and doctors from ethnic minorities are finding a place in medicine in larger numbers and proportions than hitherto. Alongside all this, in Britain at any rate, reforms in medical education will mean doctors qualifying at younger ages. This means that medicine can no longer carry its gendered cultural baggage in so unthinking a way. With greater social diversity it will not be possible in future to depict medicine with a white face, a bewhiskered jaw and greying temples, eyes peering down at you over half-glasses (Davies, 1996). The structured supports which helped reinforce old professionalism by mapping it on to gender, and class and age and ethnicity are breaking down. Rosemary Pringle has given some demonstration of this in an empirical study of relations between women doctors and nurses (Pringle, 1996).

These themes are ones that I hope you will find ways of pursuing in your care project. It will be, I would predict, the younger doctors, the male nurses, those from ethnic minority backgrounds who will be the ones who can articulate unease with the old model and express hopes for a different way of being in the care professions.

My second emerging theme springs from a conviction that there is more to be done with these concepts of masculinity and femininity and with conceptualizing ways of being and forms of relationships that resist the dichotomized alternatives they represent. Ruth Purtilo's notion of a meaningful distance in a healing relationship is perhaps an example of both/and rather than either/or approach that gendered thinking offers (Purtilo, 1993). So too, perhaps is Kathleen Jones's concept of compassionate authority (Jones, 1993). I would like to draw attention to another strand of work that seems to have a potential impact on rethinking ideas of social cohesion and care from a degendered point of view.

Jodi Dean is an American political science professor who writes about changes in the feminist movement and the divisions between feminists. In this arena, she is struggling towards a concept of solidarity that can accommodate difference (Dean, 1995, 1996, 1997). Her notion of solidarity, therefore, is not the solidarity of the sisters of early second wave feminism, nor is it the traditional working-class solidarity of the brothers in the trade union. It is a concept that deliberately avoids the celebration of sameness and any knee-jerk opposition to an enemy and is based on difference. It recognizes differentiation and affirms dependency on others for recognition and connection which, she argues, brings the possibility of working together. It is true that a group will have a common purpose, a sense of 'we'ness. but to act in solidarity involves remaining open to what one can take as common beliefs and expectations. She insists that it is not the nods of affirmation and agreement that help the group to develop but the queries that allow understanding to evolve. If you prefer her language, 'we' is performatively constituted through the communicative efforts of different 'I's' (1997: 251). The solidarity that is created is a reflective solidarity; the outcome is a new outcome.

Dean pursues her argument by detailed reference to the work of Mead and of Habermas, which I will not examine here. She notes, however, that in reflective solidarity the key thing is that the relationship is valued by those in the group. Positions are recognized as unique and nuanced. They are not guessed at and discounted before they are articulated. And because agreement is created through communication, it is never fixed. In the relationship that is reflective solidarity, each of us may arrive at a position we were not previously in − a position we could not have reached by dint of struggle on our own, or by dint of seeking support from those whose histories and perspectives are similar. In Dean's terms, there is a recognition of the *fallibility of discourse*. Jodi Dean points out that our capacity for reflexivity and for expanding our concepts of ourselves is thus enhanced by movement within and between groups that work in a solidary way.

There is an important element of degendering in this concept. First, the idea of reflective solidarity *affirms the value of the other*. It bypasses binary othering. The other is not not-A but B, whose perspective it is worth struggling to understand and accommodates different, interesting, potential world-view-changing possibilities for A. There is something in it for us to accord trust and respect to the other. Secondly, and relatedly, it *challenges the bounded individual* who by dint of mastery of knowledge and logic of thought can produce the clinching argument or the perfect strategy where the role of the

Table 34.2 Two models of collaboration

Concept of the individual	bounded (A/A, A/not-A)	connected (A/B)
Group process/style	formal adversarial 'explaining'	relaxed co-operative 'exploring'
Outcomes	resolution is imposed assumption of finality	agreement is tried expectation of change
	vindication and elation or defeat and despair	enhanced commitment stronger bonds personal renewal

group is to admire and accept. Because it acknowledges interdependence it *values the relationship beyond the business of whether at some particular point we agree or not*. Finally and since it is based on the notion that there is no overarching privileged knowledge, it regards all knowledge as *situated knowledge* (to use Donna Haraway's (1988) important concept). Bringing situated knowledges into relation with each other can widen the perception of the issue and lead to the enhancement of each.

Reflective solidarity cannot come from a view of the world as composed of hostile strangers, or a notion of the knowledge project as mastery and possession. For me this concept of reflective solidarity is important in that it gives expression to some of the most powerful and energizing moments in social life. For another purpose recently (Davies, 1998), I have tried to summarize and perhaps formalize Dean's ideas, contrasting A and B once again and focusing on a model of strong collaboration (Table 34.2).

Preparing this chapter has pushed me towards seeing reflective solidarity as perhaps relevant also to the relationships of care and to the new professionalism theme I expressed earlier as creating 'an active community in which a solution can be negotiated' (Davies, 1995b: 150). I am not sure there is a lot written about the sustained professional encounter as a situation of reflective solidarity in this way – one in which all present, including the professionals, shift their positions, enlarge their perspectives, value the insights of the other and come to see the world in a slightly different way.

Reflective solidarity, then, may be an important key for developing what Kari Waerness in her classic paper as long ago as 1984 called 'the rationality of caring' (Waerness, 1984) and for nurturing the kind of caring encounters that are so difficult when we live with and work within the gendered institutional logics of bureaucracy and professionalism. Solidarity, at first sight a long way from care, ultimately may be part of the conceptual glue that brings care and organization together.

References

Bologh, R.W. (1990) *Love or Greatness: Max Weber and Masculine Thinking – a Feminist Inquiry*, London: Unwin Hyman.

Davies, C. (1983) 'Professions and bureaucracy', in R. Dingwall and P. Lewis (eds) *The Sociology of Professions: Lawyers, Doctors and Others*, London: Macmillan.

Davies, C. (1995a) 'Competence versus care? Gender and caring work revisited', *Acta Sociologica*, 38: 17–31.

Davies, C. (1995b) *Gender and the Professional Predicament in Nursing*, Buckingham: Open University Press.

Davies, C. (1996) 'New woman, new nurse, new NHS – the changing fact of health care professionalism in Britain', plenary address at the Second Nursing History and the Politics of Welfare Conference, University of Nottingham, September (unpublished).

Davies, C. (1998) 'Reinventing ourselves: the universities, the state and the health care professions', inaugual lecture, Milton Keynes, Open University, 4 February.

Dean, J. (1995) 'Reflective solidarity', *Constellations*, 2 (1): 114–40.

Dean, J. (1996) *Solidarity of Strangers: Feminism after Identity Politics*, Berkeley, CA: University of California Press.

Dean, J. (1997) 'The reflective solidarity of democratic feminism', in J. Dean (ed.) *Feminism and the New Democracy: Resiting the Political*, London: Sage.

Freidson, E. (1970a) *Professional Dominance*, New York: Atherton.

Freidson, E. (1970b) *Profession of Medicine*, New York: Dodd, Mead.

Freidson, E. (1994) *Professionalism Reborn*, Cambridge/Oxford: Polity Press/Blackwell.

Haraway, D. (1988) 'Situated knowledges: the science question in feminism and the privilege of partial perspective', *Feminist Studies*, 14 (3): 575–99.

Harrison, S. (1988) *Managing the NHS, Shifting the Frontier*? London: Chapman and Hall.

Hochschild, A. Russell (1983) *The Managed Heart: Commercialization of Human Feeling*, Los Angeles: University of California Press.

Hugman, R. (1991) *Power in the Caring Professions*, London: Macmillan.

Illich, I. (1975) *Medical Nemesis*, London: Calder and Boyars.

Illich, I. et al. (1977) *Disabling Professions*, London: Marion Boyars.

Jones, K. (1993) *Compassionate Authority: Democracy and the Representation of Women*, London: Routledge.

Pateman, C. (1988) *The Disorder of Women*, Stanford, CA: Stanford University Press.

Pringle, R. (1989) *Secretaries Talk: Sexuality, Power and Work*, London: Verso (first published 1988, Sydney, Allen and Unwin).

Pringle, R. (1996) 'Nursing a grievance: women doctors and nurses', *Journal of Gender Studies*, 5 (2): 157–68.

Purtilo, R. (1993) 'Meaningful distances', in J. Walmsley, J. Reynolds, P. Shakespeare and R. Wolfe (eds) *Health, Welfare and Practice*, London: Sage.

Stacey, M. (1992) *Regulating British Medicine: The General Medical Council*, Chichester: Wiley.

Waerness, K. (1984) 'Caring as women's work in the welfare state', in H. Holter (ed.) *Patriarchy in a Welfare State*, Oslo: Universitetsforlaget.

PART VI

CREATING: A BETTER FUTURE?

If users are empowered and practitioners are reflective, if collaboration between co-workers is fully established, and all are able to cope with challenges from a diversity of others, if the opportunities and constraints of contexts are understood – what will the new relationships of care look like? Can we set out the direction of travel – or at least glimpse a new destination for the future?

There are three chapters in this final part. Marion Barnes and David Prior, writing before the Labour government came to power and began to talk in earnest about the 'Third Way', not only prefigure contemporary arguments but also link together many of the themes of this book by putting into words the need for a new social basis for welfare – a new kind of 'public trust'. They identify six elements of trust in interpersonal relations and six components of a framework for embedding and institutionalising these. They build their new vision out of a profound dissatisfaction with the market relationships that were a feature of the Thatcher era and out of a commitment to prioritize the user. Barnes and Prior's message is an inspiring one that echoes much of what has gone before in this book. It affirms the importance of creating conditions for collaboration, as discussed in Part III. It has a strong yet practical commitment to inclusiveness – the need that they identify for what we might call a 'presumption of competence' in interpersonal relations, is particularly striking. At the end of the chapter, Barnes and Prior warn that bringing about this new vision will be difficult and not cost free, but they are convinced that theirs is the direction in which to travel.

Simon Biggs is not so sure. Much of what he writes, with its focus on new professional identities, can be seen as a reprise of Part V. But he is also keen to paint overall themes of change on a broader canvas of modernity and postmodernity and to grapple with what he is all too aware is an off-putting 'intellectual sophistry' that the latter concept brings. He sees cause for immense optimism insofar as there are chances for interprofessionalism and user involvement to flourish in a world where old certainties have been undermined. (In this context, he might question our organizing concepts, especially 'constructing' and 'creating' as relics of the modern in a postmodern age.) Yet he also paints a bleaker picture – of a fluid and shifting world which offers us no footholds, one in which withdrawal, rigidity and 'sequestration' may result. Simon Biggs has thus added an important further layer of complexity. In the end, however, he is dissatisfied with his own analysis – wanting to offer something pragmatic and practical, yet seeing the bonuses of fluidity and wondering what can be done once we have accepted that the world is forever uncertain and that ways forward are always provisional.

We have given the last word to Michael Clarke and John Stewart. They remind us that it is not always possible or desirable to seek to arrive at a final resolution of policy dilemmas. Some issues are 'wicked issues' – thoroughly intractable, repeatedly revisited, never fully resolved. And we should expect that this will be so. We should acknowledge that our understanding is partial, deliberately draw others in and welcome the reframing of issues that will result from a more inclusive process. We should expect indeed that tomorrow's way of looking at things will be different as new groups and interests form and find expression. There are parallels between 'holding' issues in the way these authors propose and creating structures which are 'robust' in the assumptions they make about the motivation of others, as Le Grand suggested in Chapter 4. In the end, perhaps we need both the visions and the humility to recognize that even visions are partial and will change. 'If we could get the hang of it entirely,' said poet Louis McNeice, 'it would take too long.'

35

M. Barnes and D. Prior

From Private Choice to Public Trust: A New Social Basis for Welfare

. . . How do relationships of trust function within British welfare services? Consideration of the principal services that comprise the welfare state indicates a very substantial ambivalence about the extent to which users are trusted as active participants in the service relationship (see Table 35.1).

Across the range of market-oriented public welfare services, trust relationships between consumers and providers are highly ambiguous. Seen from the perspective of 'trust', there is a considerable variation between different services in the nature of the welfare consumer's identity. It seems clear that, despite the assumptions underpinning the Citizen's Charter strategy for service reform, the public service user is not an undifferentiated 'customer' who approaches each service in the same way and is treated by each service in the same way. Rather, the user appears at different points along a dimension of trust and distrust depending on the service in question, and therefore experiences quite different degrees of involvement with, and responsibility for, the way services are delivered.

One significant effect of this ambiguity is the generation of confusion, lack of confidence and cynicism among users – especially among those who are ill-equipped to compete with other consumers for scarce resources, but evident also among more middle-class consumers as their expectations are not met. The result is a vicious spiral, as people's willingness to put *their* trust in public services is further eroded, and services are forced further into crisis. A clear example is provided by parents choosing to send their children to schools outside the areas in which they live because they do not trust the local comprehensive to provide an adequate education. One result is a concentration within inner-city schools of children from poorer families with fewer resources to support their children's education,

First published in *Public Money & Management*, October–December: 51–7 (Blackwell, 1996). Abridged.

Table 35.1 *Trust relationships in British welfare services*

	Use of service		Management of service	
	Indicators of trust	Indicators of distrust	Indicators of trust	Indicators of distrust
Education	Parental choice of school	Education compulsory; core curriculum prescribed	Parents as governors	State control of resources
Health	Patient decides whether to accept prescribed treatment	Diagnosis and treatment determined by professionals	Patients' councils, but very limited influence	Managed by professionals and appointed boards
Community care	Family carers relied on for main resource	Need for service decided by professionals	Degree of partnership with users	Little user participation in resource management
Housing	People encouraged to make their own provision		Public sector tenants given self-management responsibilities	
Social security		Needs criteria defined and tested by officials; high presumption of fraud		No user participation in management

and less influence to secure appropriate state resourcing of such
schools.

A resolution of this dilemma for policy can be found in the recognition that public service users themselves have a dual identity, they are simultaneously:

- *consumers* of particular services;
- *citizens* with a general interest in public service provision.

As citizens, users have a voice in decision-making about the production of public services as well as their consumption. This focuses attention on the nature of the trust that is invested in citizens.

Citizenship is itself a highly contested concept. One approach, associated with the political drive to marketize public services, tends to collapse citizenship into consumerism: this approach is part of the contradiction that we are trying to resolve and thus offers no way forward. An alternative conception views the citizen as a participant in a political process and as an active contributor to the determination of public interests and outcomes (Prior et al., 1995). Crucially, in this approach, the citizen is trusted to look beyond individual self-interest to the interests of the policy as a whole.

We wish to argue for the rebuilding of public service management and provision around the assumption that people must be trusted as citizens to participate in the determination of public ends and in the allocation and management of public resources to meet those ends. Trust should become an explicit feature of the relationship between providers and users of services; but to enable this to happen – for users to be able to act as citizens and for providers to be able to engage with users as citizens – a new institutional framework which supports public trust between the citizen and the state is required. Such a framework needs to exist at a local level, where users come into direct contact with public services, and at the level of national policy-making. For example older people who fear that the state has broken its promise of a cradle to grave health service by drawing back from the provision of long-term care funded from the public purse will find it difficult to have confidence in the decisions made by local health care providers.

Characteristics of public trust

A key part of our argument is that public welfare services function both at an *individual* level (in the face-to-face transactions between providers and users through which services are produced and consumed) and at a *collective* level (in the aggregate social outcomes that are the consequence of public services and in which people have an interest as citizens). Institutions should be generating trust at both levels. In attempting to define such institutions, it is helpful to consider what is required for trust to exist between individuals, since it is in the context of interpersonal relationships that the concept of trust is most familiar.

Six distinct elements are required for personal trust to function between individuals (Jordan, 1987: 19–30; and Giddens, 1991: 36–42 are helpful sources for this analysis):

- *acceptance* of the validity of the other's experiences, knowledge and interpretations (but note that acceptance does not automatically entail belief in the other's viewpoint);
- *confidence* that the other has the capacity to make appropriate judgements about how to act in varying circumstances;
- *respect* for the role of the other as an active contributor to the relationship;
- *honesty* towards the other in a willingness to share all relevant information about the relationship;
- *reciprocity of duty*, recognizing that each partner in the relationship has responsibilities toward the other;

- *reciprocity of interest*, recognizing that each partner has their own goals which they will want to pursue through the relationship.

The requirement for these elements to be present in relationships of trust between individuals has specific implications when applied to the relationship between individual providers and users of public services. Their existence is likely to be contingent on a number of factors affecting both those using and those providing the service. For the user, willingness and capacity to trust officials will be mediated by factors such as:

- previous experience of that particular service, or public services in general;
- the experience of exclusion or oppression resulting from poverty, disability or discrimination;
- the impact of experiences such as abuse which can impair the basic capacity to trust.

The ability of individual providers to adopt the open approach necessary to the establishment of trust between themselves and service users may be affected by their sense of security of employment, their ability to control or influence the way in which they work, and the extent to which their skills and knowledge are valued within and beyond the organization. From both perspectives it is apparent that structural factors create macro conditions within which relationships of trust between consumers and providers, citizens and state, can generate or inhibit a more co-operative approach to public service.

With this assessment of the conditions for personal trust in mind, we can now sketch the core components of an institutional framework for public trust: dialogue, competence, participation, openness, accountability and negotiation.

Dialogue

Acceptance of the validity of the experiences, understandings and knowledges of others is achievable where the possibility of dialogue and deliberation exists. Establishment of means of dialogue is a prerequisite for mutual understanding and learning. Such means must provide opportunities for speaking ('voice') and a guarantee of being listened to. Both speaking to assist deliberation and listening are skilled activities, and there is thus an underlying requirement for people to be supported in developing such skills. However, one of the benefits of relationships based in mutual trust is that they provide a supportive environment in which to develop communication skills.

Competence

Confidence in others as partners in relationships of trust requires that all partners have the opportunity to develop competence in making judgements for themselves. These judgements concern both the needs and interests of the individual and the needs and interests of the collective. Competence in judging us in part formed through experience of other institutional elements of public trust, especially dialogue and participation; but for trust to be present at the outset requires an assumption of competence on the part of all those involved, even if this competence is relatively underdeveloped. The assumption of mutual competence helps counter assumptions of the automatic authority of certain kinds of knowledge or experience over others.

Participation

Respect for the roles of others as contributors to the relationship requires that all partners have the opportunity to participate actively and equally in decision-making. This is not a requirement that all *must* participate, rather it is a requirement that the opportunity be genuinely and clearly present and that it is possible for anyone, through participation, to influence the outcome of decisions. Equality of opportunity to participate is therefore important, and (along with a number of the other elements of the institutional framework) is a provision against domination by particular individuals or groups with privileged access to power or resources.

Openness

The principle of honesty requires the establishment of procedures to ensure that openness exists in the relationship and that full information is mutually available. Information, in this context, covers both information about the issues under consideration and information about the management of the relationship itself; thus it includes access of all partners to full information about the rules and procedures which govern the relationship. This is, in effect, a means of overcoming inclinations towards secrecy. Moreover, the principle requires that information be provided in a form which is comprehensible to all, thereby guarding against the possibility of deception.

Accountability

The existence of mutual responsibilities requires arrangements for ensuring the accountability of partners to each other. Each must be prepared to give an account of their actions and intentions to other partners, and processes are required that enable partners to hold

Conditions of public service use	MET BY	Elements of public trust
Inadequate information for decision-making		Openness Accountability
No influence over options available and restricted range of options		Participation Negotiation
No grounds for confidence that needs will be met		Accountability Participation
Lack of experience/skill in making choices		Dialogue Competence
Crisis situations		Accountability Competence
Dilemmas of risk		Openness Dialogue
Duress or coercion		Dialogue Accountability

Figure 35.1 *Elements of public trust which would resolve the difficulties encountered by the users of welfare services*

others to account. This is both a further safeguard against deception and an incentive to act in ways that secure trust. In addition, it helps ensure full understanding of the reasons why particular actions are taken and, therefore, enables the validity and appropriateness of those reasons to be debated and considered by those who are affected by them.

Negotiation

Recognition that partners will have their own interests and purposes requires that procedures and conditions for negotiation of mutually acceptable outcomes are in place. It is in this context that choice becomes a useful concept. Each partner should have the opportunity to exercise choices, but they are choices that are shaped and modified in the process of debate and negotiation over possible options.

The starting point for our analysis of the potential of an institutional framework of public trust as a more effective approach to the management of welfare services was the identification of a number of circumstances in which services are actually used, and which reveal the consumerist policy emphasis on private choices to be unhelpful or even damaging to users. Having outlined the elements of public trust, it is important to check whether such an approach does hold the promise of a more relevant response to the conditions of public service use in which users may be disadvantaged. We believe that it does, and in Figure 35.1 we show which elements of public trust provide the principal means of resolving the various difficulties encountered by users of public welfare services.

Building public trust

Our description of elements of a model of public trust clearly represents an ideal view: it provides a model to be aspired to in the design of new public service institutions, rather than a set of conditions which have to be attained. It is also clear that the model of public trust we propose has much in common with models of participative democracy, and we have borrowed explicitly from a number of proponents of such models (Dryzek, 1990; Fishkin, 1991; Gastil, 1993). Indeed, we would suggest that the attempt to develop public service institutions based on reciprocal relations of public trust will not be fully successful unless they are located within a broader project of *improving the quality of democracy* in the polity. (Such a project must be accompanied by a systematic approach to *reducing structural inequalities which exclude groups from participation* within the polity, although we cannot address this second requirement here.)

This project in turn rests on the promotion of four distinct processes of change within public services:

1 *Democratization* – creating opportunities for greater citizen involvement in decisions on the design and delivery of public services through a broader range of mechanisms for public consultation and involvement. This implies both better access to information to enable citizens to engage meaningfully in decision-making, and a reinvigoration of the representative system of political control so that elected representatives are more adequately informed by the views of the citizens they represent. A range of innovatory practices which contribute to greater democracy within public services have been developed, in this country but more so in others, and the need now is for these to be more widely applied and tested (Stewart, 1996).
2. *Decentralization* – moving the processes of decision-making and service delivery closer to the people affected by them. This requires the maximum devolution of political and managerial responsibility for services, so that people know where and by whom decisions are being taken. It is about improving the visibility and accessibility of those who are publicly accountable for services, and at the same time increasing the likelihood of decisions being made which are responsive to actual local needs. However, decentralization should not be concerned just with geographical proximity, it must also aim for a closer relationship

with citizens and service users who have needs arising from common interests or identities, for example ethnic groups or disabled people.

3. *Learning from user groups* – encouraging formal service organizations to learn from the experience of user groups in developing their own understandings of their needs and circumstances. One of the characteristics of 'social movements', of which service user groups are an example, is the development of forms of knowledge and skill which challenge the professional or official knowledge of formal organizations (Barnes and Prior, 1996). The dominance of formal or 'expert' knowledge, and the assumption of its superiority, is one of the factors excluding lay people from exercising an effective voice in their relationships with service providers. A key component of public trust must be the willingness of providers to accept the collective understanding and knowledge generated by user groups as a legitimate basis for dialogue and negotiation.

4. *Creating social capital* – recognizing as a specific objective of public policy the encouragement of groups, networks and organizations among citizens and users which seek to build trust and mutual confidence. A range of very different types of organization have been formed by service users around activities of self-help, consciousness raising and campaigning. Such activities demonstrate awareness of the value of trust between members and provide an important experience of inclusion and participation for many who have frequently been excluded from processes which affect them (Wann, 1995). By strengthening collective confidence and competence, these activities contribute to the creation of a resource of social responsibility and capacity with which service providers (and state organizations generally) can engage as trusted partners.

Conclusion

One way of summarizing the shift that we advocate from a welfare system built on the principle of private choice to one that is based on public trust is to describe it as a process of replacing market mechanisms of decision-making – which are necessarily *exclusive* of certain groups of 'consumers' – with democratic mechanisms of decision-making which aim for *inclusion* of all citizens. Such a shift cannot be cost-free: the price includes the transformation of the attitudes and practices of many officials and professionals, the learning of new skills and the development of new and difficult processes. We believe, however, that the long-term benefits to be gained are substantial: for service users in terms of better services and real empowerment; for service providers through a more effective deployment of resources; and for society generally through the generation of greater social cohesion and solidarity.

References

Barnes, M. and Prior, D. (1996) 'Trust and the competence of the welfare consumer', unpublished paper, School of Public Policy, University of Birmingham.

Dryzek, J. (1990) *Discursive Democracy*, Cambridge University Press: Cambridge.

Fishkin, J. (1991) *Democracy and Deliberation*, Yale University Press: New Haven.

Gastil, J. (1993) *Democracy in Small Groups*, New Society Publishers: Philadelphia.

Giddens, A. (1991) *Modernity and Self-Identity*, Polity Press: Cambridge.

Jordan, B. (1987) *Rethinking Welfare*, Basil Blackwell: Oxford.

Prior, D., Stewart, J. and Walsh, K. (1995) *Citizenship: Rights, Community and Participation*, Pitman: London.

Stewart, J. (1996) 'Innovation in democratic practice in local government, *Policy and Politics*, 24 (1): 29–41.

Wann, M. (1995) *Building Social Capital: Self-Help in a Twenty-First Century Welfare State*, IPPR: London.

36

S. Biggs

User Voice, Interprofessionalism and Postmodernity

. . . There is a growing acknowledgement within the social sciences that the context in which attempts at identity management are played out may be dramatically changing. This change may not simply be one of policy or ideology, but a more profound shift in social relations which it may be worth taking some space to explain. These changes have been characterized as a movement away from conditions of modernity to something else, which has been called variously: late capitalism (Jameson, 1984), high modernity (Giddens, 1993) or post-modernity (Featherstone, 1991; Smart, 1993).

Whereas the guiding principles of modernity can be thought of as a belief in progress, technical expertise, order and values that are universal, postmodernity is marked by a suspicion of big science, that progress from one perspective may mean calamity from another, an awareness of diversity that sometimes verges on fragmentation and a sense of riskiness and uncertainty pervading social life. In other words, modernity refers to the idea of 'mass' society in which boundaries are relatively impermeable and identities are more or less fixed by the larger social groups that one belongs to (such as race, gender and class), each of which confers certain expectations on the conduct of relationships between groups and individuals. An example from health services would be a rigid distinction between active healers and passive patients. Postmodernity, on the other hand, marks a shift towards a much more fluid state of affairs in which certain identities might be chosen in order to enter certain forms of relationship with others, but then discarded as other situations and opportunities make themselves available. Similarly, boundaries between groups become more permeable, allowing greater awareness of interconnectedness and movement between institutional systems (a greater awareness, for example, that chief executives can also be

First published in the *Journal of Interprofessional Care*, 11(2): 195–203 (Carfax Publishing, 1997). Abridged.

patients and that service users with disabilities have active lives and identities independent of medical conditions).

Moves toward user participation and interprofessionalism might both reflect and contribute to this momentum, away from old certainties and toward a situation that is more ambiguous and in many cases more ambivalent as well. However, rather than being an offputting form of intellectual sophistry, an analysis of postmodernity could provide a framework by which to examine what is happening in the helping services and the direction they may go in future. How far, for example, will postmodernity give birth to a new openness and how far will it result in simply redrawing boundaries along different lines, with new people 'in' and new ones 'out', with new identities legitimized, but others excluded?

There can be little doubt that much of the traditional identity of professional groupings rests on what can now be identified as 'modern' foundations. Medicine and nursing, for example, have drawn heavily on technical/scientific knowledge to justify their expert status; whilst social work has been closely identified with notions of universality and equity. Both health and welfare professions have been seen as part and parcel of a great movement for progress characteristic of much of the twentieth century. Postmodernity questions these foundations by pointing to the arbitrariness of professional divisions, the unforeseen risks associated with scientific progress and the possibility of choosing identities that may not be governed by ascribed roles and hierarchies. Central to the question of identity in this context would be the degree to which professional groupings have depended upon rigid distinctions between self and other, insider and outsider, healer and patient, and helper and client. By contrast, user participation suggests an increasing permeability of boundaries between professionals and non-professionals, whilst interprofessionalism presents a similar challenge to distinctions within the professional arena.

I will, then, approach the relationship between interprofessionalism and user participation from the perspective of identity management. I am not saying that this is the only, or for that matter the most salient, determinant of collaboration between those who work in a particular helping agency and those who require its services. Identity is, however, an important factor in the way that the self is experienced in relation to the lived environment and day to day communication. For workers and users, it is closely related to expectations arising from social policy. In this sense, the study of identities that different professions, players, stakeholders and interests adopt serves as a bridge to understanding the relationship between the personal and broader social and political forces. The permeability of these identities, in other words how far power can be shared and the barriers between various groups reduced, depends on a tension between maintaining a particular identity intact and the possibility of merger. A balance has to be found which both respects expertise and formal responsibility and concomitantly recognizes interests and qualities shared with others (see Biggs, 1997, for a more detailed discussion of this point).

Postmodern health and welfare?

The nature of health and welfare has been changing. These changes are not simply driven by the internal demands of the health and welfare system, the requirements of the populations being served, nor the particular funding arrangements within national economies, though each of these plays a part. Indeed changes in social policy may themselves reflect fundamental adjustments being made to the way 'Western' societies work, which itself influences how social realities are created and their durability is reflected in professional practice. It has been suggested above that these adjustments constitute a move away from modernity toward postmodernity, referring to a shift in the way that power becomes manifest and the balance between fixed and chosen identity. Modernist notions, such as a belief in progress through scientific know-how and adherence to all-explaining 'grand narratives' (e.g. rationalism, psychoanalysis, marxism, economic liberalism), reliance on roles and relationships that are relatively fixed and predictable and a struggle to maintain a stable core identity, it is argued, no longer hold sway.

One result of the above transition would be that social life is infused with diversity which has both positive and negative consequences (Smart, 1993), changes that have implications for identities claimed by various professional groups and by those who use services. On the one hand there is increased choice, brought on by the impermanence of ascribed role relationships. In the current context such factors would include a demise of professionalized identities, themselves maintained through a rigid split between professionals and service users. Users may be expert, for example, in other contexts, or indeed in aspects of helping situations themselves, and professionals may be increasingly aware that they are themselves users of services. A flattening out of hierarchy and greater individual choice about the identity one adopts in any one context would suggest that both interprofessionalism and user participation might be considerably easier to achieve.

On the other hand, a world containing (or, more accurately, failing to contain) increased uncertainty and fragmentation might provoke what Giddens (1993) has called a 'sequestration of experience'. By this Giddens means that social institutions have responded to an uncertain world by becoming increasingly self-referential and inward-looking in order to minimize externally generated disturbance. Certain experiences are thereby sequestered, isolated, set apart, invalidated, in order to preserve coherence within the boundaries that define what is 'inside' and therefore made valid. He seems to be suggesting here a societal dynamic that is not dissimilar to psychological defence mechanisms such as splitting off or denial of unpalatable aspects of the self. The implications for identity and boundary management would be a reaction against, rather than an embracing of, fluidity occasioned by postmodern conditions. Boundaries could change but would become more rigid rather than more permeable. Such a re-ordering of social relationships would result in a reorganization of legitimacy. In certain new areas, certain new voices and alliances would be given voice; others would, at the same time, be denied legitimacy. In other words, sequestration is an attempt to manage uncertainty by denying a voice to the unmanageable. A sense of professional and institutional embattlement (Pahl, 1994), a focus on internal administration and migration away from direct care towards 'co-ordination' (Biggs, 1991) might all be interpreted as evidence of increased sequestration.

Thus, one reading of postmodernity would suggest that boundaries become increasingly fluid and identities increasingly interchangeable, whilst another would indicate the development of new rigidities, forged in the service of maintaining some form of stability for personal identity in an uncertain work. It is in this sense that the question arises: is the postmodern glass half full or half empty? Can participation and collaboration enhance the goals of improved well-being or are they simply another shuffling of those tired chairs on the deck of a millennial *Titanic*?

Interprofessional discourse and user voices

The difference that postmodernity would demand in an understanding of interprofessionalism and user participation can be explored by examining two views of identity negotiation which are fairly typical of an essentially 'modernist' approach to miscommunication in interprofessional settings. Pietroni's (1991) paper on perceptions amongst health care students contains a number of valuable and amusing observations on interprofessional stereotyping. It is proposed that the formation of a core professional identity is central to both personal and professional integrity and progresses along a series of stereotyped lines. These stereotypes – the doctor as hero, the nurse as great mother and the social worker as scapegoat – correspond to certain archetypal forms that both anchor the identity of the other and give shape to the identity desired by the self.

Similarly, Stokes (1994) has examined the characteristic defence mechanisms that different professional groups might use in interprofessional settings. Using Bion's (1961) analysis of basic assumptions that drive group behaviour, he notes that whilst health workers operate in ways characteristic of dependency relations, welfare workers are much more likely to employ a strategy of fight or flight. Both Pietroni (1991) and Stokes (1994) suggest that interprofessional miscommunication is driven by these different core strategies for sustaining individual or group identity. Under postmodern conditions, it would be argued that such an analysis, regardless of the valuable insights it might reveal, is fallible on a number of counts. First, it is assumed that the key source of conflict in interprofessional situations lies in misperception due to the use of different strategies for maintaining core identities and that professional identity is central to personal identity formation. Under postmodern conditions, it would be argued, professionality would simply be one among many competing options for identity management. So, no single identity choice is core and other possible identities may allow common ground to be found with other stakeholders.

Second, it is assumed that this discourse is exclusively the consequence of negotiation between professional groups and as such assumes a 'grand narrative' of professional supremacy; which itself discounts the value and influence of other voices such as those of the people upon whom professional skills are practised. Under postmodern conditions, boundaries are much more permeable, allowing the sound of many more voices. The function of 'playing professions', or 'reading' what is going on in terms of professionality, may be employed, however, to legitimize only a limited range of voices. In other words, interprofessionalism is itself exclusive if it simply legitimizes more professional voices at the expense of alternatives. Finally, but by no means exclusively, a sense of common or correct purpose is assumed to underlie social behaviour. This is explicit in Bion's (1961) model, where basic assumptions are distinguished from the functional work of the group, and implicit in Pietroni's (1991) work, where it is assumed that archetypal frameworks in some way obscure a more effective level of interpersonal perception. Postmodernity would pose a significant challenge to the idea of progress toward a common and superior goal. A postmodern framework would highlight health and welfare as a landscape of competing stakeholders in which conceptions of progress or decline are continually contested. Recognition of diversity, then, has been bought at the cost of a single, dominant direction.

So, these two (modernist) approaches have privileged professionality, through locating service problems on the boundaries between professional groups, and have simultaneously underemphasized the wider boundary encircling professional discourse and excluding non-professional voices. A consideration of postmodernity, however, shifts our focus to the negotiation of increasingly permeable and multi-faceted boundary issues. . . .

To understand more fully the implications of postmodern change for service relationships, it is necessary to explore the positive and negative elements of a postmodern environment in more detail.

The half-full glass

Featherstone (1983, 1991) has emerged as a key social theorist in this area. He notes that an emphasis on lifestyle and consumer culture is typical of the changes influencing contemporary social relationships and identity. People are, according to this view, far more likely to express themselves through different modes of consumption than through their relationship to production; a phenomenon that has been made possible by what Featherstone (1991) identifies as 'post-scarcity values'. So, the foundations of identity have moved away from occupation and hierarchy and toward self-expression through the consumption of various goods and services. Choice in consumption becomes choice of identity and what appeared previously to be signifiers of social distinction become blurred.

Consumer culture, it is argued, has led to:

> a profusion of images which cannot be ultimately stabilized, or hierarchized into a system which correlates to fixed social divisions . . . (and) . . . would further suggest the irrelevance of social divisions and ultimately the end of the social as a significant reference point. (Featherstone, 1991: 83)

This postmodern perspective would seem to suggest that identity is no longer a stable phenomenon and that pre-existing 'modern' hierarchies, such as that between 'senior' professions and professions related to them and between those who control the allocation of services and those who need and receive them, are in some way breaking down. We become what we consume, we shop therefore we are, and we can choose which identity to buy into. Many of the trends associated with health and welfare reform would seem to resonate with this analysis, at least at the level of policy on interprofessionalism. Developments such as the blurring of distinctions between medicine and advanced nursing practice and the movement of staff from a variety of professional backgrounds into management positions could both be interpreted as evidence of postmodern change.

Bauman (1995) has argued that postmodern conditions point to quite different questions around the management of identity from those that helping institutions are familiar with and have reflected in their own traditional structures:

> If the modern 'problem of identity' was how to construct an identity and keep it solid and stable, the postmodern 'problem of identity' is primarily how to avoid fixation and keep the options open. In the case of identity, as

in other cases, the catchword of modernity was 'creation'; the catchword of postmodernity is 'recycling'. (Bauman, 1995: 81)

Thus, under modern conditions (and it must be remembered that the welfare state with its beliefs in progress, science, universalism and that social problems can thereby be solved, is a distinctly 'modern' project in this respect) professional boundaries and a clear distinction between helper and helped would be part and parcel of keeping service systems stable and predictable. Under postmodern conditions one would expect positions to become more flexible and, indeed, interchangeable. The identities of people who make up the system would change, chameleon-like, depending on the situation in which they found themselves. Service users become persons in need in one context, experts in the consumption of services in another and decision-makers in yet another. Professional workers would similarly become specialists, advocates, purchasers, providers and consumers of services depending on the circumstances. Identities and the boundaries that describe them should be becoming more flexible, interchangeable and less fixed.

Crook et al. (1991) have outlined a process characteristic of the move out of modernity and into postmodernity. It is one which immediately suggests parallels with the trend toward interprofessionalism and user participation. They indicate that 'value spheres', which might include anything from organizational and professional cultures through to personal identities, mutate from a situation of differentiation through hyperdifferentiation and toward dedifferentiation. The first of these, differentiation, would refer to a separating out of particular groups. These might, for example, include the different professions of medicine, nursing, psychology, social work and so on. Differentiation might also describe a clearer distinction being made between professionals and users. Historically, for example, differentiation could be seen in the development of midwifery out of a predominantly informal community of women concerned with birthing. The growth of professional social work and the demise of community activity and mutual help might also be seen in this way. Differentiation allows the concretion of particular groupings of expertise and closer communication within groups with the same specialist knowledge. These concretions would contribute to professional identities based by degrees on the increasing specification of identifiably distinct and differentiated patient or client groups.

However, as it gathers pace distinctions become hyperdifferentiated. Specialisms become so marked and so circumscribed that it is difficult for members of the same professional group to communicate meaningfully with each other. One of the consequences of this hyperdifferentiated specialization is that it is as easy to communicate with someone in a completely different field, or in markedly different circumstances, as it is to restrict communication to an exclusively intraprofessional discourse. Communication then becomes 'dedifferentiated'. For current purposes this would mean that professionals begin to share ideas across 'modern' professional boundaries, and it becomes easier for users and workers to share in decision-making. Crook et al. (1991) are careful to point out that hyperdifferentiation and dedifferentiation may not always happen in a fixed order (as good postmodernists they would not want to be accused of suggesting that things happen in ways that are linear, progressive or predictable). The abolition of old identities suggested by dedifferentiation should not get in the way of a diversity of 'open ended' identities made possible through hyperdifferentiation.

From this perspective, changes to health and welfare, such as increased emphasis on monitoring and co-ordination, the breakdown of professional barriers and the participation of users, become local manifestations of broader social currents toward diversity and recombination. It would also suggest new opportunities for users and professionals to work together in the space created by the breakdown of old divisions and increased permeability of boundaries and openness to alternative perspectives.

The glass half empty

The view described above is at once familiar and puzzlingly awry as a description of contemporary health and welfare. If this is a utopian vision of the postmodern welfare state, there are discordant and distinctly dystopian possibilities lurking beneath its celebration of surface relationships. Problems also arise as a result of the 'free floating' identities that postmodern thinkers have suggested. Central amongst these are the notions of fragmentation and changeability – that it is no longer certain where boundaries should be drawn and how stable (and thus reliable) those boundaries are. This uncertainty would affect both professional and user positions.

Difficulties arising from the postmodern scenario have been noted by Howe. Using the example of social work, he notes:

> A child of modernity, social work now finds itself in a postmodern world, uncertain whether or not there are any deep and unwavering principles which define the essence of its character and hold it together as a coherent enterprise. (Howe, 1994: 513)

. . . So, what is happening to those boundaries that describe legitimacy? Whilst there is movement toward fluidity, is there not also the sequestration of experience that Giddens (1993) has warned us about? To understand the nightmare that circles sharklike beneath the postmodern dream, the particular forms, the local constellations of power, that have occurred within health and welfare need to be explored as sites on which general postmodern influences have been played out. It is also here that we return to the nature of boundary changes that have occurred.

The reforms of health and welfare legitimized by the 1990 NHS and Community Care Act have been marked by a number of distinguishing features. First, there has been a 'hollowing out' of the state. This has included a migration from what was thought to be the primary function of helping agencies (direct care) toward the regulation of a space in which informal or privatized care takes place. Professional workers are now engaged in a sort of dance around this hollow centre, which has at one and the same time been evacuated by the state and inhabited by the citizenry, once they find themselves in need. A number of concrete policy initiatives can, in retrospect, be seen as contributing to changed practice in this direction. These would include the inspection of services delivered outwith the state, whose role has been reduced to a sort of enabling surveillance, plus the co-ordination of services rather than their direct delivery.

Second, as a consequence of this hollowing out, there has been a shift of attention toward transaction across boundaries and away from processes occurring within boundaries. Interprofessionalism and participation both fit within this trend in so far as concern is refocused on what happens on the boundaries of service systems. Boundary transactions would occur through the negotiations that take place as different professions collaborate or when users enter, exit or are consulted about services. Whilst this focus allows a certain flexibility of chosen identity, it is also less concerned with content, is less relevant and purposeful, less connected to the primary tasks of cure or relief. It allows, in other words, the creation of an abstract world, less bounded by content and consequence, but infused with feelings of freedom and that 'something' is being done.

Third, it is impossible to discuss these changes without acknowledging the power of market models on identity and boundary management. The market model assumes that one is well, solvent and articulate as a precondition to participation or, at least, makes few allowances if one is not. The consumer of health and welfare has thus to masquerade as simultaneously independent and autonomous (i.e. not ill or poor) and in distress. The market analogy is not concerned with history, culture and circumstance (Biggs, 1991), but rather with two individuals coming together to agree a bargain, both of whom then return to their own private domains. This process would tend to disguise imbalances in power between parties and encourage the fragmentation of identity.

Each of these factors – a hollowing out of primary tasks, a migration to boundaries of systems and a fantasy of autonomy – contributes to a considerable scepticism that the postmodern dream can be substantiated for both professionals and service users. Whilst professional workers may be able to blur identities in the great melting-pot of interprofessionalism, it is hard to see how 'post-scarcity values' have permeated down to the old, the sick and the poor. In other words, flexibility of identity may be monopolized by those finding themselves inside the boundary describing interprofessionalism, whilst others still find themselves outside and are afforded the stereotyping that fixes their seeming unmanageability.

This second reading places postmodernity within the logic of late capitalism as applied to welfare. A sort of *faux* egalitarianism, implied by the dissolution of boundaries between professional groupings and between professionals and users, simply hides the pillaging of the welfare state. There is, in other words, no guarantee that the blurring of boundaries will result in greater egalitarianism, responsibility or predictability in service systems. Repeated reorganization, consultation, and interprofessional negotiation take on a different significance when looked at through this half-empty glass. They may exemplify a tendency to 'keep on the move', in order to sustain fluidity and escape responsibilities that would otherwise tie stakeholders down.

Conclusions

It has been my intention that reading this chapter should help identify interprofessionalism and user participation as both reflecting and contributing to changes in social behaviour, grouped together under the head of postmodernity. The consequences and shape of these developments describe possibilities that are variously utopian and dystopian.

In writing such a piece, I have been aware that the product reflects its subject in so far as the content has tended to 'float' without the clarity of direction that a modern, pragmatic and directly practical piece of writing would usually have. This is, I feel, partly a reflection of the nature of the postmodern beast. It also draws attention to a significant danger implied by a postmodern world and one with direct relevance to the relationship between these two areas of service development. Where, in this world which would seen to include both boundaryless swamps and Himalayan divides, is the moral centre? Featherstone (1991) and Bauman (1995) indicate that we are moving towards a society, and thus a health and welfare system, without fixed groupings. This is increasingly leading stakeholders to ignore structural difference, which would include not just status, but also specialist skills and particular requirements and which is constantly on the move so that yesterday's decisions are forgotten tomorrow and responsibility is increasingly difficult to locate. In such a situation, the temptation to divert attention from problems external to the swamp towards dancing lights that denote seductive yet ultimately insubstantial 'identity games' is very great. Whether health and welfare systems can be developed in ways that recognize the diversity of positions emerging through collaboration and participation, yet evolve a clear sense of shared direction and purpose, emerges as the core question for contemporary identity and boundary management. To fail to do so would be (to paraphrase Lyotard, 1986) to imagine a world, one half of which is confronted with interprofessional complexity, the other with the terrible, ancient task of survival.

References

Bauman, S. (1995) *Life in Fragments: Essays in Postmodern Morality*, Oxford: Blackwell.

Biggs, S. (1991) 'Consumers, case managers and inspection: obscuring deprivation and need?', *Critical Social Policy*, 30: 23–38.

Biggs, S. (1997) 'Interprofessional collaboration: problems and prospects', in A. Thompson, P. Mathias and S. Øvretiet (eds) *Handbook of Interprofessional Work*, London: Ballière, Tindall. p. 26.

Bion, W. (1961) *Experiences in Groups*, London: Tavistock.

Crook, S., Pakulski, J. and Waters, M. (1991) *Postmodernization*, London: Sage.

Featherstone, M. (1983) 'Consumer culture', *Theory, Culture and Society*, 1: 4–10.

Featherstone, M. (1991) *Consumer Culture and Postmodernism*, London: Sage.

Giddens, A. (1993) *Modernity and Self-identity*, Cambridge: Polity.

Howe, D. (1994) 'Modernity, postmodernity and social work', *British Journal of Social Work*, 24: 513–33.

Jameson, F. (1984) 'Postmodernism, or the cultural logic of late capitalism', *New Left Review*, 146: 53–92.

Lyotard, J.-F. (1986) 'Defining the postmodern', *Postmodern Documents, 4*, London: ICA.

Pahl, J. (1994) 'Like the job but hate the organisation', *Social Policy Review*, 6: 190–210.

Pietroni, P.C. (1991) 'Stereotypes or archetypes? A study of perceptions amongst health care students', *Journal of Interprofessional Care*, 5: 61–9.

Smart, B. (1993) *Postmodernity: Key Ideas*, London: Routledge.

Stokes, J. (1994) 'Problems in interdisciplinary teams: the unconscious at work', *Journal of Social Work Practice*, 8: 161–8.

37

M. Clarke and J. Stewart

Handling the Wicked Issues

What are the 'wicked issues'?

The idea of the 'wicked issue' has become part of the contemporary currency of public administration and management. The words are used to refer to a variety of policy challenges. The sense they convey is of something different to the conventional issues of public policy which are solved or, at least are capable of solution, by a mixture of common sense and ingenuity. They suggest a special class of policy problem; one without an obvious or established (or even common-sense) solution, defying normal understanding – and often not sitting conveniently within the responsibilities of any one organization. . . .

Why are some issues called 'wicked'? The word is used, not in the sense of evil, but as a crossword puzzle addict or a mathematician would use it – suggesting an issue (or problem) difficult to resolve. The phrase seems first to have been used by Horst Rittel and Melvin Webber in the USA. They wrote of wicked problems:

> We are calling them 'wicked' not because these properties are themselves ethically deplorable. We use the term 'wicked' in a meaning akin to that of 'malignant' (in contrast to 'benign') or 'vicious' (like a circle) or 'tricky' (like a leprechaun) or 'aggressive' (like a lion, in contrast to the docility of a lamb). (Rittel and Webber, 1973: 160)

Wicked problems are distinguished from tamed problems, some of which may themselves have been wicked before they were tamed. A tame problem is one which one can be readily defined and for which a solution is easily found.

Wicked problems, on the other hand, are those for which there is no obvious or easily found solution. They seem intractable. . . . There can be hope that wicked problems will be solved over time, but that requires learning of the nature of the problems and of their causes. They require a capacity to derive and design new approaches for their resolution and to learn of their impact. They are likely to be resolved

---

First published as a discussion paper, *Handling the Wicked Issues: a Challenge for Government* (School of Public Policy, University of Birmingham, 1997). Abridged.

not directly but through an iterative process – learning, trying and learning.

In reality, of course, there is probably a continuum of issues from the wicked to the tame. Along the continuum will be issues which were wicked but which are on the way to solution or ones which have been resolved so that they are now tame. Widespread disease, apparently incapable of solution in the mid-nineteenth century, gave way to sanitation, concern for public health and control – and a set of issues tamed.

Almost by definition, wicked problems cannot be dealt with as management has traditionally dealt with public policy problems. They challenge existing patterns of organization and management. Organizations are usually structured by – or themselves structure – problems and defined solutions. For the wicked problems there is no accepted solution; what is required is a learning approach which must not be confined and should be prepared to think and accept the unthinkable. Where there is a tamed problem there is a solution or a set of known skills that are required to solve the problem. People can then be trained to find and apply the solution; they can be fitted into an appropriate organizational context.

Wicked problems cannot be dealt with like that. The issues need to be framed and reframed. The problems are not fully understood and solutions have to be searched for in uncertainty. The skills required are often not fully appreciated. The problem is unlikely to belong to any one organization; in all likelihood it will implicate many. Indeed, awareness of the wicked nature of the problem is often associated with the fact that the problem cannot be fully understood by any one organization, never mind solved by it. . . .

However, it is important to recognize that it is not just the fact that issues overlap organizational or even conceptual boundaries which makes them wicked. The inclination to confuse the wicked with the corporate or overarching strategic issues is a mistake. The latter will usually include the former, but not vice versa. The resolution of wicked issues will almost inevitably require action not by government alone but by many individuals and organizations. The wicked issues by their nature will be enmeshed in established ways of life and patterns of thinking; they will only be resolved by changes in those ways of life and thought patterns. If society is wasteful and polluting the earth's resources, it will be because it has supported particular ways of living; these have to change if sustainable development is to be achieved. Equally, a healthy society will seem a welcome objective to all, but its achievement will require changes in the way many people live.

Trying to resolve the wicked issues will mean working through people. The changes required will be such that they are unlikely to be imposed by legislation or regulation alone; nor would such legislation be passed or regulation be accepted without public acceptance of what is required. The wicked issues are likely only to be resolved by a style of governing which learns from people and works with people. The wicked issues require a participatory style of governing because the changes have to be owned by people.

Underlying the tackling of the wicked issues is recognition that the task is not the government or management of certainty, where clearly identified problems are faced, with understood causes and for which there are accepted solutions. Rather, the task is the government or management of uncertainty. It may not be clear what the problem is – at least in the sense of understanding its causes – and it will certainly not be clear what the solution is. Politicians and officials have to respond without necessarily knowing how to respond.

Theorists and commentators have often defined government as being about learning. In tackling the wicked issues the need is to create a learning government. Such an approach starts from a recognition of uncertainty, both about the issues and how they should be handled. This means that management should be based on a recognition of the need for learning. Ways and means have to be plotted – not so much as the path to a certain destination but for an exploration in imperfectly known territory. Policy-makers may move forward – but with reflection and ready to learn and to adapt to that learning.

Tackling wicked issues therefore requires

- holistic not partial or linear thinking, capable of encompassing the interaction of a wide variety of activities, habits, behaviour and attitudes;
- a capacity to think outside and work across organizational boundaries;
- ways of involving the public in developing responses;
- embracing a willingness to think and work in completely new ways. While most people will come to this trapped or constrained by conventional organizations, labels and assumptions, what is needed is willingness to entertain the unconventional and pursue the radical. This implies
- a new style of governing for a learning society.

. . .

Holistic – not linear or partial – thinking

. . . This is thinking capable of grasping the big picture, including the interrelationships of objectives and the interaction of activities and different objectives. By their nature, the wicked issues are

imperfectly understood and so the placing of boundaries upon analysis and thought may lead to what is important in handling the
wicked issues being neglected. . . .

Recognizing interrelationships (of issues, organizations and people)
and breadth of attention are necessary to holistic thinking. There is a
need to be inclusive, not exclusive, in the search for connections and
to resist the traps of the organization perspective, of limited
experience and of reducing the complex to the simple. The problem
is the constant inclination – because of the dominance of linear
modes of thinking – to confine analysis within a framework of neat
certainty. Not to do so is uncomfortable. This problem is exacerbated
by the fact that, inevitably, we use formal organizations to tackle
public policy issues – and most organizational design is premised on
the need to focus, simplify and order; and, in contemporary vogue, to
operate efficiently and economically as well as effectively. We do not
dispute the value of such an approach for problems easily identified
and to which solutions are easily found; the danger lies in its
dominance. Organizations in the public domain need a capacity to
work in different ways. They need a capacity for holistic thinking
both within and across organizations, as well as for linear thinking
within.

Thinking and working across organizational boundaries

A crucial part of handling wicked issues involves crossing organizational boundaries and drawing many organizations into the frame.
The need to think and work across organizational boundaries raises
issues both between organizations and within them. Organizations
cannot work effectively together if they do not work effectively within
themselves. Inter-organizational working will be limited by the
inadequacy of intra-organizational working. Again it is important to
think in a holistic way. In seeking to build inter-organizational
working between levels of government or agencies and parts of
government the focus easily becomes limited.

For example, a concern for building a healthy society tends to
concentrate on those whose contribution is most obvious. This is most
clearly seen at the local level with a focus on the social services
department and the health agencies. Such a focus does not realize the
full potential of local authorities for building a healthy society.
Functions as diverse as education, housing, planning and leisure
services all have a contribution to make. Then there are contributions
from a wide range of agencies, across levels of government and from
individual citizens which need to be taken into account. Neglect of
such contributions reflects linear thinking, limiting involvement to
the obvious, rather than taking a holistic view. Too narrow a focus

will fail to encompass the potential contribution to be made by many services and agencies to a healthy society. Similarly, limited vision will ignore the contribution the health agencies can make to dealing with other wicked issues such as urban and rural deprivation, poverty, public safety, the environment and the like. . . .

Whilst working across external boundaries is important because wicked issues, almost by definition, will involve many organizations in their understanding and search for solution, the capacity to think and work across internal boundaries is also crucial. The problem of working across boundaries within an organization is that the boundaries usually mark out specified tasks or ways of working, most governmental organizations being structured on functional lines. Structures and procedures will be designed to ensure a necessary organizational focus on those tasks. The problem is how to ensure a focus on issues which cut across those internal organizational boundaries – especially when those issues are not clearly defined. It is relatively easy, for example, for an organization to identify an issue such as the environment as a priority for the organization. The difficulty comes in ensuring that the priority is carried forward into action by all who should be involved. This requires the issue to receive continuing attention – when the main structures and processes will focus attention on the ongoing tasks of the organization. Such focus may be especially narrow where internal divisions have broken the organization down into service units or devolved cost centres and where there is an emphasis on performance management, with clear targets related to specific tasks and assessment of success in meeting them.

Day-to-day work can easily crowd out the non-routine so that wicked issues are easily forgotten or considered only spasmodically. It is not just that each part of the organization has specified tasks to be carried out – and that these assume priority – it is also that wicked issues are often not easily defined or understood and that they may need constant reframing. It is difficult for the organization to ensure that it gives them priority and to encourage holistic rather than linear thinking – and action – within its artificial boundaries. However, there are a number of things that can be done.

An issue can be made the *responsibility of an existing department or unit*. The advantage of this is to identify clarity and leadership. However, such a move carries with it the danger that the issue will be seen from the dominant perspective of one part of the organization with the potential contribution of other parts – and the holistic view – not being fully realized. Moreover, it may not even be clear where the appropriate lead comes from as the exploration – and reframing – of an issue may identify the need for a new emphasis. This may be enough to outweigh the focus and energy derived from clear responsibility within the established organizational framework.

An alternative, conventional response to using an existing part of the organization is to set up a *new unit or department* whose role is to focus on the issue. Such a unit might be free-standing or attached to an existing part of the organization, for example to a chief executive or similar person. The problem for such a unit is how to have an impact on the rest of the organization and to ensure interest and involvement. There is the danger that it seeks to be over-interventionist, causing resistance rather than co-operation. There is an equal danger that such a unit will become peripheral to the work of the organization and in practice have little impact. Clearly a middle way has to be sought. Such departments or units can be valued as a focus for attention and expertise, but only if they are taken notice of and their expertise used. A variant is to give the leadership for internal working to an established *policy unit* at the centre of the organization – Downing Street or in the chief executive's office in a local authority or executive agency.

Another approach is to bring together members of different departments as a *task force* concerned with the issue who would, then, also act as champions for the issue in their departments. The issue here is to ensure that there is sufficient commitment both of time and attitude to make the task force effective and that the staff involved have sufficient authority. Much depends upon the weight given to the task force and its membership. A key may be the involvement of a minister (or senior councillor or board member) to give the task force adequate clout. . . . At senior management level there is a case for particular officials accepting responsibility as *guardians* of the issue, available to give support to units or task forces concerned with the wicked issue and ensure its presence in the corporate workings of the organization. This will only be effective if there is commitment to the issue; simply to hand out issues to senior managers on the basis that 'you must all have one', as happens in some organizations, is self-defeating. . . .

Developing a capacity to work across both internal and external boundaries raises a number of people issues. The need to raise awareness of the importance of a wicked issue(s) *implies a commitment to development and training*. These activities should be designed, in part, to give knowledge and to build understanding of the issue. But they should, equally, be used to draw on the understandings, experience and knowledge of the staff of the organization. After all, problems of the environment, of health, of discrimination or of safety can impinge on many activities and on many staff. Drawing them in builds ownership of the issue. It also recognizes that these are issues in which the understanding given by any one perspective is limited, even when those perspectives claim to embrace the whole of the issue. Organizational and personal development and training can be part of strategic search as groups explore the interrelationship between their own activities and the issue. Training can then itself be part of organizational learning. The culture of the organization should encourage holistic thinking, and training should nurture it.

Development and training have to be reinforced by *communication*. A focus on the wicked issues, with the imperative of crossing internal and/or external organizational boundaries, requires openness, debate and information. If the wicked issues are to be understood and tackled – and an appropriate culture developed – they have to be sustained by communication sideways, upwards and downwards. . . .

Part of building the capacity for thinking and working across boundaries is the need to identify and promote particular *skills and style*. Thinking laterally and not being constrained by linear models or trapped by experience or organization is important; equally, the ability to span organization boundaries is vital. Some people will be better at these things than others. However, training, development and varied experience and career progression will play their part. Senior managers and officials will need to be especially adept at these things as they should play a key role in identifying, exploring, defining and handling wicked issues. While the position inevitably varies from government organization to government organization, many will probably suffer from a deficit in these skills and competences. Correcting this will be a key contribution to public policy, given our suggestion that the wicked issues are not only more important but will increasingly dominate the public policy agenda. A starting point would be identification of the skills required and then an audit of the organization.

Involving the public

An important part of handling many wicked issues will be finding ways of drawing in the public. Many of the traditional processes of representative democracy are inadequate in this context, because they have tended to assume the passive citizen. In these processes the role of the citizen is often reduced to no more than that of the elector making a choice between competing parties every few years. The process of representation has been reduced to the passive roles of electing or being a representative rather than involvement in an active process of deliberation between the representative and those represented. It is all too easy to see the handling of wicked issues as a top-down process. Learning and problem-solving may come as well – or better – from the bottom up. . . .

There are two problems here, and both have to be tackled. On the one hand increasing amounts of governmental activity and public policy formation and delivery take place at a distance from the representative democratic institutions of Westminster and town hall;

and, on the other, too little has been done to surround the traditional institutions of democracy with ways of involving the public other than through the ballot box. More needs to be done to develop means of accountability and to open up opportunities for debate and involvement.

These are serious issues. Wicked issues require the involvement of citizens for two reasons. Because the wicked issues represent intractable problems imperfectly understood, it is important that they are widely discussed, both to deepen understanding and to draw upon *the experience of those who face these problems* at their point of greatest impact. The voices of those who live in crime-ridden areas, of those who know discrimination, or of those who face poverty, have to be heard if the reality of the issues is to be understood.

Secondly, many of the wicked issues, as we have said, require *changes in the way people behave*. Those changes cannot readily be imposed on people. Thus the changes that may be required to meet the threats to the environment will require ways of life that are less wasteful of non-renewable resources or that cause less pollution. Behaviour will be changed only if issues are widely understood, discussed and owned. Public participation is a necessary part of gaining this and so of handling the wicked issues.

Both of these things remind us of the importance of handling wicked issues at the local level. It is here that it is much easier to involve people – both for them to learn and for public policy to learn from their experience and involvement. It is, of course, the local level which also most readily lends itself to experiment and the development of a variety of approaches – a necessary part of trying to handle and solve uncertain and intractable issues. . . .

Conclusion: a new style of governing

Handling the wicked issues requires a new style of governing. It involves a capacity to work across organizational boundaries, to think holistically and to involve the public. However, underlying these requirements must be a recognition of the intractability of the issues faced. As we have repeated, the wicked issues are imperfectly understood, their causes are far from clear and the responses to them are uncertain. This does not make the task of governing impossible, but it cannot be based on certainty of responses.

The style of governing should not be based on the assumption that a clear and final programme of action will quickly become obvious or that the management task is to carry out such a programme as effectively and efficiently as possible. Such is the task of managing tame issues and the government of certainty. Here the task is the government of uncertainty.

Equally, it should not be assumed that action is impossible, that nothing can be done and that problems are intractable in an absolute sense. Action is possible and initiatives should be encouraged. But government cannot assume it knows the answers to the problem. Comprehensive plans will be inappropriate. . . .

The style is not so much that of a traveller who knows the route, but more that of an explorer who has a sense of direction but no clear route. Search and exploration, watching out for possibilities and interrelationships, however unlikely they may seem, are part of the approach. There are ideas as to the way ahead, but some may prove abortive. What is required is a readiness to see and accept this, rather than to proceed regardless on a path which is found to be leading nowhere or in the wrong direction. There will be a need, too, to ensure that wicked issues are not crowded out by the more routine and mundane.

This suggests that what is required in dealing with the wicked issues is a style that encourages initiative, but recognizes the need for learning – not merely in government but in society. Public learning should underlie the initiatives, which should be about expanding understanding, opening the working of organizations, policy-makers and public to research, and to views and ideas. Learning should guide the process of exploration. . . . Handling the wicked issues of public policy requires different modes of thinking and action to dealing with the tamed ones (and that does even for the tame ones which require inter-organizational working). It means different ways of:

- *understanding* which recognize that understanding is partial at best; seeing from a variety of perspectives; being wary of apparent certainty and accepting uncertainty;
- *thinking* which pursue the holistic and are not being seduced by the linear; looking for the interactions and interrelationships;
- *working* which refuse to be trapped by the obvious and conventional; tolerate not knowing; and accept different perspectives, approaches and styles;
- *involving* which are inclusive, drawing in as wide a range of organizations and interests as possible and open to public participation. 'Outsiders' will being new insight and thinking and many wicked issues will involve new attitudes and behaviours as well as government action;
- *learning* about the issues and about the responses, encouraging experiment and diversity and requiring reflection. Learning government is a prerequisite for handling wider issues.

These different ways of working make a crucial point. Wicked issues are handled by government through and between organizations. Here is a paradox. Most organizations are designed – and find it easier – to handle linear thinking and tame problems. Perspectives can be more limited, routines more readily accepted and focus more closely set. The wicked issues demand that these things are set aside. As we have shown, organizational means are needed, but organizational form and experience must not be allowed to subvert. Issues which are improperly understood cannot be handled by organizations which assume understanding. Holding on to that paradox is at the heart of the challenge to government in handling the wicked issues. Organizations which seem instinctively more comfortable with the conventional and the secure need to be able to espouse the unconventional and the radical.

Reference

Rittel, Horst W.J. and Webber, Melvin (1973) 'Dilemmas in a general theory of planning', *Policy Sciences*.

Index

accountability:
administrative, 22; crisis,
26; definitions, 222;
doctor–nurse roles,
327–31; public
administration model,
21–2, 25–6; public trust,
361–2; social work,
222–9
accreditation: bodies, 243–6;
participants, 246;
participants' motivation,
247; participants'
perceptions of benefits,
253–5; preparing for,
248–9; report and
recommendations, 252–3;
standards, 249–50; survey
visit, 250–2
adoption placements, 124–8,
322
alternative therapists,
312–14
anti-racist theorists, 113,
114–15, 322
audit *see* medical audit
Audit Commission, 22, 33
autonomy (patient), 106–7,
336; versus safety,
258–60, 262
autonomy (professional) *see*
professional practice
autonomy (voluntary sector
boards), 281–2

BASW *see* British
Association of Social
Workers
Beveridge Report, 8, 12–13,
14
black and ethnic minorities:
adoption placements,
124–8, 322; health and
culture, 132–4; health
service users, 134–6,
138–9; maternity services,
39, 43; men with learning
disabilities, 202; nursing
staff, 139; social work,
114–15, 118, 123–4, 322

boundary issues:
interprofessionalism, 369,
370, 371–4; sexual
boundaries, 207–9; *see
also* accountability;
confidentiality
British Association of Social
Workers (BASW), 323, 324
bureaucracies, 14; and
gender, 347–8;
motivations of, 51–2;
public administration
model, 19–20, 23–4;
versus professionalism,
305

carers: interaction and
scripts, 91–4; pain and
vulnerability, 94–5;
personal development,
98–9; perspectives on risk
management, 258–61,
262; psychodynamics of
dementia care, 95–8
caring *see* feminist
perspectives; nursing
Central Council for
Education and Training in
Social Work (CCETSW),
112, 113, 125, 126, 322,
323
Changing Childbirth (DOH),
37, 41, 42, 43, 44–5
charities, 277; *see also*
voluntary organizations
child care, 319, 320
Child Poverty Action Group,
13
child protection, 323
'child' within, 96–8
Children Acts, 125–6, 128,
320, 322
Citizen's Charter, 25
collaboration *see* team
collaboration
College of Occupational
Therapists, 100, 104
communication, service
users–professionals,
191–3, 360, 369–73, 374

community care *see*
independent sector
community care providers;
voluntary organizations
Community Care [Direct
Payments] Act, 189
community mental health
teams (CMHTs) study,
172–9
competence and public trust,
361
complexity, 302, 303
confidentiality issues:
predictive tests, 336–41;
social work, 221–9
conflict *see* team conflict
Conservative governments,
27, 32, 34–5, 126; *see also*
'New Right'; Thatcher,
Margaret
consumer rights, 15,
115–16
consumerism, 25, 28, 371,
374
contract culture, 24
costs crisis, 11–12
critical theory, 67–8,
217–19
cultural safety and
professional practice,
136–8, 140
cultural sensitivity/factfiles,
134–6; *see also* black and
ethnic minorities

decentralization, 363–4
dementia care,
psychodynamics of, 95–8
democratization, 363
dentists, 310
Department of Health, 37,
128, 196, 231, 242, 323
dialectical materialism,
69–70
dialectical versus analytical
reason, 69, 70
disability: defining quality of
life, 181–3; service
approaches, 183–6; social
model of, 193–5